HANLEY & BELFUS PERIODICALS

Journals

- *Biomedical Technology Today*, bimonthly
- *Journal of General Internal Medicine*, bimonthly
- *Journal of Hand Therapy*, quarterly
- *Medical Decision Making*, quarterly
- *Medical Problems of Performing Artists*, quarterly

State of the Art Reviews (STARS)

- CARDIAC SURGERY (STAR), triannually
- NEUROSURGERY (STAR), triannually
- OCCUPATIONAL MEDICINE (STAR), quarterly
- PHYSICAL MEDICINE AND REHABILITATION (STAR), quarterly
- SPINE (STAR), triannually
- SURGICAL ONCOLOGY (STAR), triannually

DICTIONARY OF MEDICAL ACRONYMS & ABBREVIATIONS

jablonski

1987

HANLEY & BELFUS, INC./Philadelphia
THE C.V. MOSBY COMPANY/St. Louis • Toronto • London

Publisher: HANLEY & BELFUS, INC.
                  210 South 13th Street
                  Philadelphia, PA 19107
                  (215) 546-7293

North American and worldwide sales and distribution:

                  THE C.V. MOSBY COMPANY
                  11830 Westline Industrial Drive
                  St. Louis, MO 63146

In Canada: THE C.V. MOSBY COMPANY
                  5240 Finch Avenue East
                  Unit 1
                  Scarborough, Ontario M1S 4P2
                  Canada

DICTIONARY OF MEDICAL   ISBN 0-932883-02-8
ACRONYMS & ABBREVIATIONS

Last digit is the print number: 9 8 7 6 5 4 3 2

PREFACE

Acronyms and abbreviations are used extensively in medicine, science and technology for good reason–they are more essential in such fields. It would be difficult to imagine how one could write down chemical and mathematical formulas and equations without using abbreviations or symbols. In medicine, they are used as a convenient shorthand in writing medical records, instructions, and prescriptions, and as space-saving devices in printed literature. It is easier and more economical to write down the acronyms HETE and RAAS than their full names 12-L-hydroxy-5,8,10,14-eicosatetraenoic acid and renin-angiotensin-aldosterone system, respectively.

The main reason for abbreviations is said to be economy. Some actually save space in print, such as acronyms for the names of institutions and organizational units, as well as being convenient to use. Many are used for other reasons, as for instance, when trying to be delicate, we may euphemistically refer to bowel movement as BM, an unprincipled individual as SOB, and body odor as BO. Also, it is sometimes difficult to fathom the reasoning of bureaucratic acronym makers, who have created some tongue-twisting monstrosities, such as ADCOMSUBORDCOMPHIBSPAC (for Administrative Command, Amphibious Forces, Pacific Fleet, Subordinate Command).

Abbreviations and acronyms used in medicine can be grouped into two broad categories. The first consists of official abbreviations and symbols used in chemistry, mathematics, and other sciences, and those designating weights and measures, whose exact form, capitalization, and punctuation have been determined by official governing bodies. In this category, they mean only one thing (e.g., kg is the symbol for kilogram and Hz for hertz), and their form, capitalization, and punctuation have been established by the International System of Units (Système International d'Unités). Abbreviations in the second group, on the other hand, may appear in a variety of forms, the same abbreviation having a different number of letters, sometimes capitalized, at other times not, with or without punctuation. Moreover, they may also have numerous meanings. The abbreviation AP may mean alkaline phosphatase, acid phosphatase, action potential, angina pectoris, and many other things.

Editors of individual scientific publications make an effort to standardize the form of abbreviations and symbols in their journals and books, but they generally vary from one publication to another.

This dictionary lists acronyms and abbreviations occurring with a reasonable frequency in the medical literature that were identified by a systematic scanning of collections of books and periodicals at the National Library of Medicine. Except as they take the form of Greek letters, pure geometric symbols are not included. Although we have attempted to be as inclusive as possible, a book such as this one can never be complete, in spite of the most diligent effort, and it is expected that some abbreviations and acronyms may have escaped detection and others have been introduced since completion of the manuscript.

ACKNOWLEDGMENTS

I wish to express my appreciation to the following members of the staff of the National Library of Medicine for their assistance in the preparation of this Dictionary: Mary Hantzes, Robert Mehnert, Edith Calhoun, Regina Broadhurst, Daniel Carangi, and especially, Dr. Maria Farkas.

Stanley Jablonski
Bethesda, Maryland

HISTORICAL NOTES

Abbreviations, acronyms, and symbols have been used from the time when man made his first efforts to write. The first written message was probably done by a primitive man in the form of a clumsy picture drawn on sand in an effort to express an idea that his limited vocabulary would not have allowed him to do verbally. These early pictographs, or more specifically, ideograms, depicted only broad ideas and objects, and were gradually replaced by more sophisticated symbols, or phonograms, which represented specific sounds in speech, or phonemes, thus leading to the eventual development of the alphabet.

Even though pictographs gave way to letters of the alphabet, the concept of using symbols depicting ideas that are difficult to express verbally is still very much in use. Symbols such as those showing mathematical functions, electronic circuitry, or international road signs are not dissimilar to some Egyptian hieroglyphs, at least in the conceptual sense. They are also clearer, express ideas more economically, and are understood more readily by persons speaking different languages than those written in letters.

The history of abbreviations has been lost somewhere in antiquity. One of the oldest abbreviations is the symbol for the name of God. Since Jews were forbidden by their religion from uttering the name of God, they created the substitute Tetragrammaton, a word made from four Hebrew letters, usually transliterated as YHWH and which is pronouncible as Jehovah or Yahweh. A somewhat later nonreligious abbreviation is the Roman initialism SPQR, for *Senatus Populosque Romanus* (Senate and the Roman People). D.O.M., for *Domino Optimo Maximo* (To Almighty God), is an abbreviation seen over the portals of many old European cathedrals and churches. I.H.S., for *Iesus Hominum Salvator* (Jesus, the Savior of men), is another common old Christian abbreviation.

A good example of how abbreviations were used in medieval writings can be found in a ninth century Irish illuminated manuscript of the Gospels, the *Book of Kells*. The abbreviations, usually contractions, were used in the manuscript with high frequency and in a very uniform manner; for example, DNS (for Dominus), sps (for Spiritus), and scs (for Sanctus). These and other examples of medial abbreviations persisted until Gutenberg's invention of movable type.

It would appear that the introduction of the printing machine and, especially, word-processing and computer-assisted printing, would have eliminated the need for abbreviating words or, at least, diminished the practice. This did not occur, and abbreviations of all kinds continue to be used with a constantly increasing frequency.

FYI

The purpose of this dictionary is obvious to anyone who has struggled with medical writing or dictation or oral reports that contained undefined acroynms or abbreviations, and far too many do. It is a reality of medicine and science that the number of acronyms and abbreviations, far from being a stable collection, is increasing exponentially. Despite the efforts of teachers and editors to contain them, clinicians and researchers constantly introduce new ones, as any perusal of a current journal demonstrates. It is impossible to comprehend some specialties (i.e., pulmonary medicine) without access to a reference such as this one.

The author and publisher recognize that the corpus of medical acroynms and abbreviations is a moving target. Despite our best efforts, almost every reader will identify a few favorites that either are too recent to be included or that have been omitted for one reason or another. In order to provide the reader opportunity to "customize" this dictionary, a few pages at the back of the book have been provided for write-ins. We would like to know about the omissions in order to consider them for future reprintings, and a page at the very end is addressed to the publisher. Please photocopy or cut out and send in your suggestions.

–A–

A absolute temperature; absorbance; acceptor; accommodation; acetum; acidophil, acidophilic; *Actinomyces*; activity [radiaion]; adenine; adenosine; admittance; adrenalin; adult; age; akinetic; alanine; albino [guinea pig]; allergy, allergologist; alpha [cell]; alveolar gas; ampere; amphetamine; ampicillin; anaphylaxis; androsterone; anesthetic; angstrom, Ångström unit; anode; *Anopheles*; anterior; aqueous; area; argon; artery [Lat. *arteria*]; atomic weight; atrium; atropine; auricle; axial; blood group A; ear [Lat. *auris*]; mass number; subspinale; total acidity; water [Lat. *aqua*]; year [Lat. *annum*]

A **[band]** the dark-staining zone of a striated muscle

Å Ångstrom unit

Ā cumulated activity; antinuclear antibody

A₂ aortic second sound

A₂P₂ aortic second sound; pulmonary second sound

AI, AII, AIII angiotensin I, II, III

a absorptivity; acceleration; accommodation; ampere; anode; anterior; arterial blood; artery [Lat. *arteria*]; atto-; thermodynamic activity; total acidity water [Lat. *aqua*]

A see *alpha*

α see *alpha*

AA acetic acid; achievement age; active avoidance; acupuncture analgesia; adenine arabinoside; adrenal androgen; agranulocytic angina; Alcoholics Anonymous; alopecia areata; amino acid; amyloid A; aplastic anemia; arachidonic acid; ascending aorta; atomic absorption; autoanalyzer; axonal arborization; so much of each [Gr. *ana*]

aa arteries [*arteriae*]; so much of each [Gr. *ana*]

aA abampere

AAA abdominal aortic aneurysm/ aneurysmectomy; acquired aplastic anemia; acute anxiety attack; American Academy of Allergy; American Association of Anatomists; androgenic anabolic agent; aneurysm of ascending aorta; Area Agency on Aging

AAAHE American Association for the Advancement of Health Education

AAALAC American Association for Accreditation of Laboratory Animal Care

AAAS American Association for the Advancement of Science

AAB American Association of Bioanalysts

AABB American Association of Blood Banks

AABCC alertness (consciousness), airway, breathing, circulation, cervical spine

AAC antibiotic-associated pseudomembranous colitis; antimicrobial agent– induced colitis

AACA acylaminocephalosporanic acid

AACC American Association for Clinical Chemistry

AACCN American Association of Critical Care Nurses

AACHP American Association for Comprehensive Health Planning

AACIA American Association for Clinical Immunology and Allergy

AACN American Association of Colleges of Nursing

AACP American Academy of Cerebral Palsy; American Association of Colleges of Pharmacy

AACPDM American Academy for Cerebral Palsy and Developmental Medicine

AACSH adrenal androgen corticotropic stimulating hormone

AAD alloxazine adenine dinucleotide; alpha-1-antitrypsin deficiency

AADC amino acid decarboxylase

AADE American Association of Dental Editors; American Association of Dental Examiners

AADGP American Academy of Dental Group Practice

(A–a)D_{N2} difference in the nitrogen tension between mixed alveolar gas and mixed arterial blood

(A-a)D_{O2} difference in the partial pressures of oxygen in mixed alveolar gas and mixed arterial blood

AADP American Academy of Denture Prosthetics; amyloid A-degrading protease

AADPA American Academy of Dental Practice Administration

AADR American Academy of Dental Radiology

AADS American Academy of Dental Schools

AAE active assistive exercise; acute allergic encephalitis; American Association of Endodontists; annuloaortic ectasia

AAEE American Association of Electromyography and Electrodiagnosis

AAEH Association to Advance Ethical Hypnosis

AAF acetylaminofluorene; ascorbic acid factor

AAFP American Academy of Family Physicians

AAG alpha-1-acid glycoprotein

AAGP American Academy of General Practice; American Association for Geriatric Psychiatry

AAHD American Association of Hospital Dentists

AAHE Association for the Advancement of Health Education

AAHPER American Association for Health, Physical Education, and Recreation

AAI American Association of Immunologists; atrial inhibited [pacemaker]

AAIB alpha-1-aminoisobutyrate

AAID American Academy of Implant Dentures

AAIN American Association of Industrial Nurses

AAL anterior axillary line

AALAS American Association of Laboratory Animal Science

AALL American Association for Labor Legislation

AAM American Academy of Microbiology

AAMA American Academy of Medical Administrators; American Association of Medical Assistants

AAMC American Association of Medical Clinics; Association of American Medical Colleges

AAMD American Association of Mental Deficiency

AAMFT American Association for Marriage and Family Therapy

AAMI Association for the Advancement of Medical Instrumentation

AAMIH American Association for Maternal and Infant Health

AAMMC American Association of Medical Milk Commissioners

AAMP American Academy of Maxillofacial Prosthetics; American Academy of Medical Prevention

AAMR American Academy of Mental Retardation

AAMRL American Association of Medical Record Librarians

AAMRS automated ambulatory medical record system

AAMS acute aseptic meningitis syndrome

AAMSI American Association for Medical Systems and Informatics

AAN alpha-amino nitrogen; American Academy of Neurology; American Academy of Nursing; American Academy of Nutrition; American Association of Neuropathologists; amino acid nitrogen; analgesic-associated nephropathy; attending's admission notes

AANA American Association of Nurse Anesthetists

AANM American Association of Nurse-Midwives

AANPI American Association of Nurses Practicing Independently

AAO American Academy of Ophthalmology; American Academy of Optometry; American Academy of Osteopathy; American Academy of Otolaryngology; American Association of Ophthalmologists; American Association of Orthodontists; amino acid oxidase

AAofA Ambulance Association of America

AAOM American Academy of Oral Medicine

AAOO American Academy of Ophthalmology and Otolaryngology

AAOP American Academy of Oral Pathology

AAOS American Academy of Orthopedic Surgeons

AAP American Academy of Pediatrics; American Academy of Pedodontics; American Academy of Periodontology; American Academy of Psychoanalysts; American Academy of Psychotherapists; American Association of Pathologists; Association for the Advancement of

Psychoanalysis; Association for the Advancement of Psychotherapy; Association of American Physicians

AAPA American Academy of Physician Assistants; American Association of Pathologist Assistants

AAPB American Association of Pathologists and Bacteriologists

A–aP$_{CO2}$ alveolar-arterial carbon dioxide difference

AAPF anti-arteriosclerosis polysaccharide factor

AAPHD American Association of Public Health Dentists

AAPHP American Association of Public Health Physicians

AAPMC antibiotic-associated pseudomembranous colitis

AAPM&R American Academy of Physical Medicine and Rehabilitation

AAPS American Association of Plastic Surgeons; Association of American Physicians and Surgeons

AAR active avoidance reaction; acute articular rheumatism; antigen-antiglobulin reaction

AAROM active assertive range of motion

AART American Association for Rehabilitation Therapy; American Association for Respiratory Therapy

AAS American Academy of Sanitarians; American Analgesia Society; aneurysm of atrial septum; anthrax antiserum; aortic arch syndrome; atomic absorption spectrophotometry

AASD American Academy of Stress Disorders

AASH adrenal androgen stimulating hormone

AASP acute atrophic spinal paralysis; American Association of Senior Physicians

AASS American Association for Social Security

AAT Aachen Aphasia Test; academic aptitude test; alanine aminotransferase; alpha-1-antitrypsin; atrial triggered [pacemaker]; auditory apperception test

AATS American Association for Thoracic Surgery

AAU acute anterior uveitis

AAV adeno-associated virus

AAVMC Association of American Veterinary Medical Colleges

AAVP American Association of Veterinary Parasitologists

AB abnormal; abortion; aid to the blind; alcian blue; antibody; asbestos body; asthmatic bronchitis; axiobuccal; Bachelor of Arts [Lat. *Artium Baccalaureus*]; blood group AB

A/B acid-base ratio

A>B air greater than bone [conduction]

Ab abortion; antibody

ab abortion; antibody; from [Lat.]

3AB 3-aminobenzamide

ABA abscissic acid; allergic bronchopulmonary aspergillosis; antibacterial activity

ABB Albright-Butler-Bloomberg [syndrome]; American Board of Bioanalysis

abbr abbreviation, abbreviated

ABC absolute basophil count; acid balance control; aconite-belladonna-chloroform; airway, breathing, and circulation; alum, blood, and clay [sludge deodorizing method]; American Blood Commission; antigen-binding capacity; aspiration biopsy cytology; atomic, biological, and chemical [warfare]; axiobuccocervical

ABCC Atomic Bomb Casualty Commission

ABCDE botulism toxin pentavalent

ABCIL antibody-mediated cell-dependent immunolympholysis

ABD aged, blind, and disabled; aggressive behavioral disturbance; average body dose

Abd abdomen, abdominal; abduction, abductor

abd abdomen, abdominal

abdom abdomen, abdominal

ABDPH American Board of Dental Public Health

ABE acute bacterial endocarditis; American Board of Endodontics; botulism equine trivalent antitoxin

ABEPP American Board of Examiners in Professional Psychology

ABG arterial blood gas; axiobuccogingival

ABL abetalipoproteinemia; Albright-

Butler-Lightwood [syndrome]; antigen-binding lymphocyte; Army Biological Laboratory; automated biological laboratory; axiobuccolingual

ABLB alternate binaural loudness balance

ABMS American Board of Medical Specialties

ABMT autologous bone marrow transplantation

Abn, abn abnormal; abnormality(ies)

abnor abnormal

ABO absent bed occupancy; American Board of Orthodontists; blood group system consisting of groups A, AB, B, and O

ABOHN American Board for Occupational Health Nurses

ABOMS American Board of Oral and Maxillofacial Surgery

ABOP American Board of Oral Pathology

Abor abortion

ABP American Board of Pedodontics; American Board of Periodontology; American Board of Prosthodontists; antigen-binding protein; arterial blood pressure

ABPA allergic bronchopulmonary aspergillosis

ABPC antibody-producing cell

ABPE acute bovine pulmonary edema

ABR abortus Bang ring [test]; absolute bed rest; auditory brainstem response

ABr agglutination test for brucellosis

Abras abrasion

ABS abdominal surgery; acute brain syndrome; Adaptive Behavior Scale; admitting blood sugar; adult bovine serum; alkylbenzene sulfonate; amniotic band sequence; at bed side

abs absent; absolute

abs feb while fever is absent [Lat. *absente febre*]

abst, abstr abstract

abt about

ABV actinomycin D–bleomycin-vincristine; arthropod-borne virus

ABVD Adriamycin, bleomycin, vinblastine, and dacarbazine

ABY acid bismuth yeast [medium]

AC abdominal circumference; acetate; acetylcholine; acromioclavicular; activated

charcoal; acupuncture clinic; acute; adenocarcinoma; adenylate cyclase; adrenal cortex; air conduction; alternating current; anodal closure; antecubital; anterior chamber; anterior commissure; antibiotic concentrate; anticoagulant; anticomplement; antiphlogistic corticoid; aortic closure; atriocarotid; auriculocarotid; axiocervical; before meals [Lat. *ante cibum*]

A-C adult-versus-child

A/C anterior chamber of eye ˙

Ac accelerator [globulin]; acetyl; actinium

aC abcoulomb

ac acute; alternating current; before meals [Lat. *ante cibum*]

5-AC azacitidine

ACA adenocarcinoma; American Chiropractic Association; American College of Allergists; American College of Anesthesiologists; American College of Angiology; American College of Apothecaries; American Council on Alcoholism; aminocephalosporanic acid; anterior cerebral artery; anticentromere antibody; anticomplement activity; anticytoplasmic antibody; Automatic Clinical Analyzer

ACACN American Council of Applied Clinical Nutrition

Acad academy

A-CAH autoimmune chronic active hepatitis

ACAO acyl coenzyme A oxidase

ACB antibody-coated bacteria; aortocoronary bypass; arterialized capillary blood; asymptomatic carotid bruit

ACBE air contrast barium enema

ACBG aortocoronary bypass graft

ACC acetyl coenzyme A carboxylase; acinic cell carcinoma; accommodation; adenoid cystic carcinoma; administrative control center; adrenocortical carcinoma; alveolar cell carcinoma; ambulatory care center; anodal closure contraction; articular chondrocalcinosis

Acc adenoid cystic carcinoma; acceleration

acc accident; accommodation

ACCESS Ambulatory Care Clinic Effectiveness Systems Study

ACCH Association for the Care of Children's Health

AcCh acetylcholine

AcChR acetylcholine receptor

AcCHS acetylcholinesterase

ACCL, Accl anodal closure clonus

ACCME Accreditation Council for Continuing Medical Education

AcCoA acetyl coenzyme A

accom accommodation

ACCP American College of Chest Physicians; American College of Clinical Pharmacology

ACD absolute cardiac dullness; acid-citrate-dextrose [solution]; actinomycin D; adult celiac disease; allergic contact dermatitis; American College of Dentists; anterior chest diameter

AC-DC, ac/dc alternating current or direct current

ACE acetonitrile; acute coronary event; adrenocortical extract; alcohol, chloroform, and ether; angiotensin-converting enzyme

ace acentric

ACED anhydrotic congenital ectodermal dysplasia

ACEH acid cholesterol ester hydrolase

ACEP American College of Emergency Physicians

AcEst acetyl esterase

acetyl-CoA acetyl coenzyme A

ACF accessory clinical findings; acute care facility

ACFO American College of Foot Orthopedists

ACFS American College of Foot Surgeons

ACG accelerator globulin; American College of Gastroenterology; angiocardiography, angiocardiogram; aortocoronary graft; apexcardiogram

AC-G, AcG accelerator globulin

ACGME Accreditation Council for Graduate Medical Education

ACGP American College of General Practitioners

ACGPOMS American College of General Practitioners in Osteopathic Medicine and Surgery

ACH active chronic hepatitis; adrenocortical hormone; amyotrophic cerebellar hypoplasia; arm girth, chest depth, and hip width [nutritional index]

ACh acetylcholine

ACHA American College of Hospital Administrators

AChE acetylcholinesterase

AChR acetylcholine receptor

AC&HS before meals and at bedtime [Lat. *ante cibum & hora somni*]

ACI acoustic comfort index; acute coronary infarction; acute coronary insufficiency; adenylate cyclase inhibitor; anticlonus index

ACID Arithmetic, Coding, Information, and Digit Span

ACIF anticomplement immunofluorescence

ACIP acute canine idiopathic polyneuropathy

ACIR Automotive Crash Injury Research

AcK francium [actinium K]

ACL anterior cruciate ligament

ACl aspiryl chloride

ACLA American Clinical Laboratory Association

ACLD Association for Children with Learning Disabilities

ACLM American College of Legal Medicine

ACLPS Academy of Clinical Laboratory Physicians and Scientists

ACLS advanced cardiac life support

ACM acute cerebrospinal meningitis; albumin-calcium-magnesium; Arnold-Chiari malformation

ACMA American Occupational Medical Association

ACME Advisory Council on Medical Education

ACMR Advisory Committee on Medical Research

ACMS American Chinese Medical Society

ACMT artificial circus movement tachycardia

ACN acute conditioned neurosis; American College of Neuropsychiatrists; American College of Nutrition

ACNM American College of Nuclear Medicine; American College of Nurse-Midwives

ACNP American College of Nuclear Physicians

ACO acute coronary occlusion; anodal closure odor

ACoA anterior communicating artery

ACOG American College of Obstetricians and Gynecologists

ACOHA American College of Osteopathic Hospital Administrators

ACO-HNS American Council of Otolaryngology–Head and Neck Surgery

ACOI American College of Osteopathic Internists

ACOMS American College of Oral and Maxillofacial Surgeons

ACOOG American College of Osteopathic Obstetricians and Gynecologists

ACOP American College of Osteopathic Pediatricians

ACORDE A Corsortium on Restorative Dentistry Education

ACOS American College of Osteopathic Surgeons

Acous acoustics, acoustic

ACP accessory conduction pathway; acid phosphatase; acyl carrier protein; American College of Pathologists; American College of Pharmacists; American College of Physicians; American College of Prosthodontists; American College of Psychiatrists; Animal Care Panel; anodal closure picture; aspirin-caffeine-phenacetin; Association for Child Psychiatrists; Association of Clinical Pathologists; Association of Correctional Psychologists

ACPA American Cleft Palate Association

AC-PH acid phosphatase

ACPM American College of Preventive Medicine

ACPP adrenocortical polypeptide

ACR absolute catabolic rate; acriflavine; adenomatosis of colon and rectum; American College of Radiology; anticonstipation regimen

Acr acrylic

ACRF ambulatory care research facility

ACRM American Congress of Rehabilitation Medicine

ACS acrocephalosyndactyly; American Cancer Society; American Chemical Society; American College of Surgeons; anodal closure sound; antireticular cytotoxic serum; aperture current setting; Association of Clinical Scientists

ACSM American College of Sports Medicine

ACSV aortocoronary saphenous vein

ACT achievement through counseling and treatment; actinomycin; activated clotting time; advanced coronary treatment; anticoagulant therapy

act actinomycin; activity, active

ACTA automatic computerized transverse axial [scanning]

Act-C actinomycin C

Act-D actinomycin D

ACTe anodal closure tetanus

ACTH adrenocorticotropic hormone

ACTH-RF adrenocorticotropic hormone releasing factor

ACTN adrenocorticotropin

ACTP adrenocorticotropic polypeptide

ACV acyclovir; atrial/carotid/ventricular

ACVB aortocoronary venous bypass

ACVD acute cardiovascular disease

AD accident dispensary; acetate dialysis; addict, addiction; adenoid degeneration [agent]; admitting diagnosis; alcohol dehydrogenase; Aleutian disease; Alzheimer dementia; Alzheimer disease; analgesic dose; anodal duration; anterior division; antigenic determinant; arthritic dose; Associate Degree; atopic dermatitis; attentional disturbance; autonomic dysreflexia; average deviation; axiodistal; axis deviation; right ear [Lat. *auris dextra*]

A/D analog-to-digital [converter]

A&D ascending and descending

Ad adrenal

ad add [Lat. *adde*]; let there be added [up to a specified amount]; [Lat. *addetur*]; axiodistal; right ear [Lat. *auris dextra*]

ADA adenosine deaminase; American Dental Asociation; American Dermatological Association; American Diabetes Association; American Dietetic Association; anterior descending artery; antideoxyribonucleic acid antibody

ADAA American Dental Assistants Association

ADAMHA Alcohol, Drug Abuse, and Mental Health Administration

ADAP American Dental Assistant's Program; Assistant Director of Army Psychiatry

ADase adenosine deaminase

ADAU adolescent drug abuse unit

ADB accidental death benefit

ADC Aid to Dependent Children; albumin, dextrose, and catalase [medium]; ambulance design criteria; analog-to-digital converter; anodal duration contraction; average daily census; axiodistocervical

AdC adenylate cyclase; adrenal cortex

ADCC antibody-dependent cell-mediated cytotoxicity

ADD adduction; adenosine deaminase; attentional deficit disorder

add add [Lat. *adde*]; addition; adductor, adduction; let there be added [Lat. *addatur*]

add c trit add trituration [Lat. *adde cum tritu*]

ad def an to the point of fainting [Lat. *ad defectionem animi*]

ad deliq to fainting [Lat. *ad deliquium*]

addend to be added [Lat. *addendus*]

ADDH attention deficit disorder with hyperactivity

addict addiction, addictive

ADDS American Digestive Disease Society

ADDU alcohol and drug dependence unit

ADE acute disseminated encephalitis; antibody-dependent enhancement; apparent digestible energy

Ade adenine

AdeCbl adenosyl cobalamine

ADEE age-dependent epileptic encephalopathy

ad effect until effective [Lat. *ad effectum*]

ADEM acute disseminated encephalomyelitis

ad feb fever being present [Lat. *adstante febre*]

ADG atrial diastolic gallop; axiodistogingival

ad gr acid to an agreeable acidity [Lat. *ad gratum aciditatem*]

ad gr gust to an agreeable taste [Lat. *ad gratum gustum*]

ADH Academy of Dentistry for the Handicapped; adhesion; alcohol dehydrogenase; antidiuretic hormone

ADHA American Dental Hygienists Association

adhib to be administered [Lat. *adhibendus*]

ADI Academy of Dentistry International; acceptable daily intake; axiodistoincisal

ad int meanwhile [Lat. *ad interim*]

ADK adenosine kinase

ADL activities of daily living

ADLC antibody-dependent lymphocyte-mediated cytotoxicity

ad lib as desired [Lat. *ad libitum*]

ADM administrative medicine; Adriamycin

AdM adrenal medulla

adm administration; admission

Admin administration

admov let there be applied [Lat. *admove, admoveatur*]

ADN antideoxyribonuclease; aortic depressor nerve

ad naus to the point of producing nausea [Lat. *ad nauseam*]

ADN-B antideoxyribonuclease B

ad neut to neutralization [Lat. *ad neutralizandum*]

ADO adolescent medicine; axiodisto-occlusal

Ado adenosine

Ad-OAP Adriamycin, vincristine, cytarabine, and prednisone

ADOD arthrodentosteodysplasia

AdoDABA adenosyldiaminobutyric acid

AdoHcy *S*-adenosylhomocysteine

AdoMet *S*-adenosylmethionine

Adox oxidized adenosine

ADP adenosine diphosphate; administrative psychiatry; approved drug product; automatic data processing

ad part dolent to the painful parts [Lat. *ad partes dolentes*]

ADPKD autosomal dominant polycystic kidney disease

ADPL average daily patient load

ad pond om to the weight of the whole [Lat. *ad pondus omnium*]

ADPR adenosine diphosphate ribose

ADR Adriamycin; adverse drug reaction

Adr adrenalin; Adriamycin

adr adrenal, adrenalectomy

ADS acute diarrheal syndrome; alternative delivery system; anonymous donor's sperm; antibody deficiency syndrome; antidiuretic substance; Army Dental Service

ad sat to saturation [Lat. *ad saturandum*]

adst feb while fever is present [Lat. *adstante febre*]

ADT Accepted Dental Therapeutics; adenosine triphosphate; admission, discharge, transfer; agar-gel diffusion test; alternate day therapy; any, what you desire, thing (a placebo); Auditory Discrimination Test

ADTA American Dental Trade Association

ADTe anodal duration tetanus

ad us according to custom [Lat. *ad usum*]

ad us ext for external application [Lat. *ad usum externum*]

Adv adenovirus

adv against [Lat. *adversum*]

ad 2 vic at two times, for two doses [Lat. *ad duas vices*]

ADVIRC autosomal dominant vitreo-retinochoroidopathy

A5D5W alcohol 5%, dextrose 5%, in water

ADX adrenalectomized

AE above elbow; acrodermatitis enteropathica; adult erythrocyte; after-effect; agarose electrophoresis; air embolism; air entry; alcoholic embryopathy; anoxic encephalopathy; antitoxic unit [Ger. *Antitoxineinheit*]

A+E accident and emergency [department]

AEA alcohol, ether, and acetone [solution]

AEB avian erythroblastosis

AEC ankyloblepharon, ectodermal defects, and cleft lip [syndrome]; at earliest convenience; Atomic Energy Commission

AED antiepileptic drug

AEE atomic energy establishment

AEF allogenic effect factor; amyloid enhancing factor

AEG air encephalography, air encephalogram

aeg patient [Lat. *aeger, aegra*]

AEGIS Aid for the Elderly in Government Institutions

AEM analytical electron microscopy; avian encephalomyelitis

AEMIS Aerospace and Environmental Medicine Information System

AEN aseptic epiphyseal necrosis

AEP artificial endocrine pancreas; auditory evoked potential; average evoked potential

AEq age equivalent

aeq equal [Lat. *aequales*]

AER acoustic evoked response; aldosterone excretion rate; auditory evoked response; average electroencephalic response; average evoked response

AERE Atomic Energy Research Establishment

AERP atrial effective refractory period

AES acetone-extracted serum; American Electroencephalographic Society; American Encephalographic Society; American Endocrine Society; American Endodontic Society; American Epidemiological Society; American Equilibration Society; anti-embolic stockings; Auger's electron spectroscopy

AEST aeromedical evacuation support team

AET absorption-equivalent thickness; S-(2-aminoethyl) isothiuronium

aet age [Lat. *aetas*]

aetat aged [Lat. *aetatis*]

aetiol etiology [Brit. *aetiology*]

AEV avian erythroblastosis virus

AF abnormal frequency; acid-fast; aflatoxin; albumose-free; aldehyde fuchsin; amaurosis fugax; aminophylline; amniotic fluid; antibody-forming; aortic flow; Arthritis Foundation; ascitic fluid; atrial fibrillation; atrial flutter; attributable fraction; audio frequency; auricular fibrillation

aF abfarad

af audio frequency

AFA alcohol-formaldehyde-acetic [fixative]

AFAR American Foundation for Aging Research

AFB acid-fast bacillus; aflatoxin B; aortofemoral bypass

AFC antibody-forming cell

AFCR American Federation for Clinical Research

AFD accelerated freeze drying

AFDC Aid to Families with Dependent Children

AFDH American Fund for Dental Health

AFF atrial fibrillation; atrial filling fraction; atrial flutter

aff afferent

AFG aflatoxin G; amniotic fluid glucose

AFI amaurotic familial idiocy

AFib atrial fibrillation

AFIP Armed Forces Institute of Pathology

AFL atrial flutter

AFLNH angiofollicular lymph node hyperplasia

AFM aflatoxin M

AFNC Air Force Nurse Corps
AFND acute febrile neutrophilic dermatosis
AFO ankle-foot orthrosis
AFP alpha-fetoprotein; anterior faucial pillar; atypical facial pain
aFP alpha-fetoprotein
AFPP acute fibropurulent pneumonia
AFQ aflatoxin Q
AFR aqueous flare response; ascorbic free radical
AFRD acute febrile respiratory disease
AFRI acute febrile respiratory illness
AFS American Fertility Society; anti-fibroblast serum
AFSAM Air Force School of Aviation Medicine
AFSP acute fibrinoserous pneumonia
AFT aflatoxin; agglutination-flocculation test
AFTA American Family Therapy Association
AG agarose; analytical grade; antigen; antiglobulin; antigravity; atrial gallop; attached gingiva; axiogingival; azurophilic granule
AG, A/G albumin-globulin [ratio]
Ag antigen; silver [Lat. *argentum*]
ag antigen
AGA accelerated growth area; American Gastroenterological Association; American Genetic Association; American Geriatrics Association; American Goiter Association; antiglomerular antibody; appropriately grown for gestational age
Ag-Ab antigen-antibody complex
AGAG acidic glycosaminoglycans
AGBAD Alexander Graham Bell Association for the Deaf
AGC absolute granulocyte count; automatic gain control
AGCT Army General Classification Test
AGD agar gel diffusion; agarose diffusion
AGDD agar gel double diffusion
AGE angle of greatest extension
AGED automated general experimental device
AGEPC acetyl glyceryl ether phosphorylcholine
AGF angle of greatest flexion
ag feb when the fever is coming on [Lat. *aggrediente febre*]
AGG agammaglobulinemia

agg agglutination; aggravation; aggregation
agglut agglutination
aggred feb while the fever is coming on [Lat. *aggrediente febre*]
AGGS anti-gas gangrene serum
agit shake [Lat. *agita*]
agit ante sum shake before taking [Lat. *agita ante sumendum*]
agit vas the vial being shaken [Lat. *agitato vase*]
AGL acute granulocytic leukemia; aminoglutethimide
AGMK African green monkey kidney [cell]
AGMkK African green monkey kidney [cell]
AGN acute glomerulonephritis; agnosia
VIII$_{AGN}$ factor VIII antigen
AgNOR silver-staining nucleolar organizer region
AGOS American Gynecological and Obstetrical Society
AGP acid glycoprotein; agar gel precipitation
AGPA American Group Practice Association; American Group Psychotherapy Association
AGPT agar-gel precipitation test
AGR aniridia, genitourinary abnormalities, and mental retardation; anticipatory goal response
agri agriculture
AGS adrenogenital syndrome; American Geriatrics Society; audiogenic seizures
AGT acute generalized tuberculosis; antiglobulin test
agt agent
AGTH adrenoglomerulotropic hormone
AGTT abnormal glucose tolerance test
AGV aniline gentian violet
AH abdominal hysterectomy; absorptive hypercalciuria; accidental hypothermia; acetohexamide; acute hepatitis; after hyperpolarization; amenorrhea and hirsutism; aminohippurate; anterior hypothalamus; antihyaluronidase; arcuate hypothalamus; Army Hospital; arterial hypertension; artificial heart; ascites hepatoma; astigmatic hypermetropia; autonomic hyperreflexia
A/H amenorrhea-hyperprolactinemia
A+H accident & health [policy]

A·h ampere hour
aH abhenry
ah hyperopic astigmatism
AHA acetohydroxamic acid; acquired hemolytic anemia; acute hemolytic anemia; American Heart Association; American Hospital Association; anterior hypothalamic area; anti-heart antibody; antihistone antibody; area health authority; aspartyl-hydroxamic acid; Associate, Institute of Hospital Administrators; autoimmune hemolytic anemia
AHC acute hemorrhagic conjunctivitis; acute hemorrhagic cystitis
AHCA American Health Care Association
AHCy adenosyl homocysteine
AHD antihypertensive drug; arteriosclerotic heart disease; atherosclerotic heart disease; autoimmune hemolytic disease
AHDMS automated hospital data management system
AHDP azacycloheptane diphosphonate
AHE acute hemorrhagic encephalomyelitis
AHEC area health education center
AHES artificial heart energy system
AHF acute heart failure; American Health Foundation; American Hepatic Foundation; American Hospital Formulary; antihemophilic factor; Argentinian hemorrhagic fever; Associated Health Foundation
AHFS American Hospital Formulary Service
AHG aggregated human globulin; antihemophilic globulin; antihuman globulin
AHGG antihuman gammaglobulin; aggregated human gammaglobulin
AHGS acute herpetic gingival stomatitis
AHH alpha-hydrazine analog of histidine; anosmia and hypogonadotropic hypogonadism [syndrome]; arylhydrocarbon hydroxylase; Association for Holistic Health
AHI active hostility index; Animal Health Institute; apnea-plus-hypopnea index
AHIP assisted health insurance plan
AHIS automated hospital information system
AHLE acute hemorrhagic leukoencephalitis

AHLG antihuman lymphocyte globulin
AHLS antihuman lymphocyte serum
AHM allied health manpower; ambulatory Holter monitor
AHMA American Holistic Medicine Association
AHMC Association of Hospital Management Committees
AHN Army Head Nurse; assistant head nurse
AHO Albright's hereditary osteodystrophy
AHP acute hemorrhagic pancreatitis; after hyperpolarization; air at high pressure; Assistant House Physician
AHPA American Health Planning Association
AHPO anterior hypothalamic preoptic [area]
AHR Association for Health Records
AHRA American Hospital Radiology Administration
AHRF American Hearing Research Foundation
AHS Academy of Health Sciences; African horse sickness; alveolar hypoventilation syndrome; American Hearing Society; American Hospital Society; assistant house surgeon
AHSDF area health service development fund
AHSN Assembly of Hospital Schools of Nursing
AHT aggregation half time; antihyaluronidase titer; augmented histamine test
AHTG antihuman thymocyte globulin
AHTP antihuman thymocyte plasma
AHU acute hemolytic uremic [syndrome]
AHV avian herpes virus
AI accidental injury; accidentally incurred; adiposity index; aggregation index; allergy and immunology; angiogenesis inhibitor; anxiety index; aortic incompetence; aortic insufficiency; apical impulse; articulation index; artificial insemination; artificial intelligence; atherogenic index; atrial insufficiency; axioincisal
AIA allylisopropylacetamide; amylase inhibitor activity
AIB aminoisobutyrate; avian infectious bronchitis
AIBA aminoisobutyric acid

AIBS American Institute of Biological Sciences
AIC aminoimidazole carboxamide; Association des Infirmières Canadiennes
AICA anterior inferior cerebellar artery
AICAR aminoimidazole carboxamide ribonucleotide
AICF autoimmune complement fixation
AID acquired immunodeficiency disease; acute infectious disease; acute ionization detector; Agency for International Development; argon ionization detector; artificial insemination donor; autoimmune deficiency; autoimmune disease; automatic implantable defibrillator
AIDS acquired immune deficiency syndrome
AIDS-KS acquired immune deficiency syndrome with Kaposi's sarcoma
AIE acute inclusion body encephalitis; acute infectious encephalitis, acute infectious endocarditis
AIEP amount of insulin extractable from pancreas
AIF anemia-inducing factor; anti-invasion factor
AIG anti-immunoglobulin
AIH American Institute of Homeopathy; artificial insemination, homologous; artificial insemination by husband
AIHA American Industrial Hygiene Association; autoimmune hemolytic anemia
AIHC American Industrial Health Conference
AIL acute infectious lymphocytosis; angiocentric immunoproliferative lesion; angioimmunoblastic lymphadenopathy
AILD angioimmunoblastic lymphadenopathy with dysproteinemia
AIM Abridged Index Medicus; acute transverse myelopathy; artificial intelligence in medicine
AIMS abnormal involuntary movement scale
AIN acute interstitial nephritis; American Institute of Nutrition
A Insuf aortic insufficiency
AION anterior ischemic optic neuropathy
AIP acute idiopathic pericarditis; acute infectious polyneuritis; acute intermittent porphyria; automated immunoprecipi-

tation; average intravascular pressure; integral anatuberculin, Petragnani
AIPS American Institute of Pathologic Science
AIR amino-imidazole ribonucleotide
AIRA anti-insulin receptor antibody
AIRF alterations in respiratory function
AIS androgen insensitivity syndrome; anterior interosseous nerve syndrome; anti-insulin serum
AISA acquired idiopathic sideroblastic anemia
AIS/MR Alternative Intermediate Services for the Mentally Retarded
AITT arginine insulin tolerance test
AIU absolute iodine uptake; antigen-inducing unit
AIUM American Institute of Ultrasound in Medicine
AIVR accelerated idioventricular rhythm
AJ, A/J ankle jerk
AJCCS American Joint Committee on Cancer Staging
AK above knee; adenosine kinase; adenylate kinase
A/K above knee
AKA above knee amputation; also known as; antikeratin antibody
AK amp above knee amputation
AKE acrokeratoelastoidosis
A/kg amperes per kilogram
AKP alkaline phosphatase
AKS auditory and kinesthetic sensation
AL acute leukemia; adaptation level; albumin; alcoholism; alignment mark; amyloidosis; antihuman lymphocytic [globulin]; avian leukosis; axiolingual; left ear [Lat. *auris laeva*]
Al allantoic; aluminum
al left ear [Lat. *auris laeva*]
ALA American Laryngological Association; American Lung Association; amino-levulinic acid
ALa axiolabial
Ala alanine
AL-Ab antilymphocyte antibody
ALAD abnormal left axis deviation
ALAD, ALA-D aminolevulinic acid dehydrase
ALAG, ALaG axiolabiogingival
ALAL, ALaL axiolabiolingual
ALARA as low as reasonably achievable [radiation exposure]

ALAS aminolevulinic acid synthetase

ALAT alanine aminotransferase

ALB albumin; avian lymphoblastosis

alb albumin; white [Lat. *albus*]

ALC acute lethal catatonia; Alternative Lifestyle Checklist; approximate lethal concentration; avian leukosis complex; axiolinguocervical

alc alcohol, alcoholism, alcoholic

ALCAPA anomalous origin of left coronary artery from pulmonary artery

ALcR, alcR alcohol rub

AlCr aluminum crown

ALD adrenoleukodystrophy; alcoholic liver disease; aldolase; anterior latissimus dorsi

Ald aldolase

ALDH aldehyde dehydrogenase

Aldo, ALDOST aldosterone

ALEP atypical lymphoepithelioid cell proliferation

ALF American Liver Foundation

ALFT abnormal liver function test

ALG antilymphocytic globulin; axiolinguogingival

ALGOL algorithmic oriented language

ALH anterior lobe hormone; anterior lobe of hypophysis

ALIP abnormal localized immature myeloid precursor

ALK, alk alkaline; alkylating

ALK-P alkaline phosphatase

ALL acute lymphoblastic leukemia; acute lymphocytic leukemia

all allergy, allergic

ALLA acute lymphocytic leukemia antigen

ALLO atypical *Legionella*-like organism

ALM aerial lentiginous melanoma

ALME acetyl-lysine methyl ester

ALMI anterior lateral myocardial infarct

ALMV anterior leaflet of the mitral valve

ALN anterior lymph node

ALO average lymphocyte output; axiolinguo-occlusal

ALOS average length of stay

ALP alkaline phosphatase; anterior lobe of pituitary; antilymphocytic plasma

α Greek letter alpha; angular acceleration; first [carbon atom next to the carbon atom bearing the active group in organic compounds]; optical rotation; probability of type I error; solubility coefficient

alpha-GLUC alpha-glucosidase

alpha₂M alpha$_2$-macroglobulin

ALPS angiolymphoproliferative syndrome

ALROS American Laryngological, Rhinological, and Otological Society

ALS acute lateral sclerosis; advanced life support; amyotrophic lateral sclerosis; angiotensin-like substance; anticipated life span; antilymphocyte serum

ALT alanine aminotransferase; avian laryngotracheitis

Alt, alt alternate; altitude

ALTB acute laryngotracheobronchitis

alt dieb every other day [Lat. *alternis diebus*]

ALTEE acetyl-*L*-tyrosine ethyl ester

alt hor every other hour [Lat. *alternis horis*]

alt noct every other night [Lat. *alternis nocta*]

ALU arithmetic and logic unit

ALV adeno-like virus; avian leukosis virus

Alv alveolus, alveolar

alv adst when the bowels are constipated [Lat. *alvo adstricta*]

alv deject discharge from the bowels [Lat. *alvi dejectiones*]

ALV M alveolar mucosa

ALW arch-loop whorl

ALWMI anterolateral wall myocardial infarct

AM actomyosin; acute myelofibrosis; aerospace medicine; alveolar macrophage; alveolar mucosa; ambulatory; amethopterin; ametropia; ammeter; amperemeter; ampicillin; amplitude modulation; anovular menstruation; arithmetic mean; arousal mechanism; aviation medicine; axiomesial; before noon [Lat. *ante meridiem*]; Master of Arts [Lat. *artium magister*]; meter angle; myopic astigmatism

Am americium; amnion; amyl

A/m amperes per meter

A-m² ampere-square meter

am ametropia; before noon [Lat. *ante meridiem*]; meter angle; myopic astigmatism

AMA against medical advice; American Medical Association; antimitochondrial antibody; antimyosin antibody; Australian Medical Association

AMA-DE American Medical Association Drug Evaluation

AMAP as much as possible

A-MAT amorphous material

AMB avian myeloblastosis; amphotericin B

amb ambient; ambiguous; ambulance; ambulatory

ambig ambiguous

AMBL acute megakaryoblastic leukemia

ambul ambulatory

AMC Animal Medical Center; antimalaria campaign; arm muscle circumference; Army Medical Corps; arthrogryposis multiplex congenita; automated mixture control; axiomesiocervical

AMCHA aminomethylcyclohexane-carboxylic acid

AMD acid maltase deficiency; acromandibular dysplasia; alpha-methyldopa; Association for Macular Diseases; axiomesiodistal

AMDS Association of Military Dental Surgeons

AME aseptic meningoencephalitis

AMEA American Medical Electroencephalographic Association

AMEDS Army Medical Service

AMEGL, AMegL acute megakaryoblastic leukemia

AMet adenosyl-*L*-methionine

AMF antimuscle factor

AMG amyloglucosidase; antimacrophage globulin; axiomesiogingival

AMH automated medical history

Amh mixed astigmatism with myopia predominating

AMHA Association of Mental Health Administrators

AMHT automated multiphasic health testing

AMI acquired monosaccharide intolerance; acute myocardial infarction; amitriptyline; anterior myocardial infarction; Association of Medical Illustrators; axiomesioincisal

AML acute monocytic leukemia; acute myeloblastic leukemia; acute myelocytic leukemia; anterior mitral leaflet

AMLB alternate monoaural loudness balance [test]

AMLR autologous mixed lymphocyte reaction

AMLS antimouse lymphocyte serum

AMM agnogenic myeloid metaplasia; ammonia; antibody to murine cardiac myosin; World Medical Association [Fr. *Association Médicale Mondiale*]

AMML acute myelomonocytic leukemia

AMMoL acute myelomonoblastic leukemia

ammon ammonia

AMN adrenomyeloneuropathy; alloxazine mononucleotide

AMO assistant medical officer; axiomesio-occlusal

A-mode amplitude modulation

AMOL acute monoblastic leukemia

amor amorphous

AMP accelerated mental processes; acid mucopolysaccharide; adenosine monophosphate; amphetamine; ampicillin; ampule; amputation; average mean pressure

amp ampere; amplification; ampule; amputation, amputee

AMPA American Medical Publishers Association

AMPAC American Medical Political Action Committee

AMP-c cyclic adenosine monophosphate

amp-hr ampere-hour

A-M pr Austin-Moore prosthesis

AMPS abnormal mucopolysacchariduria; acid mucopolysaccharide

AMPT alpha-methylparatyrosine

ampul ampule

AMR activity metabolic rate; alternate motion rate; alternating motion reflex

AMRA American Medical Record Association

AMRL Aerospace Medical Research Laboratories

AMRNL Army Medical Research and Nutrition Laboratory

AMRS automated medical record system

AMS acute mountain sickness; aggravated in military service; altered mental status; American Microscopical Society; amylase; antimacrophage serum; Army Medical Service; Association of Military

Surgeons; auditory memory span; automated multiphasic screening

ams amount of a substance

AMSA acridinylamine methanesulfon-m-anisidide; American Medical Society on Alcoholism; American Medical Students Association

AMSC Army Medical Specialist Corps

AMSRDC Army Medical Service Research and Development Command

AMT acute miliary tuberculosis; alpha-methyltyrosine; American Medical Technologists; amethopterin; amphetamine

amt amount

AMU Army Medical Unit

amu atomic mass unit

AmuLV Abelson murine leukemia virus

AMV avian myeloblastosis virus

AMVI acute mesenteric vascular insufficiency

AMWA American Medical Women's Association; American Medical Writers' Association

AMY amylase

AN acanthosis nigricans; acne neonatorum; acoustic neuroma; adult, normal; aneurysm; anisometropia; anode; anorexia nervosa; antenatal; anterior; antineuraminidase; aseptic necrosis; atrionodal; avascular necrosis

A/N as needed

An actinon; anisometropia; anode, anodal

A$_n$ normal atmosphere

ANA acetylneuraminic acid; American Narcolepsy Association; American Neurological Association; American Nurses Association; anesthesia [*anaesthesia*]; antibody to nuclear antigens; antinuclear antibody; aspartyl naphthylamide

ANAE alpha-naphthyl acetate esterase

anal analgesia, analgesic; analysis, analytic

ANAP agglutination negative, absorption positive [reaction]

anast anastomosis

Anat, anat anatomy, anatomist

ANC absolute neutrophil count; acid neutralization capacity; antigen-neutralizing capacity; Army Nurse Corps

ANCC, AnCC anodal closure contraction

AND algoneurodystrophy; anterior nasal discharge

ANDA Abbreviated New Drug Application

ANDTE, AnDTe anodal duration tetanus

anes, anesth anesthesia, anesthetic

ANESR apparent norepinephrine secretion rate

AnEx, an ex anodal excitation

ANF alpha-naphthoflavone; American Nurses' Foundation; antinuclear factor

ang angiography, angiogram; angle, angular

Ang GR angiotensin generation rate

anh anhydrous

ANIT alpha-naphthyl-isothiocyanate

ank ankle

ANL acute nonlymphoblastic leukemia

ANLL acute nonlymphocytic leukemia

Ann annual

ann fib annulus fibrosus

ANuA antinuclear antibody

ANOC, AnOC anodal opening contraction

ANOVA analysis of variance

ANP A-norprogesterone; atrial natriuretic peptide

A-NPP absorbed normal pooled plasma

ANRC American National Red Cross

ANS acanthion; American Nutrition Society; 8-anilino-1-naphthalene-sulfonic acid; anterior nasal spine; antineutrophilic serum; antirat neutrophil serum; Army Nursing Service; arterionephrosclerosis; Associate in Nursing Science; autonomic nervous system

ANSCII American National Standard Code for Information Interchange

ANSI American National Standards Institute

ANT acoustic noise test; aminonitro-thiazole

ant anterior; antimycin

AntA antimycin A

antag antagonist

anti-HB$_c$ antibody to hepatitis B core antigen

anti-HB$_s$ antibody to hepatitis B surface antigen

anti-PNM Ab anti-peripheral nerve myelin antibody

ant jentac before breakfast [Lat. *ante jentaculum*]

ANTR apparent net transfer rate

ANTU alpha-naphthylthiourea

ANUG acute necrotizing ulcerative gingivitis

AO abdominal aorta; acid output; acridine orange; anodal opening; anterior oblique; aortic opening; atomic orbital; atrioventricular valve opening; auriculoventricular valve opening; axio-occlusal

A&O alert and oriented

AOA Administration on Aging; American Optometric Association; American Orthopedic Association; American Orthopsychiatric Association; American Osteopathic Association

AOAA amino-oxyacetic acid

AOAC Association of Official Agricultural Chemists

AOAP as often as possible

AOAS American Osteopathic Academy of Sclerotherapy

AOB accessory olfactory bulb; alcohol on breath

AOBS acute organic brain syndrome

AOC amyloxycarbonyl; anodal opening contraction; area of concern

AOCA American Osteopathic College of Anesthesiologists

AOCD American Osteopathic College of Dermatology

AOCl anodal opening clonus

AOCPA American Osteopathic College of Pathologists

AOCPR American Osteopathic College of Proctology

AOCR American Osteopathic College of Radiology; American Osteopathic College of Rheumatology

AOD Academy of Operative Dentistry; Academy of Oral Dynamics; adult onset diabetes; arterial occlusive disease; auriculo-osteodysplasia

AODM adult onset diabetes mellitus

AODME Academy of Osteopathic Directors of Medical Education

AOHA American Osteopathic Hospital Association

AOL acro-osteolysis

AOM azoxymethane

AOMA American Occupational Medical Association

AOO anodal opening odor; atrial asynchronous (competitive, fixed-rate) [pacemaker]

AOP anodal opening picture; aortic pressure

AOPA American Orthotics and Prosthetics Association

AOS American Ophthalmological Society; American Otological Society; anodal opening sound; anterior [o]esophageal sensor

AOSSM American Orthopedic Society for Sports Medicine

AOT Association of Occupational Therapists

AOTA American Occupational Therapy Association

AOTe anodal opening tetanus

AOU apparent oxygen utilization

AP accessory pathway; acid phosphatase; action potential; acute proliferative; adolescent psychiatry; alkaline phosphatase; alum precipitated; aminopeptidase; angina pectoris; antepartal [Lat. *ante partum*]; anterior pituitary; anteroposterior; antidromic potential; aortic pressure; apical pulse; apothecary; appendectomy; appendicitis; appendix; area postrema; arithmetic progression; arterial pressure; artificial pneumothorax; assessment and plans; association period; atrial pacing; atrioventricular pathway; axiopulpal; before dinner [Lat. *ante prandium*]; before parturition [Lat. *ante partum*]

A&P anterior and posterior; assessment and plans; auscultation and percussion

Ap apex

APA aldosterone-producing adenoma; American Pancreatic Association; American Pharmaceutic Association; American Physiotherapy Association; American Podiatric Association; American Psychiatric Association; American Psychoanalytic Association; American Psychological Association; American Psychopathological Association; American Psychotherapy Association; aminopenicillanic acid; antipernicious anemia [factor]

APAF antipernicious anemia factor

APAP acetaminophen

APB atrial premature beat

APC acetylsalicylic acid, phenacetin, and caffeine; adenoidal-pharyngeal-conjunctival [agent]; adenomatous polyposis coli; antigen-presenting cell;

antiphlogistic corticoid; aperture current; apneustic center; aspirin-phenacetin-caffeine; atrial premature contraction

APCC aspirin-phenacetin-caffeine-codeine

APCF acute pharyngoconjunctival fever

APCG apex cardiogram

APD action potential duration; antero-posterior diameter; atrial premature depolarization; autoimmune progesterone dermatitis; automated peritoneal dialysis

A-PD anteroposterior diameter

APE acetone powder extract; acute polioencephalitis; acute psychotic episode; aminophylline, phenobarbital, and ephedrine; anterior pituitary extract; avian pneumoencephalitis

APECED autoimmune polyendocrinopathy-candidosis-ectodermal dystrophy

APF acidulated phosphofluoride; American Psychological Foundation; animal protein factor; antiperinuclear factor

APG acid-precipated globulin; animal pituitary gonadotropin

APGAR American Pediatric Gross Assessment Record

APGL alkaline phosphatase activity of granular leukocytes

APH antepartum hemorrhage; anterior pituitary hormone; Association of Private Hospitals

APHA American Protestant Hospital Association; American Public Health Association

APhA American Pharmaceutical Association

APHP anti-Pseudomonas human plasma

API alkaline protease inhibitor; Analytical Profile Index; atmospheric pressure ionization

APIC Association for Practitioners in Infection Control

APIE assessment, plan, implementation, and evaluation

APIM Association Profesionnelle Internationale des Médecins

APIP additional personal injury protection

APIVR artificial pacemaker-induced ventricular rhythm

APKD adult-onset polycystic kidney disease

APL abductor pollicis longus; accelerated painless labor; acute premyelocytic leukemia; animal placenta lactogen; anterior pituitary-like

APM Academy of Parapsychology and Medicine; Academy of Physical Medicine; Academy of Psychosomatic Medicine; acid precipitable material; aspartame; Association of Professors of Medicine

APMR Association for Physical and Mental Retardation

APN average peak noise

APO apomorphine

apoth apothecary

APP alum-precipitated pyridine; amino-pyrazolopyrimidine; antiplatelet plasma; avian pancreatic polypeptide

app appendix

APPA American Psychopathological Association

appar apparatus

APPG aqueous procaine penicillin G

appl appliance; application, applied

approx approximate

appt appointment

appy appendectomy

APR abdominoperineal resection; absolute proximal reabsorption; amebic prevalence rate; anterior pituitary reaction

aprax apraxia

APRL American Prosthetic Research Laboratory

AProL acute promyelocytic leukemia

APRP acidic proline-rich protein; acute phase reactant protein

APRT adenine phosphoribosyl transferase

APS adenosine phosphosulfate; American Pediatric Society; American Physiological Society; American Proctologic Society; American Prosthodontic Society; American Psychological Society; American Psychosomatic Society

APSGN acute poststreptococcal glomerulonephtitis

APSQ Abbreviated Parent Symptom Questionnaire

APSS Association for the Psychophysiological Study of Sleep

APT alum-precipitated toxoid

APTA American Physical Therapy Association

APTD Aid to Permanently and Totally Disabled

APTT, aPTT activated partial thromboplastin time

APUD amine precursor uptake and decarboxylation

AQ achievement quotient; any quantity

aq water [Lat. *aqua*]

aq ad add water [Lat. *aquam ad*]

aq bull boiling water [Lat. *aqua bulliens*]

aq cal hot water [Lat. *aqua calida*]

aq dest distilled water [Lat. *aqua destillata*]

aq ferv hot water [Lat. *aqua fervens*]

aq frig cold water [Lat. *aqua frigata*]

aq pur pure water [Lat. *aqua pura*]

AQS additional qualifying symptoms

aq tep tepid water [Lat. *aqua tepida*]

aqu aqueous

AR achievement ratio; actinic reticuloid [syndrome]; active resistance; adherence ratio; airway resistance; alarm reaction; allergic rhinitis; alloy restoration; analytical reagent; androgen receptor; anterior root; aortic regurgitation; apical-radial; Argyll Robertson [pupil]; arsphenamine; articulare; artificial respiration; at risk; atrophic rhinitis; autoradiography; autosomal recessive

Ar argon; articulare

A/R apical/radial

A&R advised and released

ARA Academy of Rehabilitative Audiometry; acetylene reduction activity; American Rheumatism Association; antireticulin antibody; Associate of the Royal Academy

ara-A adenine arabinoside

ara-C cytosine arabinoside

ARAMIS American Rheumatism Association Medical Information System

ARAS ascending reticular activating system

ARB adrenergic receptor binder

arb arbitrary unit

ARBOR arthropod-borne [virus]

ARC accelerating rate calorimetry; acquired immunodeficiency syndrome–related complex; active renin concentration; AIDS-related complex; American Red Cross; anomalous retinal corres-

pondence; Arthritis Rehabilitation Center; Association for Retarded Children

ARCA acquired red cell aplasia

ARCI Addiction Research Center Inventory

ARCS Associate of the Royal College of Science

ARD absolute reaction of degeneration; acute respiratory disease; adult respiratory distress; anorectal dressing; arthritis and rheumatic diseases; atopic respiratory disease

ARDS adult respiratory distress syndrome

AREDYLD acrorenal field defect, ectodermal dysplasia, lipoatrophic diabetes

ARF acute renal failure; acute respiratory failure; acute rheumatic fever; Addiction Research Foundation; area resource file

ARFC active rosette-forming T-cell

ARG, Arg arginine

arg silver [Lat. *argentum*]

ARI acute respiratory illness; airway reactivity index

ARIA automated radioimmunoassay

ARL average remaining lifetime

ARLD alcohol related liver disease

ARM adrenergic receptor material; Armenian [hamster]; artificial rupture of membranes; atomic resolution microscopy

ARN acute renal necrosis; acute retinal necrosis; Association of Rehabilitation Nurses

ARNMD Association for Research in Nervous and Mental Diseases

ARNP Advanced Registered Nurse Practitioner

ARO Associate for Research in Ophthalmology

AROM active range of motion; artificial rupture of membranes

ARP absolute refractory period; American Registry of Pathologists; assimilation regulatory protein; at risk period; automaticity recovery phase

ARPES angular resolved photoelectron spectroscopy

ARPT American Registry of Physical Therapists

ARRC Associate of the Royal Red Cross

ARRS American Roentgen Ray Society

ARRT American Registry of Radiologic Technologists

ARS alizarin red S; American Radium Society; American Rhinologic Society; antirabies serum

Ars arsphenamine

ARSA American Reye's Syndrome Association

ARSC Associate of the Royal Society of Chemistry

ARSM acute respiratory system malfunction

ARSPH Associate of the Royal Society for the Promotion of Health

ART absolute retention time; Accredited Record Technician; algebraic reconstruction technique; automated reagin test; automaticity recovery time

art artery, arterial; articulation; artificial

artic articulation, articulated

artif artificial

ARV AIDS-associated retrovirus

AS acetylstrophanthidin; acoustic stimulation; active sleep; Adams-Stokes [disease]; Alport syndrome; anal sphincter; androsterone sulfate; ankylosing spondylitis; anovulatory syndrome; antiserum; antistreptolysin; anxiety state; aortic stenosis; aqueous solution; aqueous suspension; arteriosclerosis; artificial sweetener; astigmatism; asymmetric; atropine sulfate; audiogenic seizure; left ear [Lat. *auris sinistra*]

As arsenic; astigmatism

A·s ampere second

A x s ampere per second

aS absiemens

as left ear [Lat. *auris sinistra*]

ASA acetylsalicylic acid; Adams-Stokes attack; American Society of Anesthesiologists; American Standards Association; American Surgical Association; argininosuccinic acid; arylsulfatase-A; aspirin-sensitive asthma

ASAAD American Society for the Advancement of Anesthesia in Dentistry

ASAHP American Society of Allied Health Professions

ASAIO American Society for Artificial Internal Organs

ASAP American Society for Adolescent Psychology; as soon as possible

ASAT aspartate aminotransferase

ASB American Society of Bacteriologists; anesthesia standby; asymptomatic bacteriuria

ASC acetylsulfanilyl chloride; American Society of Cytology

asc ascending

ASCH American Society of Clinical Hypnosis

ASCI American Society for Clinical Investigation

ASCII American Standard Code for Information Interchange

ASCLT American Society of Clinical Laboratory Technicians

ASCMS American Society of Contemporary Medicine and Surgery

ASCO American Society of Clinical Oncology; American Society of Contemporary Ophthalmology

ASCP American Society of Clinical Pathologists; American Society of Consulting Pharmacists

ASCR American Society of Chiropodical Roentgenology

ascr ascribed to [Lat. *ascriptum*]

ASCVD arteriosclerotic cardiovascular disease; atherosclerotic cardiovascular disease

ASD aldosterone secretion defect; antisiphon device; arthritis syphilitica deformans; atrial septal defect

ASDC American Society of Dentistry for Children; Association of Sleep Disorders Centers

ASDH acute subdural hematoma

ASE acute stress erosion

ASF African swine fever; aniline-sulfur-formaldehyde [resin]

ASFR age-specific fertility rate

ASG American Society for Genetics; Army Surgeon General

ASGE American Society for Gastrointestinal Endoscopy

AS/GP antiserum, guinea pig

ASH American Society of Hematology; antistreptococcal hyaluronidase; asymmetrical septal hypertrophy

AsH astigmatism, hypermetropic

ASHA American School Health Association; American Social Health Association; American Speech and Hearing Association

ASHBM Associate Scottish Hospital Bureau of Management

ASHD arteriosclerotic heart disease

ASHET American Society for Health Manpower Education and Training

ASHG American Society for Human Genetics

ASHI Association for the Study of Human Infertility

AS/Ho antiserum, horse

ASHP American Society of Hospital Pharmacists; American Society for Hospital Planning

ASHPA American Society for Hospital Personnel Administration

ASI anxiety status inventory

ASII American Science Information Institute

ASIM American Society of Internal Medicine

ASIS anterior superior iliac spine

ASK antistreptokinase

ASL antistreptolysin

ASLIB Association of Special Libraries and Information Bureau

ASLM American Society of Law and Medicine

ASLO antistreptolysin O

ASLT antistreptolysin test

ASM American Society for Microbiology; anterior scalenus muscle

AsM astigmatism, myopic

ASMD atonic sclerotic muscle dystrophy

ASME Association for the Study of Medical Education

ASMI anteroseptal myocardial infarct

As/Mk antiserum, monkey

ASMPA Armed Services Medical Procurement Agency

ASMR age-standardized mortality ratio

ASMT American Society for Medical Technology

ASN alkali-soluble nitrogen; American Society of Nephrology; American Society of Neurochemistry; arteriosclerotic nephritis; asparagine; Associate in Nursing

Asn asparagine

ASO antistreptolysin O; arteriosclerosis obliterans

ASOS American Society of Oral Surgeons

ASOT antistreptolysin-O test

ASP African swine pox; aged substrate plasma; alkali-stable pepsin; American Society of Parasitology; ankylosing spondylitis; aortic systolic pressure; area

systolic pressure; asparaginase; aspartic acid

Asp aspartic acid; asparaginase

ASPA American Society of Physician Analysts; American Society of Podiatric Assistants

ASPDM American Society of Psychosomatic Dentistry and Medicine

ASPG antispleen globulin

ASPM American Society of Paramedics

ASPO American Society for Psychoprophylaxis in Obstetrics

ASPP Association for Sane Psychiatric Practices

ASPRS American Society of Plastic and Reconstructive Surgeons

ASR aldosterone secretion rate

AS/Rab antiserum, rabbit

ASRT American Society of Radiologic Technologists

ASS acute serum sickness; anterior superior spine

ASSC acute splenic sequestration crisis

ASSO American Society for the Study of Orthodontics

Assoc association, associate

AST angiotensin sensitivity test; anterior spinothalamic tract; aspartate aminotransferase (SGOT); Association of Medical Technologists; atrial overdrive stimulation rate; audiometry sweep test

Ast astigmatism

ASTA anti-alpha-staphylolysin

Asth asthenopia

ASTHO Association of State and Territorial Health Officers

ASTI antispasticity index

ASTM American Society for Testing and Materials

ASTMH American Society of Tropical Medicine and Hygiene

ASTO antistreptolysin O

as tol as tolerated

ASTZ antistreptozyme

ASV anodic stripping voltammetry; antisiphon valve; antisnake venom; avian sarcoma virus

ASVO American Society of Veterinary Ophthalmology

ASVPP American Society of Veterinary Physiologists and Pharmacologists

Asx amino acid that gives aspartic acid after hydrolysis

asym asymmetry, asymmetric

AT achievement test; Achilles tendon; adjunctive therapy; air temperature; aminotransferase; amitriptyline; anaerobic threshold; antithrombin; antitrypsin; applanation tonometry; ataxia-telangiectasia; atrial tachycardia; axonal terminal; old tuberculin [Gr. *alt Tuberkulin*]
AT old tuberculin [Gr. *alt Tuberkulin*]
A-T ataxia telangiectasia
AT₁₀ dihydrotachysterol
AT III antithrombin III
At astatine; atrium, atrial
at air tight; atom, atomic
ATA alimentary toxic aleukia; American Thyroid Association; antithymic activity; anti-thyroglobulin antibody; anti-Toxoplasma antibody; atmosphere absolute; aurintricarboxylic acid
ATB at the time of the bomb [A-bomb in Japan]
ATC activated thymus cell
ATCC American Type Culture Collection
ATD Alzheimer-type dementia; androstatrienedione; anthropomorphic test dummy; asphyxiating thoracic dystrophy
ATDC Association of Thalidomide Damaged Children
ATE adipose tissue extract; autologous tumor extract
ATEE N-acetyl-1-tyrosyl-ethyl ester
ATF ascites tumor fluid
At Fib atrial fibrillation
ATG antihuman thymocyte globulin; antithrombocyte globulin; antithymocyte globulin; antithyroglobulin
ATGAM antithymocyte gamma-globulin
AT/GC adenine-thymine/guanine-cytosine [ratio]
ATH acetyl-tyrosine hydrazide
ATh Associate in Therapy
Athsc atherosclerosis
ATL Achilles tendon lengthening; adult T-cell leukemia; antitension line
ATLA adult T-cell leukemia virus-associated antigen
ATLS Advanced Trauma Life Support Program
ATLV adult T-cell leukemia virus
ATM acute transverse myelopathy
atm standard atmosphere
ATMA antithyroid plasma membrane antibody

atmos atmospheric
ATN acute tubular necrosis; augmented transition network
ATNC atraumatic normocephalic
at no atomic number
ATNR asymmetric tonic neck reflex
ATP adenosine triphosphate; ambient temperature and pressure
A-TP adsorbed test plasma
ATPase adenosine triphosphatase
ATP-2Na adenosine triphosphate disodium
ATPS ambient temperature and pressure, saturated
ATR Achilles tendon reflex
atr atrophy
ATS Achard-Thiers syndrome; acid test solution; American Thoracic Society; American Trudeau Society; American Trauma Society; antirat thymocyte serum; antitetanus serum; antithymocyte serum; anxiety tension state; arteriosclerosis
ATSDR Agency for Toxic Substances and Disease Registry
ATT arginine tolerance test; aspirin tolerance time
att attending
ATV avian tumor virus
at vol atomic volume
at wt atomic weight
AU according to custom [Lat. *ad usum*]; allergenic unit; Ångström unit; antitoxin unit; arbitrary unit; Australia antigen; azauridine; both ears together [Lat. *aures unitas*]; each ear [Lat. *auris uterque*]
Au Australia [antigen]; gold [Lat. *aurum*]
AUA American Urological Association
Au Ag Australia antigen
AUC area under the curve
aud auditory
aud-vis audiovisual
AUG acute ulcerative gingivitis
Aug increase [Lat. *augere*]
AUL acute undifferentiated leukemia
AUO amyloid of unknown origin
AUPHA Association of University Programs in Health Administration
aur, auric auricle, auricular
AUS acute urethral syndrome
AuS Australia serum hepatitis
ausc auscultation
aux auxiliary

AV anteroventral; anteversion; anticipatory vomiting; aortic valve; arteriovenous; artificial ventilation; atrioventricular; audiovisual; auriculoventricular; average; aviation medicine; avoirdupois

A-V arteriovenous; atrioventricular; auriculoventricular

A/V ampere/volt

Av average; avoirdupois

aV abvolt

AVA antiviral antibody; arteriovenous anastomosis

AV/AF anteverted, anteflexed

AVB atrioventricular block

AVC Academy of Veterinary Cardiology; associative visual cortex; Association of Vitamin Chemists; atrioventricular canal

AVCS atrioventricular conduction system

AVD aortic valvular disease; apparent volume of distribution; atrioventricular dissociation; Army Veterinary Department

avdp avoirdupois

AVE aortic valve echocardiogram

AVF antiviral factor; arteriovenous fistula

aV$_f$ unipolar limb lead on the left leg in electrocardiography

avg average

AVH acute viral hepatitis

AVI air velocity index; Association of Veterinary Inspectors

aV$_1$ unipolar limb lead on the left arm in electrocardiography

AVLINE Audiovisuals On-Line

AVM arteriovenous malformation; aviation medicine

AVMA American Veterinary Medical Association

AVN atrioventricular nodal [conduction]; atrioventricular node

AVNFRP atrioventricular node functional refractory period

AVNR atrioventricular nodal reentry

AVP ambulatory venous pressure; antiviral protein; aqueous vasopressin; arginine vasopressin

AVR accelerated ventricular rhythm; aortic valve replacement

aV$_r$ unipolar limb lead on the right arm in electrocardiography

AVRI acute viral respiratory infection

AVRP atrioventricular refractory period

AVRT atrioventricular reentrant tachycardia

AVS aortic valve stenosis; auditory vocal sequencing

AVT Allen vision test; arginine vasotocin; Aviation Medicine Technician

Av3V anteroventral third ventricle

AW above waist; abrupt withdrawal; anterior wall; atomic warfare; atomic weight

A&W alive and well

AWG American Wire Gauge

AWI anterior wall infarction

AWMI anterior wall myocardial infarction

AWP airway pressure

AWRS anti-whole rabbit serum

AWS alcohol withdrawal syndrome

AWTA aniridia-Wilms' tumor association

awu atomic weight unit

ax axillary; axis, axial

AXF advanced x-ray facility

AXT alternating exotropia

A^y yellow [mouse]

AYA acute yellow atrophy

AYF antiyeast factor

AYP autolyzed yeast protein

AZ Aschheim-Zondek [test]

Az nitrogen {Fr. *azote*]

AZA azathioprine

azg azaguanine

AZO [indicates presence of the group] –N:N–

AZQ diaziquone

AZT Aschheim-Zondek test; azidothymidine

AzUr 6-azauridine

–B–

B bacillus; bands; barometric; base; basophil, basophilic; bath [Lat. *balneum*]; Baumé scale; behavior; bel; Benoist scale; benzoate; beta; biscuspid; blood; bloody; blue; body; boils at; Bolton point; bone marrow-derived [cell or lymphocyte];

boron; bound; bovine; bregma; brother; *Brucella*; buccal; Bucky [film in cassette in Potter-Bucky diaphragm]; bursa cells; magnetic induction; supramentale [point]
b barn; base; boils at; born; brain; supramentale [point]; twice [Lat. *bis*]
B_0 constant magnetic field in nuclear magnetic resonance
B_1 radiofrequency magnetic field in nuclear magnetic resonance; thiamine
B_2 riboflavin
B_6 pyridoxine
B_7 biotin
B_8 adenosine phosphate
B_{12} cyanocobalamin
ß see beta
BA Bachelor of Arts; backache; bacterial agglutination; basion; benzyladenine; best amplitude; betamethasone acetate; bilateral asymmetrical; biliary atresia; blocking antibody; blood agar; bone age; boric acid; bovine albumin; brachial artery; breathing apparatus; bronchial asthma; buccoaxial; sand bath [Lat. *baleum arenae*]
Ba barium; basion; barium [enema];
ba basion
BAA benzoylarginine amide; branched amino acid
BAB blood agar base
Bab Babinski's reflex; baboon
BabK baboon kidney
BAC bacterial adherent colony; bacterial antigen complex; blood alcohol concentration; British Association of Chemists; bronchoalveolar cells; buccoaxiocervical
Bac, *bac Bacillus*, bacillary
BACOP bleomycin, Adriamycin, cyclophosphamide, vincristine, and prednisone
Bact, bact *Bacterium*; bacterium, bacteria
BAD biological aerosol detection; British Association of Dermatologists
BaE barium enema
BAEE benzoylarginine ethyl ester
BaEn barium enema
BAEP brainstem auditory evoked potential
BAER brainstem auditory evoked response

BAG buccoaxiogingival
BAGG buffered azide glucose glycerol
BAIB beta-aminoisobutyric [acid]
BAIF bile acid independent flow
BAIT bacterial automated identification technique
BAL blood alcohol level; British anti-lewisite; bronchoalveolar lavage
bal balance; balsam; bath [Lat. *balneum*]
bals balsam
BALT bronchus-associated lymphoid tissue
BaM barium meal
Bam benzamide
BAME benzoylarginine methyl ester
BAN British Approved Name; British Association of Neurologists
BAO basal acid output; brachial artery output
BAP bacterial alkaline phosphatase; blood-agar plate; bovine albumin in phosphate buffer; brachial artery pressure
BAPhysMed British Association of Physical Medicine
BAPI barley alkaline protease inhibitor
BAPN beta-aminoproprionitrile fumarate
BAPS British Association of Paediatric Surgeons; British Association of Plastic Surgeons
BAPT British Association of Physical Training
BAPV bovine alimentary papilloma virus
BAR bariatrics; barometer, barometric
bar barometric
BART blood-activated recalcification time
BAS balloon atrial septostomy; benzyl anti-serotinin
bas basophil, basophilic
BASH body acceleration synchronous with heart rate
BASIC Beginner's All-Purpose Symbolic Introduction Code
baso basophil
BAT brown adipose tissue
BAUS British Association of Urological Surgeons
BAV bicuspid aortic valve
BAVFO bradycardia after arteriovenous fistula occlusion
BB bad breath; bed bath; beta blockade, beta blocker; BioBreeding [rat]; blanket

bath; blood bank; blood buffer; blow bottle; blue bloaters [emphysema]; both bones; breakthrough bleeding; breast biopsy; buffer base; isoenzyme of creatine kinase containing two B subunits

bb Bolton point

BBA born before arrival

BBB blood-brain barrier; bundle branch block

BBBB bilateral bundle branch block

BBC bromobenzycyanide

BBD benign breast disease

BBE *Bacteroides* bile esculin [agar]

BBEP brush border endopeptidase

BBI Bowman-Birk soybean inhibitor

BBM brush border membrane

BBMV brush border membrane vesicle

BBS benign breast syndrome; bombesin

BBT basal body temperature

BB/W BioBreeding/Worcester [rat]

BC Bachelor of Surgery [Lat. *Baccalaureus Chirurgiae*]; bactericidal concentration; battle casualty; biliary colic; bipolar cell; birth control; blastic crisis; blood culture; Blue Cross [plan]; bone conduction; bronchial carcinoma; buccal cartilage; buccocervical

b/c benefit/cost [ratio]

BCA balloon catheter angioplasty; blood color analyzer; Blue Cross Association; branchial cleft anomaly

BCAA branched chain-enriched amino acid

BCB brilliant cresyl blue

BC/BS Blue Cross/Blue Shield [plan]

BCC basal-cell carcinoma; birth control clinic

bcc body-centered-cubic

BCCG British Cooperative Clinical Group

BCCP biotin carboxyl carrier protein

BCD binary-coded decimal

BCDDP Breast Cancer Detection Demonstration Project

BCE basal cell epithelioma; bubble chamber equipment

BCF basophil chemotactic factor

BCFP breast cyst fluid protein

BCG bacille Calmette-Guérin [vaccine] ballistocardiography, ballistocardiogram; bicolor guaiac test; bromcresol green

BCH basal cell hyperplasia

BCh Bachelor of Surgery [Lat. *Baccalaureus Chirurgiae*]

BChD Bachelor of Dental Surgery

BChir Bachelor of Surgery [Lat. *Baccalaureus Chirurgiae*]

bChl bacterial chlorophyll

BCHS Bureau of Community Health Services

BCLL B-cell chronic lymphocytic leukemia

BCLP bilateral cleft of lip and palate

BCLS basic cardiac life support

BCM birth control medication

BCME bis-chloromethyl ether

BCNS basal cell nevus syndrome

BCNU 1,3-bis-(2-chloroethyl)-1-nitrosourea

BCP birth control pill; Blue Cross Plan; bromcresol purple

BCPV bovine cutaneous papilloma virus

BCR bromocriptine

BCS battered child syndrome; blood cell separator; British Cardiac Society; Budd-Chiari syndrome

BCTF Breast Cancer Task Force

BCtg bovine chymotrypsinogen

BCtr bovine chymotrypsin

BCW biological and chemical warfare

BD barbital-dependent; barbiturate dependence; base deficit; base of prism down; basophilic degeneration; Batten's disease; behavioral disorder; belladonna; bicarbonate dialysis; bile duct; binocular deprivation; black death; block design [test]; blue diaper [syndrome]; borderline dull; bound; buccodistal

Bd board

bd twice a day [Lat. *bis die*]

BDA British Dental Association

BDAC Bureau of Drug Abuse Control

BDC burn-dressing change

BDE bile duct examination

BDentSci Bachelor of Dental Science

BDG buccal developmental groove; buffered desoxycholate glucose

BDI Beck Depression Inventory

BDL below detectable limits

BDLS Brachmann-de Lange syndrome

BDS Bachelor of Dental Surgery; biological detection system

bds to be taken twice a day [Lat. *bid in die summendus*]

BDSc Bachelor of Dental Science
BDUR bromodeoxyuridine
BDW buffered distilled water
BE bacillary emulsion; bacterial endocarditis; barium enema; base excess; below-elbow; bile-esculin [test]; bovine enteritis; brain edema; bread equivalent; breast examination; bronchoesophagology
Be beryllium
BEA bromoethylamine
BEAM brain electrical activity monitoring
BEAR biological effects of atomic radiation
BEC bacterial endocarditis; blood ethyl alcohol; bromo-ergocryptine
BEE basal energy expenditure
beg begin, beginning
beh behavior, behavioral
BEI back-scattered electron imaging; butanol-extractable iodine
BEIR biological effects of ionizing radiation
BEK bovine embryonic kidney [cells]
BEL blood ethanol level
ben well [Lat. *bene*]
BEP brain evoked potential
BER basic electrical rhythm
BES balanced electrolyte solution
BESP bovine embryonic spleen [cells]
BET Brunauer-Emmet-Teller [method]
ß [Greek letter beta] an anomer of a carbohydrate; buffer capacity; carbon separated from a carboxyl by one other carbon in aliphatic compounds; a constituent of a plasma protein fraction; probability of Type II error; a substituent group of a steroid that projects above the plane of the ring
1-ß power of statistical test
ß$_2$m beta$_2$-microglobulin

BEV baboon endogenous virus
BeV, Bev billion electron volts
BF bentonite flocculation; black female; blastogenic factor; blood flow; bouillon filtrate [tuberculin] [Fr. *bouillon filtré*]; breakfast fed; buffered; burning feet [syndrome]; butter fat
bf bouillon filtrate [tuberculin]
B/F bound/free [antigen ratio]
BFB biological feedback
BFC benign febrile convulsion

BFH benign familial hematuria
BFLS Börjeson-Forssman-Lehmann syndrome
BFO blood-forming organ
BFP biologic false-positive
BFPR biologic false-positive reaction
BFR biologic false reaction; blood flow rate; bone formation rate; buffered Ringer [solution]
BFT bentonite flocculation test
BFU burst-forming unit
BFU-E burst-forming unit, erythroid
BG basal ganglion; basic gastrin; beta-galactosidase; beta-glucuronidase; bicolor guaiac [test]; blood glucose; bone graft; brilliant green; buccogingival
B-G Bordet-Gengou [agar, bacillus, phenomenon]
BGA blue-green algae
BGAV blue-green algae virus
BGC blood group class
BGE butyl glycidyl ether
BGG bovine gamma-globulin
bGH bovine growth hormone
Bg^J beige [mouse]
BGLB brilliant green lactose broth
BGP beta-glycerophosphatase
BGS blood group substance; British Geriatrics Society
BGSA blood granulocyte-specific activity
BGTT borderline glucose tolerance test
BH base hospital; benzalkonium and heparin; bill of health; board of health; Bolton-Hunter [reagent]; both hands; brain hormone; Bryan high titer; bundle of His
BH$_4$ tetrahydrobiopterin
BHA bound hepatitis antibody; butylated hydroxyanisole
BHAT Beta Blocker Heart Attack Trial
BHB beta-hydroxybutyrate
bHb bovine hemoglobin
BHBA beta-hydroxybutyric acid
BHC benzene hexachloride
BHF Bolivian hemorrhagic fever
BHI biosynthetic human insulin; brain-heart infusion [broth]; Bureau of Health Insurance
BHIA brain-heart infusion agar
BHI-ac brain-heart infusion broth with acetone

BHIB brain-heart infusion broth
BHIBA brain-heart infusion blood agar
BHIS beef heart infusion supplemented [broth]
BHK baby hamster kidney [cells]; type-B Hong Kong [influenza virus]
BHL biological half-life
BHM Bureau of Health Manpower
BHN bephenium hydroxynaphthoate; Brinell hardness number
BHP basic health profile
BHR basal heart rate
BHS Bachelor of Health Science; beta-hemolytic streptococcus
BHT beta-hydroxytheophylline; breath hydrogen test; butylated hydroxytoluene
BHU basic health plan
BHV bovine herpes virus
BH/VH body hematocrit–venous hematocrit [ratio]
BHyg Bachelor of Hygiene
BI bacterial index; base of prism in; basilar impression; biological indicator; bodily injury; bone injury; bowel impaction; burn index
Bi bismuth
BIAC Bioinstrumentation Advisory Council
bib drink [Lat. *bibe*]
biblio bibliography
BIBRA British Industrial Biological Research Association
BIC blood isotope clearance
Bic biceps
bicarb bicarbonate
BID bibliographic information and documentation; brought in dead
bid twice a day [Lat. *bis in die*]
BIDLB block in posteroinferior division of left branch
BIG 6 analysis of 6 serum components
BIGGY bismuth glycine glucose yeast
BIH benign intracranial hypertension
bihor during two hours [Lat. *bihorium*]
BIL basal insulin level; bilirubin
Bil bilirubin
bil, bilat bilateral
bili bilirubin
bili-c conjugated bilirubin
bilirub bilirubin
bin twice a night [Lat. *bis in noctus*]
biochem biochemistry, biochemical

BIOETHICSLINE Bioethical Information On-Line
biol biology, biological
biophys biophysics, biophysical
BIOSIS BioScience Information Service
BIP bacterial intravenous protein; biparietal; bismuth iodoform paraffin; Blue Cross interim payment
BIPLED bilateral, independent, periodic, lateralized epileptiform discharge
BIPM Internation Bureau of Weights and Measures [Fr. *Bureau International des Poids et Mesures*]
BIPP bismuth iodoform paraffin paste
BIR basic incidence rate; British Institute of Radiology
bis twice [Lat.]
bisp bispinous diameter
BIU barrier isolation unit
BJ Bence Jones [protein, proteinuria]; biceps jerk; Bielschowsky-Jansky [syndrome]; bones and joints
BJE bones, joints, and examination
BJM bones, joints, and muscles
BJP Bence Jones protein or proteinuria
BK below the knee; bovine kidney [cells]; bradykinin
B-K initials of two patients after whom a multiple cutaneous nevus was named [mole]
Bk berkelium
bk back
BKA below-knee amputation
BK-A basophil kallikrein of anaphylaxis
bkf breakfast
BKTT below knee to toe
BKWP below knee walking plaster
BL basal lamina; baseline; Bessey-Lowry [unit]; bleeding; blood loss; bone marrow lymphocyte; buccolingual; Burkitt's lymphoma
Bl black
B-l bursa-equivalent lymphocyte
bl blood, bleeding; blue
BLAD borderline left axis deviation
blad bladder
BLB Bessey-Lowry-Brock [method or unit]; Boothby-Lovelace-Bulbulian [oxygen mask]
BlC blood culture
BLCL Burkitt's lymphoma cell line
BLD benign lymphoepithelial disease

bld blood
BLE both lower extremities
BLEO bleomycin
BLG beta-lactoglobulin
BLI bombesin-like immunoreactivity
blk black
BLL below lower limit
BLLD British Library Lending Division
BLM bilayer lipid membrane; bimolecular liquid membrane; bleomycin
BLN bronchial lymph node
BLOBS bladder obstruction
BLOT British Library of Tape
BLP beta-lipoprotein
BlP blood pressure
BLROA British Laryngological, Rhinological, and Otological Association
BLS basic life support; blind loop syndrome; blood and lymphatic system; blood sugar; Bloom syndrome; Bureau of Labor Statistics
BLSD bovine lumpy skin disease
BLT blood-clot lysis time
BIT blood type, blood typing
BLU Bessey-Lowry unit
BLV bovine leukemia virus
BM Bachelor of Medicine; basal medium; basal metabolism; basement membrane; basilar membrane; black male; body mass; Bohr magneton; bone marrow; bowel movement; buccal mass; buccomesial
bm salt-water bath [Lat. *balneum maris*]
BMA bone marrow arrest; British Medical Association
BmA *Brugia malayi* adult antigen
BMB biomedical belt; bone marrow biopsy
BMBL benign monoclonal B cell lymphocytosis
BMC bone mineral content
BMD Becker's muscular dystrophy; Boehringer Mannheim Diagnostics; bone mineral density; bovine mucosal disease
BMDC Biomedical Documentation Center
BME basal medium Eagle; biundulant meningoencephalitis
BMed Bachelor of Medicine
BMedBiol Bachelor of Medical Biology
BMedSci Bachelor of Medical Science
BMG benign monoclonal gammopathy
BMic Bachelor of Microbiology

BMJ bones, muscles, joints; British Medical Journal
bmk birthmark
BML bone marrow lymphocytosis
BMLS billowing mitral leaflet syndrome
BMMP benign mucous membrane pemphigoid
BMN bone marrow necrosis
BMOC Brinster's medium for ovum culture
Bmod behavior modification
B-mode brightness modulation
BMP bone morphogenetic protein
BMQA Board of Medical Quality Assurance
BMR basal metabolic rate
BMS Bachelor of Medical Science; biomedical monitoring system; bleomycin sulfate; Bureau of Medical Services; Bureau of Medicine and Surgery
BMSA British Medical Students Association
BMST Bruce maximum stress test
BMT Bachelor of Medical Technology; bone marrow transplantation
BMU basic multicellular unit
BMZ basement membrane zone
BN branchial neuritis; brown Norway [rat]
BNA Basle Nomina Anatomica
BNDD Bureau of Narcotics and Dangerous Drugs
BNEd Bachelor of Nursing Education
BNF British National Formulary
BNIST National Bureau of Scientific Information [Fr. *Bureau National d'Information Scientifique*]
BNO bladder neck obstruction; bowels not opened
BNPA binasal pharyngeal airway
BNSc Bachelor of Nursing Science
BNT brain neurotransmitter
BO Bachelor of Osteopathy; base of prism out; behavior objective; body odor; bowel obstruction; bucco-occlusal
Bo Bolton point
bo bowels
B&O belladonna and opium
BOA born on arrival; British Orthopaedic Association
BOBA beta-oxybutyric acid
BOC blood oxygen capacity; butyloxycarbonyl

BOD biochemical oxygen demand
BOEA ethyl biscoumacetate
BOH board of health
bol pill [Lat. *bolus*]
BOLD bleomycin, vincristine, lomustin, and dacarbazine
BOM bilateral otitis media
BOOP bronchiolitis obliterans-organizing pneumonia
BOP buffalo orphan prototype [virus]
BOR basal optic root; before time of operation; bowels open regularly; branchio-oto-renal [syndrome]
BORR blood oxygen release rate
BOT botulinum toxin
bot bottle
BOW bag of waters
BP Bachelor of Pharmacy; back pressure; barometric pressure; basic protein; bathroom privileges; bed pan; before present; behavior pattern; Bell's palsy; benzpyrene; biotic potential; biparietal; biphenyl; birth place; blood pressure; boiling point; Bolton point; borderline personality; British Pharmacopoeia; bronchopleural; buccopulpal; bullous pemphigus; bypass
B/P blood pressure
bp base pair; boiling point
BPA blood pressure assembly; bovine plasma albumin; British Paediatric Association; bronchopulmonary aspergillosis
BPB bromphenol blue
BPC British Pharmaceutical Codex
BPD biparietal diameter; borderline personality disorder; bronchopulmonary dysplasia
BPE bacterial phosphatidylethanolamine
BPF bradykinin-potentiating factor; burst-promoting factor
BPG blood pressure gauge
BPH Bachelor of Public Health; benign prostatic hypertrophy
BPh British Pharmacopoeia
BPharm Bachelor of Pharmacy
BPHEng Bachelor of Public Health Engineering
BPHN Bachelor of Public Health Nursing
BPL benign proliferative lesion; benzyl penicilloyl-polylysine; beta-propiolactone
BPM beats per minute; breaths per minute; brompheniramine maleate

BPMF British Postgraduate Medical Federation
BPMS blood plasma measuring system
BPN bacitracin, polymyxin B, neomycin sulfate; brachial plexus neuropathy
BPO benzyl penicilloyl
BPP bovine pancreatic polypeptide; bradykinin potentiating peptide
BPPN benign paroxysmal positioning nystagmus
BPPV bovine paragenital papilloma virus
BPR blood pressure recorder
BPRS Brief Psychiatric Rating Scale; Brief Psychiatric Reacting Scale
BPS beats per second; Behavioral Pharmacological Society; bovine papular stomatitis; brain protein solvent; breaths per second
BPsTh Bachelor of Psychotherapy
BPT benign paroxysmal torticollis
BPTI basic pancreatic trypsin inhibitor; basic polyvalent trypsin inhibitor
BPV benign paroxysmal vertigo; bovine papilloma virus
BP(Vet) British Pharmacopoeia (Veterinary)
Bq becquerel
BQA Bureau of Quality Assurance
BR barrier reared [experimental animals]; bathroom; bed rest; bilirubin; biologic response
Br bregma; bridge; bromine; bronchitis; *Brucella*
br boiling range; branch; breath; brother
BRA bilateral renal agenesis
BRAC basic rest-activity cycle
Brach brachial
BRAP burst of rapid atrial pacing
BRATT bananas, rice, applesauce, tea and toast
BRBC bovine red blood cell
BRBNS blue rubber bleb nevus syndrome
BRBPR bright red blood per rectum
BRCS British Red Cross Society
BRD bladder retraining drill
BrdU bromodeoxyuridine
BrdUrd bromodeoxyuridine
BRH benign recurrent hematuria
BRIC benign recurrent intrahepatic cholestasis
Brkf breakfast

BRM biuret reactive material
BRN Board of Registered Nursing
BRO bronchoscopy
Bron bronchi, bronchial
BRP bathroom privileges; bilirubin production
Brph bronchophony
BRS Bibliographic Retrieval Services; British Roentgen Society
brth breath
Bruc *Brucella*
BS Bachelor of Science; Bachelor of Surgery; *Bacillus subtilis*; Bartter syndrome; before sleep; Behçet syndrome; bilateral symmetrical; bismuth sulfite; blood sugar; Bloom syndrome; Blue Shield [plan]; bowel sound; breaking strength; breath sounds; British Standard; Bureau of Standards
b x s brother x sister inbreeding
BSA benzenesulfonic acid; Biofeedback Society of America; bismuth-sulfite agar; bis-trimethylsilyl-acetamide; Blind Service Association; Blue Shield Association; body surface area; bovine serum albumin
bsa bovine serum albumin
BSAG Bristol Social Adjustment Guides
BSAP brief short-action potential; brief, small, abundant potentials
BSB body surface burned
BSC bedside commode; bench scale calorimeter; Biological Stain Commission; Biomedical Science Corps
BSc Bachelor of Science
BSC-1, BS-C-1 *Cercopithecus* monkey kidney cells
BSCC British Society for Clinical Cytology
BSCP bovine spinal cord protein
BSDLB block in anterosuperior division of left branch
BSE bilateral symmetrical and equal; breast self-examination
BSEP brain stem evoked potential
BSER brain stem evoked response audiometry
BSF back scatter factor; busulfan
BSG branchio-skeleto-genital [syndrome]
BSI Borderline Syndrome Index; bound serum iron; British Standards Institution
BSIF bile salt independent fraction

BSL benign symmetric lipomatosis; blood sugar level
BSM Bachelor of Science in Medicine
BSN Bachelor of Science in Nursing; bowel sounds normal
BSO bilateral salpingo-oophorectomy; British School of Osteopathy
BSP Bromsulphalein
BSp bronchospasm
BSPh Bachelor of Science in Pharmacy
BSR basal skin resistance; blood sedimentation rate; brain stimulation reinforcement
BSS Bachelor of Sanitary Science; balanced salt solution; Bernard-Soulier syndrome; black silk suture; buffered salt solution; buffered single substrate
B-SS Bernard-Soulier syndrome
BSSG sitogluside
BST blood serologic test; brief stimulus therapy
BSTFA bis-trimethylsilyltrifluoroacetamide
BT bedtime; bitemporal; bladder tumor; bleeding time; blood type, blood typing; blue tetrazolium; blue tongue; body temperature; bovine turbinate [cells]; brain tumor; breast tumor
BTA Blood Transfusion Association
BTB breakthrough bleeding; bromthymol blue
BTE bovine thymus extract
BTFS breast tumor frozen section
BTG beta-thromboglobulin
BTg bovine trypsinogen
BThU British thermal unit
BTL bilateral tubal ligation
BTM benign tertian malaria
BTMSA bis-trimethylsilacetylene
BTPABA N-benzoyl-L-tyrosyl-p-aminobenzoic acid
BTPS at body temperature and ambient pressure, and saturated with water vapor [gas]
BTR bezold-type reflex
BTr bovine trypsin
BTS blood transfusion service; bradycardia-tachycardia syndrome
bTSH bovine thyroid-stimulating hormone
BTU British thermal unit
BTV blue tongue virus
BTX-B brevetoxin-B

BU base of prism up; blood urea; Bodansky unit; bromouracil; burn unit
Bu butyl
bu bushel
BUA blood uric acid
Buc buccal
BUDR 5-bromodeoxyuridine
BUDS bilateral upper dorsal sympathectomy
BUE both upper extremities
BUF buffalo [rat]
BUG buccal ganglion
BUI brain uptake index
BULL buccal or upper lingual of lower
bull let it boil [Lat. *bulliat*]
BuMed Bureau of Medicine and Surgery
BUMP Behavioral Regression or Upset in Hospitalized Medical Patients [scale]
BUN blood urea nitrogen
BUO bleeding of undetermined origin, bruising of undetermined origin
Burd Burdick suction
BUS Bartholin, urethral and skene glands; busulfan
But, but butyrate, butyric
BV bacitracin V; biological value; blood vessel; blood volume; bronchovesicular
bv steam bath [Lat. *balneum vaporis*]
BVA Blind Veterans Association; British Veterinary Association
BVC British Veterinary Codex
BVD bovine viral diarrhea
BVDT brief vestibular disorientation test
BVE binocular visual efficiency
BVH biventricular hypertrophy
BVI blood vessel invasion
BVL bilateral vas ligation
BVM bronchovascular markings; Bureau of Veterinary Medicine
BVMOT Bender Visual-Motor Gestalt Test
BVMS Bachelor of Veterinary Medicine and Science
BVP blood vessel prosthesis; burst of ventricular pacing
BVSc Bachelor of Veterinary Science
BVU bromoisovalerylurea
BVV bovine vaginitis virus
BW bacteriological warfare; below waist; biological warfare; birth weight; bladder washout; body water; body weight
bw body weight

B&W black and white [milk of magnesia and cascara extract]
BWD bacillary white diarrhea
BWFI bacteriostatic water for injection
BWS Beckwith-Wiedemann syndrome
BWST black widow spider toxin
BWSV black widow spider venom
BWt birth weight
BX, bx bacitracin X; biopsy
BYE Barila-Yaguchi-Eveland [medium]
Bz benzoyl
BZD benzodiazepine

–C–

C ascorbic acid; bruised [Lat. *contusus*]; calcitonin-forming [cell]; calculus; calorie [large]; canine tooth; capacitance; carbohydrate; carbon; cardiovascular disease; carrier; cathode; Caucasian; Celsius; centigrade; central; central electrode placement in electroencephalography; centromeric or constitutive heterochromatic chromosome [banding]; certified; cervical; cesarean section; chest (precordial) lead in electrocardiography; chicken; clearance; clonus; *Clostridium*; closure; clubbing; coarse [bacterial colonies]; cocaine; coefficient; color sense; colored [guinea pig]; complement; compliance; component; compound [Lat. *compositus*]; concentration; conditioned, conditioning; constant; contraction; control; conventionally reared [experimental animal]; correct; coulomb; *Cryptococcus*; curie; cyanosis; cylinder; cysteine; cytidine; cytochrome; cytosine; gallon [Lat. *congius*]; hundred; large calorie; molar heat capacity; rib [Lat. *costa*]; velocity of light; with
c with [Lat. *cum*]
C1 first cervical nerve; first cervical vertebra; first component of complement
C_1 first rib
C$\overline{1}$ activated first component of complement
C1 INH inhibitor of first component of complement
CI first cranial nerve

C2 second cervical nerve; second cervical vertebra; second component of complement

C_2 second rib

$C\overline{2}$ activated second component of complement

CII second cranial nerve

C3 third cervical nerve; third cervical vertebra; third component of complement

C_3 Collins' solution; third rib

$C\overline{3}$ activated third component of complement

CIII third cranial nerve

C4 fourth cervical nerve; fourth cervical vertebra; fourth component of complement

$C\overline{4}$ activated fourth component of complement

CIV fourth cranial nerve

C5 fifth cervical nerve; fifth cervical vertebra; fifth component of complement

$C\overline{5}$ activated fifth component of complement

CV fifth cranial nerve

C6 sixth cervical nerve; sixth cervical vertebra; sixth component of complement

$C\overline{6}$ activated sixth component of complement

CVI sixth cranial nerve

C7 seventh cervical nerve; seventh cervical vertebra; seventh component of complemen

$C\overline{7}$ activated seventh component of complement

CVII seventh cranial nerve

C8 eighth component of complement

$C\overline{8}$ activated eighth component of complement

CVIII eighth cranial nerve

C9 ninth component of complement

$C\overline{9}$ activated ninth component of complement

CIX-CXII ninth to twelfth cranial nerves

°C degree Celsius

C' complement

c calorie [small]; candle; canine tooth; capacity; carat; centi-; concentration; contact; cup; curie; cyclic; meal [Lat. *cibus*] specific heat capacity; with [Lat. *cum*]

c' coefficient of portage

CA anterior commissure [Lat. *commissura anterior*]; calcium antagonist; California [rabbit]; cancer; carbonic anhydrase; carcinoma; cardiac arrest; catecholamine, catecholaminergic; cathode; cerebral aqueduct; cervicoaxial; Chemical Abstracts; cholic acid; chloroamphetamine; chronic avovulation; chronological age; clotting assay; coagglutination; coarctation of the aorta; cold agglutinin; colloid antigen; common antigen; conceptional age; coronary artery; corpora alata; corpora amylacea; cortisone acetate; croup-associated [virus]; cytosine arabinoside; cytotoxic antibody

Ca calcium; cancer, carcinoma; cathode

ca about [Lat. *circa*]; candle

C&A Clinitest and Acetest

CA-2 second colloid antigen

CAA carotid audiofrequency analysis; constitutional aplastic anemia; crystalline amino acids

CAAT computer-assisted axial tomography

CAB captive air bubble; cellulose acetate butyrate; coronary artery bypass

CABG coronary artery bypass grafting

CABGS coronary artery bypass graft surgery

CaBP calcium-binding protein

CABS coronary artery bypass surgery

CAC cardiac-accelerator center; cardiac arrest code

CaCC cathodal closure contraction

CACP cisplatin

CaCV calicivirus

CAD cold agglutinin disease; compressed air disease; computer-assisted diagnosis; coronary artery disease

Cad cadaver, cadaveric

CaDTe cathodal-duration tetanus

CAE caprine arthritis-encephalitis; cellulose acetate electrophoresis; contingent after-effects

CaE calcium excretion

CaEDTA calcium disodium ethylenediaminetetraacetate

CAEV caprine arthritis-encephalitis virus

CAF cell adhesion factor

Caf caffeine

CAG chronic atrophic gastritis; coronary angiography

CAH chronic active hepatitis; chronic aggressive hepatitis; congenital adrenal hyperplasia; cyanacetic acid hydrazide

CAHD coronary arteriosclerotic heart disease

CAHEA Committee on Allied Health Education and Accreditation

CAI complete androgen insensitivity; computer-assisted instruction

CAIS complete androgen insensitivity syndrome

CAL calcium test; calculated average life; calories; chronic airflow limitation; computer-assisted learning

Cal large calorie

cal small calorie

C$_{alb}$ albumin clearance

Calc calcium

CALD chronic active liver disease

calef make warm [Lat. *calefac*]; warmed [Lat. *calefactus*]

CALGB cancer and leukemia group B

cALL common null cell acute lymphocytic leukemia

cALLA common lymphocytic leukemia antigen

CAM cell-associating molecule; chorioallantoic membrane; contralateral axillary metastasis

C$_{am}$ amylase clearance

CAMAC computer automated measurement and control

CAMF cyclophosphamide, Adriamycin, methotrexate, fluorouracil

CAMP computer-assisted menu planning; concentration of adenosine monophosphate; cyclophosphamide, doxorubicin, methotrexate, and procarbazine

cAMP cyclic adenosine monophosphate

CaMV cauliflower mosaic virus

Can cancer

CA/N child abuse and neglect

canc cancelled

CANCERLIT Cancer Literature

CancerProj Cancer Research Projects

CANP calcium-activated neutral protease

CAO chronic airway obstruction; coronary artery obstruction

CaOC cathodal opening contraction

CAP capsule; catabolite gene activator protein; cell attachment protein; cellular acetate propionate; cellulose acetate phthalate; chloramphenicol; College of American Pathologists; complement-activated plasma; compound action potential; coupled atrial pacing; cyclosphosphamide, doxorubicin, and cisplatin; cystine aminopeptidase

cap capsule; let him take [Lat. *capiat*]

CAPA cancer-associated polypeptide antigen

CAPD continuous ambulatory peritoneal dialysis

CAPERS Computer Assisted Psychiatric Evaluation and Review System

capiend to be taken [Lat. *capiendus*]

cap moli soft capsule [Lat. *capsula mollis*]

cap quant vult to be taken as much as one wants to [Lat. *capiat quantum vult*]

CAPRCA chronic, acquired, pure red cell aplasia

CAPRI Cardiopulmonary Research Institute

caps capsule

CAPYA child and adolescent psychoanalysis

CAR Canadian Association of Radiologists; cardiac ambulation routine; chronic articular rheumatism; computer-assisted research; conditioned avoidance response

car carotid

CARB carbohydrate; coronary artery bypass graft

carb carbohydrate; carbonate

carbo carbohydrate

card cardiac

cardiol cardiology

CARF Commission on Accreditation and Rehabilitation Facilities

CAS calcarine sulcus; calcific aortic stenosis; cardiac adjustment scale; Celite-activated normal serum; Center for Alcohol Studies; Chemical Abstracts Service; cold agglutinin syndrome; congenital alcoholic syndrome; control adjustment strap; coronary artery spasm

Cas casualty

cas castration, castrated

CASA computer-assisted self assessment

CASH Commission for Administrative Services in Hospitals

CASHD coronary arteriosclerotic heart disease

CASMD congenital atonic sclerotic muscular dystrophy

CAS-REGN Chemical Abstracts Service Registry Number

CASRT corrected adjusted sinus node recovery time

CASS Coronary Artery Surgery Study

CAT capillary agglutination test; catalase; cataract; catecholamine; Children's Apperception Test; chloramphenicol acetyltransferase; chlormerodrin accumulation test; choline acetyltransferase; chronic abdominal tympany; computerized axial tomography; computer of average transients

CAT'ase catalase

CATCH Community Actions to Control High Blood Pressure

Cath cathartic; catheter, catheterize

CATLINE Catalog On-Line

CAT-S Children's Apperception Test, Supplemental

CAT scan computerized axial tomography scan

CATT calcium tolerance test

Cauc Caucasian

caud caudal

CAV congenital absence of vagina; congenital adrenal virilism; constant angular velocity; croup-associated virus

cav cavity

CAVB complete atrioventricular block

CAVD complete atrioventricular dissociation; completion, arithmetic problems, vocabulary, following directions [test]

CAVH continuous arteriovenous hemofiltration

CAVHD continuous arteriovenous hemodialysis

C$_{AW}$ airway conductance

CAVO common atrioventricular orifice

CB Bachelor of Surgery [Lat. *Chirurgiae Baccalaureus*]; carbenicillin; carotid body; chronic bronchitis; chocolate blood [agar]; code blue; compensated base

Cb niobium [columbium]

CBA chronic bronchitis and asthma; cost-benefit analysis

CBAB complement-binding antibody

CBADAA Certifying Board of the American Dental Assistants Association

CBC carbenicillin; complete blood cell count

cbc complete blood cell count

CBCL Child Behavior Checklist

CBD closed bladder drainage; common bile duct

CBF cerebral blood flow; coronary blood flow

CBG coronary bypass graft; corticosteroid-binding globulin; cortisol-binding globulin

CBGv corticosteroid-binding globulin variant

CBH cutaneous basophilic hypersensitivity

CBI continuous bladder irrigation

CBL circulating blood lymphocytes; cord blood leukocytes

Cbl cobalamin

cbl chronic blood loss

CBM capillary basement membrane

CBMMP chronic benign mucous membrane pemphigus

CBN cannabinol; Commission on Biological Nomenclature

CBOC completion bed occupancy care

CBP carbohydrate-binding protein; cobalamin-binding protein

CBR chemical, biological, and radiological [warfare]; chemically-bound residue; chronic bed rest; complete bed rest; crude birth rate

CBS chronic brain syndrome

CBT carotid body tumor

CBV central blood volume, circulating blood volume; corrected blood volume

CBVD cerebrovascular disease

CBW chemical and biological warfare

CBZ carbamazepine

CC calcium cyclamate; cardiac cycle; cardiovascular clinic; cell culture; central compartment; cerebral commissure; chief complaint; choriocarcinoma; chronic complainer; classical conditioning; clean catch [of urine]; clinical course; commission certified; compound cathartic; computer calculated; cord compression; corpus callosum; costochondral; Coulter counter; creatinine clearance; critical care; critical condition; crus cerebri; cubic centimeter; current complaint; Current Contents

Cc concave

cc concave; corrected; cubic centimeter

CCA cephalin cholesterol antigen; chick cell agglutination; chimpanzee coryza agent; choriocarcinoma; common carotid artery; congenital contractural arachnodacyly; constitutional chromosome abnormality

CCAT conglutinating complement absorption test

CCBV central circulating blood volume

CCC care-cure coordination; cathodal closure contraction; chronic calculous cholecystitis; consecutive case conference

CC&C colony count and culture

CCCC centrifugal countercurrent chromatography

CCCl cathodal closure clonus

CCCP carbonyl cyanide *m*-chlorophenyl-hydrazone

CCCR closed chest cardiac resuscitation

CCCT closed craniocerebral trauma

CCD calibration curve data; charge-coupled device; childhood celiac disease; countercurrent distribution

CCDC Canadian Communicable Disease Center

CCDN Central Council for District Nursing

CCE carboline carboxylic acid ester; chamois contagious ecthyma; clubbing, cyanosis, and edema; countercurrent electrophoresis

CCEI Crown-Crisp Experimental Index

CCF centrifuged culture fluid; cephalin-cholesterol flocculation; compound comminuted fracture; congestive heart failure; crystal-induced chemotactic factor

CCFE cyclophosphamide, cisplatin, fluorouracil, and extramustine

CCFMG Cooperating Committee on Foreign Medical Graduates

CCHD cyanotic congenital heart disease

CCHE Central Council for Health Education

CCHMS Central Committee for Hospital Medical Services

CCHP Consumer Choice Health Plan

CCHS congenital central hypoventilation syndrome

CCI chronic coronary insufficiency

CCK cholecystokinin

CCK-8 cholecystokinin octapeptide

CCK-PZ cholecystokinin-pancreozymin

CCL carcinoma cell line; certified cell line; critical carbohydrate level

CCM cerebrocostomandibular [syndrome]; craniocervical malformation

c cm cubic centimeter

CCMC Committee on the Costs of Medical Care

CCME Coordinating Council on Medical Education

CCMS clean catch midstream [urine]; clinical care management system

CCN coronary care nursing; critical care nursing

CCNU N-(2-chloroethyl)-N'-cyclohexyl-N-nitrosourea

CCP ciliocytophthoria; cytidine cyclic phosphate

CCPD continuous cycling (cyclical) peritoneal dialysis

CCPDS Centralized Cancer Patient Data System

CCR complete continuous remission

C_{cr} creatinine clearance

CCRN Critical Care Registered Nurse

CCS casualty clearing station; cell cycle specific; cloudy cornea syndrome; concentration camp syndrome; costoclavicular syndrome

CCSCS central cervical spinal cord syndrome

CCSG Children's Cancer Study Group

CCT chocolate-coated tablet; coated compressed tablet; composite cyclic therapy; controlled cord traction; coronary care team; cranial computed tomography

CCTe cathodal closure tetanus

CCTV closed circuit television

CCU cardiac care unit; Cherry-Crandall unit; coronary care unit; critical care unit

CCUP colpocystourethropexy

CCV channel catfish virus; conductivity cell volume

CCW counterclockwise

CD cadaver donor; canine distemper; carbohydrate dehydratase; cardiac disease; cardiac dullness; cardiovascular disease; Carrel-Dakin [fluid]; caudad, caudal; celiac disease; cell dissociation; cesarean delivery; circular dichroism; combination drug; common duct; communicable disease; completely denaturated; conjugata diagonalis; consanguineous donor; contact dermatitis; contagious disease; control diet; convulsive disorder; convulsive dose; corneal dystrophy; Crohn's disease; crossed diagonal; curative dose; cystic duct; diagonal conjugate diameter of the pelvis [Lat. *conjugata diagonalis*]

C/D cigarettes per day; cup to disc ratio

C&D cystoscopy and dilatation

Cd cadmium; caudal; coccygeal; condylion

cd candela

CD$_{50}$ median curative dose

CDA Canadian Dental Association; Certified Dental Assistant; chenodeoxycholic acid; ciliary dyskinesia activity; complement dependent antibody; completely denatured alcohol; congenital dyserythropoietic anemia

C&DB cough and deep breath

CDC calculated date of confinement; capillary diffusion capacity; cell division cycle; Center for Disease Control; Communicable Disease Center

CD-C controlled drinker–control

CDCA chenodeoxycholic acid

CDD certificate of disability for discharge; chronic degenerative disease; chronic disabling dermatosis

CDDP cis-diamminedichloroplatinum

CDE canine distemper encephalitis; chlordiazepoxide; common duct exploration

CDF chondrodystrophia foetalis

CDG central developmental groove

CDH ceramide dihexoside; congenital diaphragmatic hernia; congenital dysplasia of hip

CDI cell-directed inhibitor; central diabetes insipidus; Children's Depression Inventory; cranial diabetes insipidus

CDL chlordeoxylincomycin

CDLE chronic discoid lupus erythematosus

CDLS Cornelia de Lange syndrome

CDM chemically-defined medium; clinical decision making

cDNA complementary deoxyribonucleic acid

CDNB 1-chloro-2,4-dinitrobenzene

CDP collagenase-digestible protein; continuous distending pressure; coronary drug project; cytidine diphosphate

CDPC cytidine diphosphate choline

CDR calcium-dependent regulator

CDS cardiovascular surgery; catechol-3, 5-disulfonate; caudal dysplasia syndrome;

Chemical Data System; Christian Dental Society

CDSM Committee on Dental and Surgical Materials

cd-sr candela-steradian

CDSS clinical decision support system

CDT carbon dioxide therapy; Certified Dental Technician

Cdyn dynamic compliance

CE California encephalitis; cardiac enlargement; chemical energy; chick embryo; cholesterol esters; conjugated estrogens; constant error; continuing education; contractile element; cytopathic effect

Ce cerium

C-E chloroform-ether

CEA carcinoembryonic antigen; cholesterol-esterifying activity; cost-effectiveness analysis; crystalline egg albumin

CEARP Continuing Education Approval and Recognition Program

CEC ciliated epithelial cell

CED chondroectodermal dysplasia

CEEV Central European encephalitis virus

CEF centrifugation extractable fluid; chick embryo fibroblast; constant electric field

CEFMG Council on Education for Foreign Medical Graduates

CEH cholesterol ester hydrolase

CEHC calf embryonic heart cell

CEI character education inquiry; converting enzyme inhibitor

CEID crossed electroimmunodiffusion

CEJ cement-enamel junction

CEK chick embryo kidney

Cel Celsius

Cell celluloid

CELO chick embryonal lethal orphan [virus]

CEM conventional transmission electron microscope

CEN Certificate for Emergency Nursing

cen centromere; central

CENP centromere protein

cent centigrade; central

CEO chick embryo origin; Chief Executive Officer

CEOT calcifying epithelial odontogenic tumor

CEP chronic eosinophilic pneumonia;

chronic erythropoietic porphyria; continuing education program; cortical evoked potential; counter-electrophoresis

CEPH cephalic; cephalosporin

ceph cephalin

CEPH FLOC cephalin flocculation

CEQ Council on Environmental Quality

CER ceramide; conditioned emotional response

CERD chronic end-stage renal disease

CERP Continuing Education Recognition Program

Cert, cert certified

cerv cervix, cervical

CES cat eye syndrome; central excitatory state; chronic electrophysiological study

CESD cholesterol ester storage disease

CET capital expenditure threshold; congenital eyelid tetrad

CETE Central European tick-borne encephalitis

CEU congenital ectropion uveae; continuing education unit

CF calcium leucovorin; calf blood flow; calibration factor; cancer-free; carbolfuchsin; cardiac failure; carrier-free; cascade filtration; Caucasian female; characteristic frequency; chemotactic factor; chest and left leg [lead in electrocardiography]; Chiari-Frommel [syndrome]; chick fibroblast; Christmas factor; citrovorum factor; colicin factor; colonization factor; colony forming; complement fixation; constant frequency; contractile force; coronary flow; count fingers; counting finger; cycling fibroblast; cystic fibrosis

Cf californium

cf bring together, compare [Lat. *confer*]

CFA complement-fixing antibody; complete Freund's adjuvant; cryptogenic fibrosing alveolitis

CFB central fibrous body

CFC capillary filtration coefficient; colony-forming capacity; continuous flow centrifugation

CFD cephalo-facial deformity

CFF critical flicker fusion [test]; critical fusion frequency; cystic fibrosis factor; Cystic Fibrosis Foundation

cff critical flicker fusion; critical fusion frequency

CFH Council on Family Health

CFI chemotactic-factor inactivator; complement fixation inhibition

CFM chlorofluoromethane; close-fitting mask; craniofacial microsomia

CFMA Council for Medical Affairs

CFMG Commission on Foreign Medical Graduates

CFP chronic false positive; Clinical Fellowship Program; cystic fibrosis of pancreas; cystic fibrosis protein

CFR case-fatality ratio; citrovorum-factor rescue; complement-fixation reaction; cyclic flow reduction

CFS cancer family syndrome; crush fracture syndrome; Cystic Fibrosis Society

CFSE crystal field stabilization energy

CFSTI Clearinghouse for Federal Scientific and Technical Information

CFT clinical full time; complement-fixation test

CFU colony-forming unit

CFU-C colony-forming unit–culture

CFU-E colony-forming unit–erythrocyte

CFU$_{EOS}$ colony-forming unit–eosinophil

CFU-F colony-forming unit–fibroblastoid

CFU$_{GM}$ colony-forming unit–granulocyte macrophage

CFU$_L$ colony-forming unit–lymphoid

CFU$_M$ colony-forming unit–megakaryocyte

CFU$_{MEG}$ colony-forming unit–megakaryocyte

CFU$_{NM}$ colony-forming unit–neutrophil-monocyte

CFU$_S$ colony-forming unit–spleen

CFW Carworth farm [mouse], Webster strain

CFWM cancer-free white mouse

CFX cefoxitin; circumflex coronary artery

CFZC continuous-flow zonal centrifugation

CG cardiogreen; choking gas; choriogenic gynecomastia; chorionic gonadotropin; chronic glomerulonephritis; cingulate gyrus; colloidal gold; control group; cryoglobulin; cystine guanine; phosgene [choking gas]

cg center of gravity; centigram

CGA catabolite gene activator

CGAS Children's Global Assessment Scale

CGD chronic granulomatous disease

CGDE contact glow discharge electrolysis

CGFNS Commission on Graduates of Foreign Nursing Schools

CGH chorionic gonadotropic hormone

CGI chronic granulomatous inflammation; Clinical Global Impression [Scale]

CGL chronic granulocytic leukemia

c gl correction with glasses

CGM central gray matter

cgm centigram

CGMMV cucumber green mottle mosaic virus

cGMP cyclic guanosine monophosphate

CGN chronic glomerulonephritis

CGNB composite ganglioneuroblastoma

CG/OQ cerebral glucose–oxygen quotient

CGP N-carbobenzoxy-glycyl-L-phenyl-alanine; chorionic growth hormone–prolactin; choline glycerophosphatide; circulating granulocyte pool

CGS cardiogenic shock; catgut suture

CGS, cgs centimeter-gram-second [system]

CGT chorionic gonadotropin; cyclodextrin glucanotransferase

CGTT cortisone glucose tolerance test

CH Chediak-Higashi [syndrome]; cholesterol; Christchurch chromosome; communicating hydrocele; Conradi-Hünermann [syndrome]; crown-heel [length]; cycloheximide; wheelchair

C$_H$ constant domain of H chain

C&H cocaine and heroin

Ch chest; Chido [antibody]; chief; child; choline; Christchurch [syndrome]; chromosome

cH hydrogen ion concentration

ch chest; child; chronic

CHA Catholic Hospital Association; chronic hemolytic anemia; congenital hypoplastic anemia; cyclohexyladenosine; cyclohexylamine

ChA choline acetylase

CHAD cyclophosphamide; Adriamycin, cisplatin, and hexamethylmelamine

CHAMPUS Civilian Health and Medical Program of Uniformed Services

CHAMPVA Civilian Health and Medical Program of Veterans Administration

Chang C Chang conjunctiva cells

Chang L Chang liver cells

CHAP Certified Hospital Admission Program

CHARGE coloboma, heart disease, atresia choanae, retarded growth and retarded development and/or CNS anomalies, genital hypoplasia, and ear anomalies and/or deafness [syndrome]

chart paper [Lat. *charta*]

CHAS Center for Health Administration Studies

ChAT choline acetyltransferase

CHB complete heart block; congenital heart block

ChB Bachelor of Surgery [Lat. *Chirurgiae Baccalaureus*]

CHBHA congenital Heinz body hemolytic anemia

CHC community health center; community health computing; community health council

CH$_3$ CCNU semustine

CHCP correctional health care program

CHD Chediak-Higashi disease; childhood disease; chronic hemodialysis; congenital heart disease; congestive heart disease; coronary heart disease; cyanotic heart disease

ChD Doctor of Surgery [Lat. *Chirurgiae Doctor*]

ChE cholinesterase

CHEC community hypertension evaluation clinic

CHEF Chinese hamster embryo fibroblast

chem chemistry, chemical; chemotherapy

CHEMLINE Chemical Dictionary On-Line

CHERSS continuous high-amplitude EEG rhythmical synchronous slowing

CHF chick embryo fibroblast; congenital hepatic fibrosis; congestive heart failure; Crimean hemorrhagic fever

CHFV combined high-frequency ventilation

chg change, changed

CHH cartilage-hair hypoplasia

CHI closed head injury

χ Greek letter *chi*

χ² chi-squared statistic; chi-squared [test]; measure goodness of fit

χ_m magnetic susceptibility

χ_s electric susceptibility

CHILD congenital hemidysplasia with ichthyosiform erythroderma and limb defects [syndrome]

CHIP comprehensive health insurance plan

Chir Doct Doctor of Surgery [Lat. *Chirurgiae Doctor*]

CHL Chinese hamster lung; chlorambucil; chloramphenicol

Chl chloroform

CHLA cyclohexyl linoleic acid

Chlb chlorobutanol

CHLD chronic hypoxic lung disease

chlor chloride

ChM Master of Surgery [Lat. *Chirurgiae Magister*]

CHMD clinical hyaline membrane disease

CHN carbon, hydrogen, and nitrogen; child neurology; Chinese [hamster]

CHO carbohydrate; Chinese hamster ovary

Cho choline

C_{H2O} water clearance

choc chocolate

chol cholesterol

c hold withhold

CHOP cyclophosphamide, doxorubicin, vincristine, and prednisone

CHP charcoal hemoperfusion; child psychiatry; comprehensive health planning; cutaneous hepatic porphyria

ChP chest physician

chpx chickenpox

Chr *Chromobacterium*

chr chromosome; chronic

c hr candle hour

c-hr curie-hour

ChRBC chicken red blood cell

chron chronic

CHRS cerebro-hepato-renal syndrome

CHS central hypoventilation syndrome; Chediak-Higashi syndrome; chondroitin sulfate

CHSD Children's Health Services Division

CHSS cooperative health statistics system

ChTg chymotrypsinogen

ChTK chicken thymidine kinase

CHU closed head unit

CHV canine herpes virus

CI cardiac index; cardiac insufficiency; cell immunity; cell inhibition; cephalic index; cerebral infarction; chemotherapeutic index; clinical investigator; clomipramine; clonus index; coefficient of intelligence; colloidal iron; color index; confidence interval; contamination index; coronary insufficiency; corrected count increment; crystalline insulin; cytotoxic index

Ci curie

CIA chymotrypsin inhibitor activity; colony-inhibiting activity

cib food [Lat. *cibus*]

CIBD chronic inflammatory bowel disease

CIBHA congenital inclusion-body hemolytic anemia

CIC cardioinhibitor center; circulating immune complex; constant initial concentration

CICU cardiac intensive care unit; cardiovascular inpatient care unit; coronary intensive care unit

CID chick infective dose; combined immunodeficiency disease; cytomegalic inclusion disease

CIDEP chemically induced dynamic electron polarization

CIDNP chemically induced dynamic nuclear polarization

CIDS cellular immunity deficiency syndrome; continuous insulin delivery system

CIE counter-current immunoelectrophoresis; counterimmunoelectrophoresis

CIEP counterimmunoelectrophoresis

CIF cloning inhibitory factor

CIFC Council for the Investigation of Fertility Control

CIG cold-insoluble globulin

CIg intracytoplasmic immunoglobulin

cIgM cytoplasmic immunoglobulin M

CIH carbohydrate-induced hyperglyceridemia; Certificate in Industrial Health; children in hospital

ci-hr curie-hour

CII Carnegie Interest Inventory

CIIPS chronic idiopathic intestinal pseudo-obstruction syndrome

CIM cortical induction of movement; Cumulated Index Medicus

Ci/ml curies per milliliter

CIMS chemical ionization mass spectrometry

CIN cervical intraepithelial neoplasia; chronic interstitial nephritis

CIN1, CIN I cervical intraepithelial neoplasia, grade 1 (mild dysplasia)

CIN 2, CIN II cervical intraepithelial neoplasia, grade 2 (moderate-severe)

CIN 3, CIN III cervical intraepithelial neoplasia, grade 3 (severe dysplasia and carcinoma *in situ*)

C_{in} insulin clearance

CIOMS Council for International Organizations of Medical Sciences

CIP chronic idiopathic polyradiculoneuropathy

CIPN chronic inflammatory polyneuropathy

cir circular

circ circuit; circular; circumcision

CIS carcinoma in situ; catheter-induced spasm; central inhibitory state; Chemical Information Service; clinical information system

CI-S calculus index, simplified

CiS cingulate sulcus

cis-DPP cisplatin

CIT citrate; conjugated-immunoglobulin technique

cit citrate

cit disp dispense quickly [Lat. *cito dispensetur*]

CIVII continuous intravenous insulin infusion

CIXA constant infusion excretory urogram

CJD Creutzfeldt-Jakob disease

CJS Creutzfeldt-Jakob syndrome

CK calf kidney; chicken kidney; choline kinase; creatine kinase; cyanogen chloride; cytokinin

ck check, checked

CKC cold-knife conization

CKG cardiokymography

CK-PZ cholecystokinin-pancreozymin

CL cardiolipin; cell line; chemilumin-escence; chest and left arm [lead in electrocardiography]; cholesterol-lecithin; chronic leukemia; cirrhosis of liver; cleft lip; clinical laboratory; corpus luteum; critical list; cycle length; cytotoxic lymphocyte

C_L constant domain of L chain

Cl chloride; chlorine; clavicle; clear; clinic; *Clostridium*; closure; colistin

cl centiliter; cleft; clinic; cloudy

CLA Certified Laboratory Assistant; cervicolinguoaxial; contralateral local anesthesia; cyclic lysine anhydride

ClAc chloroacetyl

CLAH congenital lipoid adrenal hyperplasia

CLAS congenital localized absence of skin

class classification

clav clavicle

CLB chlorambucil; curvilinear body

CLBBB complete left bundle branch block

CLC Charcot-Leyden crystal

CLD chronic liver disease; chronic lung disease; crystal ligand field

CLDH choline dehydrogenase

cldy cloudy

CLE centrilobular emphysema; continuous lumbar epidural [anesthesia]

CLED cystine-lactose-electrolyte-deficient [agar]

CLF cholesterol-lecithin flocculation

CLH chronic lobular hepatitis; cutaneous lymphoid hyperplasia

CLI corpus luteum insufficiency

CLIA Clinical Laboratories Improvement Act

CLIF cloning inhibitory factor; *Crithidia luciliae* immunofluorescence

clin clinic, clinical

CLINPROT Clinical Cancer Protocols

CLIP corticotropin-like intermediate lobe peptide

CLL cholesterol-lowering lipid; chronic lymphatic leukemia; chronic lymphocytic leukemia; cow lung lavage

CLMA Clinical Laboratory Management Association

CLMV cauliflower mosaic virus

CLO cod liver oil

Clon *Clonorchis*

Clostr *Clostridium*
CLP cleft lip with cleft palate; paced cycle length
CIP clinical pathology
CLS Clinical Laboratory Scientist
CLSH corpus luteum stimulating hormone
CLSL chronic lymphosarcoma (cell) leukemia
CLT Certified Laboratory Technician; chronic lymphocytic thyroiditis; Clinical Laboratory Technician; clot lysis time
CLT(NCA) Laboratory Technician Certified by the National Certification Agency for Medical Laboratory Personnel
CLV constant linear velocity
CL VOID clean voided specimen [urine]
CM California mastitis [test]; calmodulin; capreomycin; carboxymethyl; cardiomyopathy; Caucasian male; center of mass; cerebral mantle; Chick-Martin [coefficient]; chloroquine-mepacrine; chopped meat [medium]; circular muscle; circulating monocyte; cochlear microphonic; complete medium; complications; conditioned medium; congenital malformation; congestive myocardiopathy; continuous murmur; contrast medium; copulatory mechanism; costal margin; cow's milk; cytometry; Master of Surgery [Lat. *Chirurgiae Magister*]; narrow-diameter endosseous screw implant [Fr. *crête manche*]
C&M cocaine and morphine
Cm curium
C$_m$ maximum clearance
cm centimeter; costal margin; tomorrow morning [Lat. *cras mane*]
cm^2 square centimeter
cm^3 cubic centimeter
CMA Canadian Medical Association; Certified Medical Assistant; cow's milk allergy; cultured macrophages
CMAP compound muscle (or motor) action potential
CMB carbolic methylene blue; Central Midwives' Board; chloromercuribenzoate
CMC carboxymethylcellulose; care management continuity; carpometacarpal; cell-mediated cytolysis; chloramphenicol; chronic mucocutaneous candidiasis; critical micellar concentration

CMCt care management continuity across settings
CMD childhood muscular dystrophy; congenital muscular dystrophy; count median diameter
CME continuing medical education; Council on Medical Education; crude marijuana extract; cystoid macular edema
CMF calcium-magnesium free; catabolite modular factor; chondromyxoid fibroma; Christian Medical Fellowship; craniomandibulofacial; cyclophosphamide, methotrexate, and fluorouracil
CMFV cyclophosphamide, methotrexate, fluorouracil, and vincristine
CMFVP cyclophosphamide, methotrexate, fluorouracil, vincristine, prednisone
CMG chopped meat glucose [medium]; cystometrography, cystometrogram
CMGN chronic membranous glomerulonephritis
CMGS chopped meat-glucose-starch [medium]
CMGT chromosome-mediated gene transfer
CMH congenital malformation of the heart
CMHC community mental health center
cmH$_2$O centimeters of water
CMI carbohydrate metabolism index; care management integration; cell-mediated immunity; cell multiplication inhibition; chronic mesenteric ischemia; Commonwealth Mycological Institute; Cornell Medical Index
CMID cytomegalic inclusion disease
c/min cycles per minute
CMIR cell-mediated immune response
CMIT Current Medical Information and Terminology
CMJ carpometacarpal joint
CMK chloromethyl ketone; congenital multicystic kidney
CML cell-mediated lymphocytotoxicity; chronic myelocytic leukemia; chronic myelogenous leukemia
CMM cell-mediated mutagenesis; cutaneous malignant melanoma
cmm cubic millimeter
CMME chloromethyl methyl ether
CMML chronic myelomonocytic leukemia

CMN cystic medial necrosis
CMN-AA cystic medial necrosis of ascending aorta
CMO cardiac minute output; Chief Medical Officer
cMO centimorgan
CMOS complementary metal-oxide semiconductor
CMP cardiomyopathy; comprehensive medical plan; cytidine monophosphate
CMPGN chronic membranoproliferative glomerulonephritis
CMR cerebral metabolic rate; crude mortality ratio
CMRG cerebral metabolic rate of glucose
CMRO$_2$ cerebral metabolic rate of oxygen
CMRR common mode rejection ratio
CMS Christian Medical Society; chronic myelodysplastic syndrome; clofibrate-induced muscular syndrome; Clyde Mood Scale
cms to be taken tomorrow morning [Lat. *cras mane sumendus*]
cm/s centimeters per second
cm/sec centimeters per second
CMSS circulation, motor ability, sensation, and swelling; Council of Medical Specialty Societies
CMT California mastitis test; cancer multistep therapy; Charcot-Marie-Tooth [syndrome]; circus movement tachycardia; continuous memory test; Council on Medical Television; Current Medical Terminology
CMTD Charcot-Marie-Tooth disease
CMU chlorophenyldimethylurea
CMUA continuous motor unit activity
CMV conventional mechanical ventilation; cool mist vaporizer; cucumber mosaic virus; cytomegalovirus
CMX cefmenoxime
CN caudate nucleus; cellulose nitrate; charge nurse; child nutrition; clinical nursing; cochlear nucleus; congenital nystagmus; cranial nerve; Crigler-Najjar [syndrome]; cyanogen; cyanosis neonatorum
C/N carbon/nitrogen [ratio]; carrier/noise [ratio]
CN⁻ cyanide anion

cn tomorrow night [Lat. *cras nocte*]
CNA calcium nutrient agar; Canadian Nurses Association
CNB cutting needle biopsy
CNCbl cyanocobalamin
CNE chronic nervous exhaustion
CNF chronic nodular fibrositis; congenital nephrotic syndrome of the Finnish [type]
CNH central neurogenic hyperpnea; community nursing home
CNHD congenital nonspherocytic hemolytic disease
CNK cortical necrosis of kidneys
CNL cardiolipin natural lecithin
CNM Certified Nurse-Midwife; computerized nuclear morphometry
CNMT Certified Nuclear Medicine Technologist
CNP community nurse practitioner; 2',3'-cyclic nucleotide 3'-phosphodiesterase
CNPase 2',3'-cyclic nucleotide 3'-phosphohydrolase
CNS central nervous system; clinical nurse specialist; sulfocyanate
cns to be taken tomorrow night [Lat. *cras nocte sumendus*]
CNSHA congenital non-spherocytic hemolytic anemia
CNS-L central nervous system leukemia
CNV choroidal neovascularization; contingent negative variation; cutaneous necrotizing vasculitis
CO carbon monoxide; cardiac output; castor oil; casualty officer; centric occlusion; cervicoaxial; choline oxidase; coenzyme; compound; control; corneal opacity; cross over
C/O check out; complains of; in care of
CO$_2$ carbon dioxide
Co cobalt
co compounded, a compound [Lat. *compositus*]
Co I coenzyme I
Co II coenzyme II
COA Canadian Ophthalmological Association; Canadian Orthopaedic Association; cervico-oculo-acusticus [syndrome]
CoA coenzyme A
COAD chronic obstructive airway disease

coag coagulation, coagulated
COAP cyclophosphamide, vincristine, cytarabine, and prednisone
CoASH uncombined coenzyme A
CoA-SPC coenzyme A-synthetizing protein complex
COB chronic obstructive bronchitis; coordination of benefits
COBOL common business oriented language
COBS cesarean-obtained barrier-sustained; chronic organic brain syndrome
COBT chronic obstruction of the biliary tract
COC cathodal opening contraction; coccygeal; combination oral contraceptive
cochl a spoonful [Lat. *cochleare*]
cochl amp a heaping spoonful [Lat. *cochleare amplum*]
cochl mag a tablespoonful [Lat. *cochleare magnum*]
cochl med a dessert spoonful [*Lat. cochleare medium*]
cochl parv a teaspoonful [Lat. *cochleare parvum*]
C O C I Consortium on Chemical Information
COCl cathodal opening clonus
coct boiling [Lat. *coctio*]
COD cause of death; chemical oxygen demand
cod codeine
CODATA Committee on Data for Science and Technology
coeff coefficient
COEPS cortical originating extra-pyramidal system
CoF cobra factor
COFS cerebro-oculo-facial-skeletal [syndrome]
COG cognitive function tests
COGTT cortisone oral glucose tolerance test
COH carbohydrate
CoHb carboxyhemoglobin
COHSE Confederation of Health Service Employees
COI Central Obesity Index
col colicin; colored; column; strain [Lat. *cola*]
colat strained [Lat. *colatus*]
COLD chronic obstructive lung disease
COLD A cold agglutinin titer

colet let it be strained [Lat. *coletur*]
coll collection, collective; college; eyewash [Lat. *collyrium*]
collut mouthwash [Lat. *collutorium*]
collyr eyewash [Lat. *collyrium*]
color let it be colored [Lat. *coloretur*]
COM College of Osteopathic Medicine; computer-output microfilm
com commitment
comb combination, combine
comf comfortable
comm, commun communicable
COMP complication
comp comparative; compensation, compensated; complaint; composition; compound, compounded; compress; computer
compd compound, compounded
compl completion, completed; complication, complicated
complic complication, complicated
compn composition
COMT catechol-O-methyltransferase
COMTRAC computer-based case tracing
CON certificate of need
Con concanavalin
con against [Lat. *contra*]
Con A concanavilin A
Con A-HRP concanavilin A-horse-radish peroxidase
conc, concentr concentrated, concentrations
concis cut [Lat. *concisus*]
cond condensation, condensed; condition, conditioned; conductivity
conf conference
cong gallon [Lat. *congius*]
congen congenital
conj conjunctiva, conjunctival
CONPA-DRI I vincristine, doxorubicin, and melphalan
CONPA-DRI III conpa-dri I plus intensified doxorubicin
CONS consultation
cons conservation; conservative; consultation; keep [Lat. *conserva*]
consperg dust, sprinkle [Lat.*consperge*]
const constant
constit constituent
cont against [Lat. *contra*]; bruised [Lat. *contusus*]; contains, contents; continue, continuation
contag contagion, contagious

conter rub together [Lat. *contere*]
contin let it be continued [Lat. *continuetur*]
contra contraindicated
contralat contralateral
cont rem let the medicine be continued [Lat. *continuetur remedium*]
contrib contributory
contrit broken down [Lat. *contritus*]
contus bruised [Lat. *contusus*]
conv convalescence, convalescent, convalescing; convergence, convergent
COOD chronic obstruction outflow disease
COOP cooperative
coord coordination, coordinated
COP capillary osmotic pressure; change of plaster; coefficient of performance; colloid oncotic pressure; colloid osmotic pressure; cyclophosphamide, Oncovin, and prednisone
COPA Council on Postsecondary Accreditation
COPC community oriented primary care
COPD chronic obstructive pulmonary disease
COPE chronic obstructive pulmonary emphysema
COP$_i$ colloid osmotic pressure in interstitial fluid
COPP cyclophosphamide, vincristine, procarbazine, and prednisone
COP$_p$ colloid osmotic pressure in plasma
COPRO coproporphyrin
CoQ coenzyme Q
coq boil [Lat. *coque*]
coq in s a boil in sufficient water [Lat. *coque in sufficiente aqua*]
coq s a boil properly [Lat. *coque secundum artem*]
COR body [Lat. *corpus*]; cardiac output recorder; conditioned orientation reflex; corrosion, corrosive; cortisone
cor coronary; correction, corrected
CORA conditioned orientation reflex audiometry
CORD Commissioned Officer Residency Deferment
cort bark [Lat. *cortex*]; cortex
COS Clinical Orthopaedic Society
COSATI Committee on Scientific and Technical Information

COSMIS Computer System for Medical Information Systems
COSTAR Computer-Stored Ambulatory Record
COSTEP Commissioned Officer Student Training and Extern Program
COT colony overlay test; content of thought; contralateral optic tectum; critical off-time
COTA Certified Occupational Therapy Assistant
COTD cardiac output by thermodilution
COTe cathodal opening tetanus
COTRANS Coordinated Transfer Application System
coul coulomb
COV cross-over value
CoVF cobra venom facator
COWS cold to opposite and warm to same side
CP candle power; capillary pressure; cardiac pacing; cardiac performance; central pit; cerebral palsy; chemically pure; chest pain; child psychiatry; child psychology; chloroquine-primaquine; chondrodysplasia punctata; chronic pain; chronic pyelonephritis; cleft palate; clinical pathology; closing pressure; cochlear potential; code of practice; cold pressor; color perception; combining power; compound; compressed; constant pressure; coproporphyrin; cor pulmonale; creatine phosphate; creatine phosphokinase; cross-linked protein; crude protein; current practice; cyclophosphamide; cyclophosphamide and prednisone; cytosol protein
C&P compensation and pension; cystoscopy and pyelography
C/P cholesterol-phospholipid [ratio]
Cp ceruloplasmin; chickenpox
C$_p$ constant pressure; phosphate clearance
cP centipoise
cp centipoise; compare
CPA Canadian Psychiatric Association; cerebellopontine angle; chlorophenylalanine; circulating platelet aggregate; costophrenic angle; cyclophosphamide; cyproterone acetate
C3PA complement 3 proactivator
CPAF chlorpropamide-alcohol flushing

C_{pah} para-aminohippurate clearance

CPAP continuous positive airway pressure

CPB cardiopulmonary bypass; cetyl-pyridinium bromide; competitive protein binding

CPBA competitive protein-binding analysis

CPBV cardiopulmonary blood volume

CPC cerebellar Purkinje cell; cerebral palsy clinic; cetylpyridinium chloride; chronic passive congestion; circumferential pneumatic compression; clinico-pathological conference

CPCL congenital pulmonary cystic lymphangiectasia

CPCP chronic progressive coccidioidal pneumonitis

CPCS circumferential pneumatic compression suit

CPD cephalopelvic disproportion; chorio-retinopathy and pituitary dysfunction; citrate-phosphate-dextrose; contact potential difference; contagious pustular derma-titis; cyclopentadiene

cpd compound

CPDA citrate-phosphate-dextrose-adenine

CPDD calcium pyrophosphate deposition disease; cis-platinum-diamine dichloride

CPDL cumulative population doubling level

CPE cardiac pulmonary edema; chronic pulmonary emphysema; compensation, pension, and education; corona-penetrating enzyme; cytopathogenic effect

CPEO chronic progressive external oph-thalmoplegia

CPF contraction peak force

CPG carotid phonoangiogram

CPGN chronic proliferative glomerulo-nephritis

CPH Certificate in Public Health; chronic paroxysmal hemicrania; chronic persistent hepatitis

CPHA Commission on Professional and Hospital Activities

CPI California Personality Inventory; Cancer Potential Index; congenital palato-pharyngeal incompetence; constitutional psychopathic inferiority; cysteine protein-ase inhibitor

CPIB chlorophenoxyisobutyrate

CPK creatine phosphokinase

CPKD childhood polycystic kidney disease

CPL caprine placental lactogen; congen-ital pulmonary lymphangiectasia

cpl complete, completed

CPLM cysteine-peptone-liver infusion medium

CPM central pontine myelinosis; chlor-pheniramine maleate; continuous passive motion; cyclophosphamide

cpm counts per minute

CPMV cowpea mosaic virus

CPN chronic polyneuropathy; chronic pyelonephritis

CPP cancer proneness phenotype; cerebral perfusion pressure; dl-2[3-(2'-chlorophenoxy)phenyl] propionic [acid]; cyclopentenophenanthrene

CPPB continuous positive pressure breathing

CPPD calcium pyrophosphate dihydrate; cisplatin

CPPV continuous positive pressure ventilation

CPR cardiac pulmonary reserve; cardiopulmonary resuscitation; centripetal rub; cerebral cortex perfusion rate; chlorophenyl red; cortisol production rate

c-PR cyclopropyl

CPRD Committee on Prosthetics Research and Development

CPRS Children's Psychiatric Rating Scale; Comprehensive Psychopathological Rating Scale

CPS carbamyl phosphate synthetase; characters per second; clinical perform-ance score; complex partial seizures; constitutional psychopathic state; conta-gious pustular stomatitis; C-polysac-charide; cumulative probability of success; current population survey

cps cycles per second

CPT carnitine palmityl transferase; chest physiotherapy; ciliary particle transport; cold pressor test; combining power test; continuous performance test; Current Procedural Terminology

CPTH chronic post-traumatic headache

CPU central processing unit

CPUE chest pain of unknown etiology

CPV canine parvovirus; cytoplasmic polyhedrosis virus

CPVD congenital polyvalvular disease

CPZ cefoperazone; chlorpromazine; Compazine

CQ chloroquine; chloroquine-quinine; circadian quotient; conceptual quotient

CQM chloroquine mustard

CR calculus removed; cardiac rehabilitation; cardiorespiratory; caries-resistant; centric relation; chest and right arm [lead in electrocardiography]; chest roentgenogram, chest roentgenography; child-resistant [bottle top]; choice reaction; chromium; clinical record; clinical research; clot retraction; coefficient of fat retention; colon resection; colony reared [animal]; complement receptor; complete remission; complete response; conditioned reflex, conditioned response; congenital rubella; controlled release; cortico-resistant; creatinine; cresyl red; critical ratio; crown-rump [measurement]

C&R convalescence and rehabilitation

Cr chromium; cranium, cranial; creatinine; crown

CRA central retinal artery

CRABP cellular retinoic acid-binding protein

cran cranium, cranial

CRAO central retinal artery occlusion

crast for tomorrow [Lat. crastinus]

CRBBB complete right bundle branch block

CRBC chicken red blood cell

CRBP cellular retinol-binding protein

CRC cardiovascular reflex conditioning; colorectal carcinoma

CrCl creatinine clearance

CRCS cardiovascular reflex conditioning system

CRD chronic renal disease; chronic respiratory disease; complete reaction of degeneration

CRE cumulative radiation effect

creat creatinine

CREST calcinosis, Raynaud's phenomenon, esophageal involvement, sclerodactyly, and telangiectasia [syndrome]

CRF chronic renal failure; chronic respiratory failure; coagulase-reacting factor; corticotropin-releasing factor

CRFK Crandell feline kidney cells

CRH corticotropin-releasing hormone

CRHL Collaborative Radiological Health Laboratory

CRHV cottontail rabbit herpes virus

CRI congenital rubella infection; cross-reaction idiotype

crit hematocrit

CRL cell repository line; Certified Record Librarian; complement receptor location; complement receptor lymphocyte; crown- rump length

CRM Certified Reference Materials; cross- reacting material

CRNA Certified Registered Nurse Anesthetist

cRNA chromosomal ribonucleic acid

CRNF chronic rheumatoid nodular fibrositis

Cr Ns cranial nerves

CRO cathode ray oscilloscope; centric relation occlusion

CROS contralateral routing of signal

CRP corneal-retinal potential; C-reactive protein; cyclic AMP receptor protein

CrP creatine phosphate

CRPA C-reactive protein antiserum

CRPF contralateral renal plasma flow

CRS caudal regression syndrome; Chinese restaurant syndrome; colon and rectum surgery; congenital rubella syndrome

CRST calcinosis, Raynaud's phenomenon, sclerodactyly, telangiectasia [syndrome]; corrected sinus recovery time

CRT cardiac resuscitation team; cathode-ray tube; choice reaction time; complex reaction time; computerized renal tomography; copper reduction test; corrected ray tube; corrected retention time; cortisone resistant thymocyte

CRTP Consciousness Research and Training Project

CRTT Certified Respiratory Therapy Technician

CRU clinical research unit

CRV central retinal vein

CRVF congestive right ventricular failure

crys, cryst crystal, crystalline

CS calf serum; campomelic syndrome; cardiogenic shock; caries-susceptible; cat scratch; central service; central supply; cerebrospinal; cervical spine; cervical stimulation; cesarean section; chest strap; chondroitin sulfate; chorionic somatomammotropin; clinical laboratory scientist; clinical stage; Cockayne syndrome; concentrated strength; conditioned stimulus; congenital syphilis; conjunctival secretion; conscious, consciousness; constant spring; control serum; convalescence, convalescent; coronary sclerosis; coronary sinus; corticoid-sensitive; corticosteroid; crush syndrome; current strength; cycloserine; cyclosporin

C&S conjunctiva and sclera; culture and sensitivity

CS IV clinical stage 4

C4S chondroitin-4-sulfate

Cs cesium

C_s standard clearance

cS centistoke

CSA canavaninosuccinic acid; chondroitin sulfate A; colony-stimulating activity; compressed spectral assay; cyclosporin A

CsA cyclosporin

CSAA Child Study Association of America

CSB contaminated small bowel

CSBF coronary sinus blood flow

CSC blow on blow (administration of small amounts of drugs at short intervals) [Fr. *coup sur coup*]; collagen sponge contraceptive; cryogenic storage container

CSCD Center for Sickle Cell Disease

CSCR Central Society for Clinical Research

CSD carotid sinus denervation; cat scratch disease; conditionally streptomycin dependent; conduction system disease; cortical spreading depression

CSE clinical-symptom/self-evaluation [questionnaire]; cross-sectional echocardiography

C sect cesarean section

CSF cancer family syndrome; cerebrospinal fluid; colony-stimulating factor; coronary sinus flow

CSFH cerebrospinal fluid hypotension

CSFV cerebrospinal fluid volume

CSF–WR cerebrospinal fluid–Wassermann reaction

CSGBI Cardiac Society of Great Britain and Ireland

CSH carotid sinus hypersensitivity; chronic subdural hematoma; cortical stromal hyperplasia

CSI cancer serum index

CSICU cardiac surgical intensive care unit

CSII continuous subcutaneous insulin infusion

CSIN Chemical Substances Information Network

CSL cardiolipin synthetic lecithin

CSLU chronic stasis leg ulcer

CSM carotid sinus massage; cerebrospinal meningitis; Committee on Safety of Medicines; corn-soy milk

CSMA chronic spinal muscular atrophy

CSMB Center for the Study of Multiple Births

CSMMG Chartered Society of Massage and Medical Gymnastics

CSN carotid sinus nerve

CS(NCA) Clinical Laboratory Scientist Certified by the National Certification Agency for Medical Laboratory Personnel

CSNRT, cSNRT corrected sinus node recovery time

CSOM chronic suppurative otitis media

CSP carotid sinus pressure; cavum septi pellucidi; cell surface protein; Chartered Society of Physiotherapy; Cooperative Statistical Program; criminal sexual psychopath; cyclosporin

CSR central supply room; Cheyne-Stokes respiration; corrected sedimentation rate; cortisol secretion rate; cumulative survival rate

CSS carotid sinus syndrome; chewing, sucking, swallowing; chronic subclinical scurvy; Churg-Strauss syndrome

CSSD central sterile supply department

CST cavernous sinus thrombosis; contraction stress test; convulsive shock therapy

C_{st} static compliance

cSt centistoke

C_{stat} static compliance

CSTI Clearinghouse for Scientific and Technical Information

CSU catheter specimen of urine; central statistical unit; clinical specialty unit

CSV chick syncytial virus

CT calcitonin; calf testis; cardiac tamponade; cardiothoracic [ratio]; carotid tracing; carpal tunnel; cell therapy; cerebral thrombosis; chicken tumor; *Chlamydia trachomatis*; chlorothiazide; cholera toxin; chymotrypsin; circulation time; classic technique; clotting time; coagulation time; coated tablet; cobra toxin; coil test; collecting tubule; compressed tablet; computed tomography; connective tissue; continue treatment; continuous-flow tub; contraction time; controlled temperature; Coombs test; corneal transplant; coronary thrombosis; corrected transposition; corrective therapy; crest time; cystine-tellurite; cytotechnologist; unit of attenuation [number]

Ct carboxyl terminal

ct carat

C$_{T-1824}$ T-1824 (Evans blue) clearance

CTA Canadian Tuberculosis Association; chromotropic acid; Committee on Thrombolytic Agents; congenital trigeminal anesthesia; cyanotrimethyl-androsterone; cystine trypticase agar; cytoplasmic tubular aggregate

Cta menses [Lat. *catamenia*]

CTAB cetyltrimethyl-ammonium bromide

CTAC Cancer Treatment Advisory Committee

ctant with the same amount [Lat. *cum tanto*]

CTAP connective tissue activating peptide

CTAT computerized transaxial tomography

CTC chlortetracycline; Clinical Trial Certificate; computer-aided tomographic cisternography

CTCL cutaneous T-cell lymphoma

ctCO$_2$ carbon dioxide concentration

CTD carpal tunnel decompression; chest tube drainage; congenital thymic dysplasia; connective tissue disease

CTE cultured thymic epithelium

CTEM conventional transmission electron microscopy

CTF cancer therapy facility; certificate; Colorado tick fever; cytotoxic factor

CTFE chlorotrifluoroethylene

CTG cardiotocography; chymotrypsinogen

CTGA complete transposition of great arteries

CTH ceramide trihexoside

CTL cytotoxic T-lymphocyte

CTLL cytotoxic lymphoid line

CTM cardiotachometer; Chlortrimeton; cricothyroid muscle

CTMM computed tomographic metrizamide myelography

cTNM TNM (*q.v.*) staging of tumors as determined by clinical noninvasive examination

CTP cytidine triphosphate; cytosine triphosphate

CTR cardiothoracic ratio; carpal tunnel release

CTS carpal tunnel syndrome

CTT cefotetan; compressed tablet triturate; computerized transaxial tomography

CTU cardiac-thoracic unit; centigrade thermal unit; constitutive transcription unit

CTW central terminal of Wilson; combined testicular weight

CTX chemotaxis; cyclophosphamide

CTx cardiac transplantation

CTZ chemoreceptor trigger zone; chlorothiazide

CU casein unit; clinical unit; chymotrypsin unit; color unit; contact urticaria; convalescent unit

Cu copper [Lat. *cuprum*]

C$_u$ urea clearance

cu cubic

CuB copper band

CUC chronic ulcerative colitis

cu cm cubic centimeter

CUG cystidine, uridine, and guanidine; cystourethrogram, cystourethrography

cu in cubic inch

cuj of which [Lat. *cujus*]

cuj lib of whatever you please [Lat. *cujus libet*]

cult culture

CUMITECH Cumulative Techniques and Procedures in Clinical Microbiology

cu mm cubic millimeter

CUP carcinoma unknown primary

cur cure, curative; current

CURN Conduct and Utilization of Research in Nursing

CUSA cavitron ultrasonic aspirator

CuTS cubital tunnel syndrome

CV cardiovascular; carotenoid vesicle; cell volume; central venous; cerebrovascular; cervical vertebra; Chikungunya virus; closing volume; coefficient of variation; color vision; concentrated volume; conduction velocity; corpuscular volume; cresyl violet; crystal violet;

tomorrow evening [Lat. *cras vespere*]; true conjugate [diameter of the pelvic inlet] [Lat. *conjugata vera*]
C/V coulomb per volt
Cv specific heat at constant volume
C$_v$ constant volume
CVA cardiovascular accident; cerebrovascular accident; chronic villous arthritis; costovertebral angle; cyclophosphamide, vincristine, and Adriamycin
CVAH congenital virilizing adrenal hyperplasia
CVAT costovertebral angle tenderness
CVC central venous catheter
CVD cardiovascular disease; cerebrovascular disease; color-vision-deviant
CVF central visual field; cobra venom factor
CVG contrast ventriculography
CVH combined ventricular hypertrophy; common variable hypogammaglobulinemia
CVI cardiovascular insufficiency; cerebrovascular insufficiency; common variable immunodeficiency
CVID common variable immunodeficiency
CVM cardiovascular monitor; cyclophosphamide, vincristine, and methotrexate
CVMP Committee on Veterans Medical Problems
CVO central vein occlusion; central venous oxygen; Chief Veterinary Officer; obstetric conjugate [of the pelvic inlet] [Lat. *conjugata vera obstetrica*]
CVOD cerebrovascular obstructive disease
CVP cell volume profile; central venous pressure; cyclophosphamide, vincristine, and prednisone
CVR cardiovascular-renal; cardiovascular-respiratory; cephalic vasomotor response; cerebrovascular resistance
CVRD cardiovascular-renal disease
CVS cardiovascular surgery; cardiovascular system; challenge virus strain; chorionic villi sampling; clean voided specimen
CVT central venous temperature; congenital vertical talus
CVTR charcoal viral transport medium
CW cardiac work; case work; cell wall; chemical warfare; chest wall; children's ward; clockwise; continuous wave; crutch walking
C/W consistent with
CWBTS capillary whole blood true sugar
CWD continuous-wave Doppler
CWDF cell wall–deficient form [bacteria]
CWF Cornell Word Form
CWI cardiac work index
CWL cutaneous water loss
CWMS color, warmth, movement sensation
CWOP childbirth without pain
CWP coal worker's pneumoconiosis
CWPEA Childbirth Without Pain Education Association
CWS chest wall stimulation; child welfare service; cold water-soluble; cotton wool spots
CWT cold water treatment
Cwt hundredweight
CX cervix; chest x-ray
Cx cervix; circumflex; clearance; convex
CXR chest x-ray
Cy cyanogen; cyclophosphamide
CyA cyclosporin A
cyath a glassful [Lat. *cyathus*]
CYC cyclophosphamide
cyc cyclazocine; cycle; cyclotron
Cyclo C cyclocytidine hydrochloride
Cyd cytidine
CYE charcoal yeast extract [agar]
CYL casein yeast lactate
cyl cylinder; cylindrical lens
CYN cyanide
CYP cyproheptadine
CYS cystoscopy
Cys cyclosporin; cysteine
Cys-Cys cystine
CYSTO cystogram
cysto cystoscopy
CYT cytochrome
Cyt cytosine
cyt cytology, cytological; cytoplasm, cytoplasmic
cytol cytology, cytological
CY-VA-DIC cyclophosphamide, vincristine, Adriamycin, and dacarbazine
CZ cefazolin
Cz central midline placement of electrodes in electroencephalography
CZI crystalline zinc insulin

–D–

D aspartic acid; cholecalciferol; coefficient of diffusion; dacryon; date; daughter; day; dead; dead air space; debye; deceased; deciduous; decimal reduction time; degree; density; dental; dermatology, dermatologist, dermatologic; deuterium; deuteron; development; deviation; dextro; diagnosis; diagonal; diameter; diarrhea; died; difference; diffusion, diffusing; diopter; diplomate; disease; distal; diuresis; diurnal; divorced; dog; donor; dorsal; dose [Lat. *dosis*]; drive; drug; duodenum, duodenal; duration; dwarf; electric displacement; give [Lat. *da*]; let it be given [Lat. *detur*]; right [Lat. *dexter*]; unit of vitamin D potency

D̄ mean dose

D₁ diagonal one; first dorsal vertebra

1-D one-dimensional

D₂ diagonal two; second dorsal vertebra

2-D two-dimensional

D₃₋₁₂ third to twelfth dorsal vertebrae

d atomic orbital with angular momentum quantum number 2; day [Lat. *dies*]; dead; deceased; deci-; decrease, decreased; degree; density; deoxy.; deoxyribose; dextrorotatory; died; diopter; distal; dose; doubtful; duration; right [Lat. *dexter*]

Δ see *delta*

δ see *delta*

DA dark agouti [rat]; degenerative arthritis; delayed action; Dental Assistant; developmental age; differentiation antigen; diphenylchlorarsine; Diploma in Anesthetics; direct agglutination; disability assistance; disaggregated; dopamine; drug addict, drug addiction; ductus arteriosus

D/A digital-to-analog [converter]; discharge and advise

D-A donor-acceptor

da daughter; day; deca-

DAAO diaminoacid oxidase

DAB 3,3'-diaminobenzidine; dysrhythmic aggressive behavior

DABA 2,4-diaminobutyric acid

DAC digital-to-analog converter; disaster assistance center; Division of Ambulatory Care

dac dacryon

DACM N-(7-diamethylamino-4-methyl-3- coumarinyl) maleimide

DACT dactinomycin

DAD diffuse alveolar damage; dispense as directed

DADDS diacetyldiaminodiphenylsulfone

DADS Director Army Dental Service

DAE diphenylanthracene endoperoxide

DAF delayed auditory feedback

DAG dianhydrogalactitol

DAH disordered action of the heart

DAHEA Department of Allied Health Education and Accreditation

DAHM Division of Allied Health Manpower

DALA delta-aminolevulinic acid

DALE Drug Abuse Law Enforcement

DAM degraded amyloid; diacetyl monoxime; diacetylmorphine

dam decameter

dAMP deoxyadenosine monophosphate; deoxyadenylate adenosine monophosphate

D and C dilatation and curettage

dand to be given [Lat. *dandus*]

DANS 1-dimethylaminonaphthalene-5-sulfonyl chloride

DAO diamine oxidase

DAP diaminopimelic acid; dihydroxyacetone phosphate; dipeptidylaminopeptidase; direct latex agglutination pregnancy [test]; Draw-a-Person [test]

DAP&E Diploma of Applied Parasitology and Entomology

DAPRU Drug Abuse Prevention Resource Unit

DAPT direct agglutination pregnancy test

DARTS Drug and Alcohol Rehabilitation Testing System

DAS delayed anovulatory syndrome; dextroamphetamine sulfate

DASH Distress Alarm for the Severely Handicapped

DAT delayed-action tablet; dementia Alzheimer's type; dental aptitude test; diet as tolerated; differential agglutination titer; Differential Aptitude Test; diphtheria antitoxin; direct agglutination test; direct antiglobulin test; Disaster Action Team

DATE dental auxiliary teacher education

DAU 3-deazauridine; Dental Auxiliary Utilization

dau daughter

DAV Disabled American Veterans; duck adenovirus

DAvMED Diploma in Aviation Medicine

DAVP deamino-arginine vasopressin

DAW dispense as written

DB data base; date of birth; dense body; dextran blue; diet beverage; direct bilirubin; disability; distobuccal; double-blind [study]; Dutch belted [rabbit]

dB, db decibel

db diabetes

DBA dibenzanthracene; *Dolichos biflorus* agglutinin

DBAE dihydroxyborylaminoethyl

DBC dye-binding capacity

DB&C deep breathing and coughing

DBCL dilute blood cot lysis [method]

DBD dibromodulcitol

DBDG distobuccal developmental groove

DBE deep breathing exercise; dibromoethane

DBED penicillin G benzathine

DBH dopamine beta-hydroxylase

DBI development at birth index; phenformin hydrochloride

DBIOC data base input/output control

dBk decibels above 1 kilowatt

DBM data base management; dibromomannitol; dobutamine

dBm decibels above 1 milliwatt

DBMS data base management systems

DBO distobucco-occlusal

db/ob diabetic obese [mouse]

DBP diastolic blood pressure; dibutylphthalate; distobuccopulpal; Döhle body panmyelopathy

DBS despeciated bovine serum; diminished breath sounds; direct bonding system; Division of Biological Standards

DBT dry bulb temperature

DBW desirable body weight

dBW decibels above 1 watt

DC daily census; data communication; decrease; deep compartment; Dental Corps; deoxycholate; diagonal conjugate; diagnostic center; diagnostic code; differentiated cell; digit copying; diphenylcyanoarsine; direct current; discharge, discharged; discontinue, discontinued; distocervical; Doctor of Chiropractic;

donor cells; dyskeratosis congenita; electric defibrillator using DC discharge

D/C discontinue

DC65 Darvon compound 65

D&C dilatation and curettage; drugs and cosmetics

dC deoxycytidine

dc direct current

DCA deoxycholate-citrate agar; deoxycholic acid; desoxycorticosterone acetate; dichloroacetate

DCC day care center; dextran-coated charcoal; N,N'-dicyclohexylcarbodimide; disaster control center; double concave

DCCMP daunomycin, cyclocytidine, 6-mercaptopurine, and prednisolone

DC$_{CO2}$ diffusing capacity for carbon dioxide

DCD Diploma in Chest Diseases

D/c'd discontinued

DCF 2'-deoxycoformycin; direct centrifugal flotation; dopachrome conversion factor

DCG deoxycorticosterone glucoside; disodium cromoglycate

DCH delayed cutaneous hypersensitivity; Diploma in Child Health

DCh Doctor of Surgery [Lat. *Doctor Chirurgiae*]

DCHEB dichlorohexafluorobutane

DCHN dicyclohexylamine nitrite

DChO Doctor of Ophthalmic Surgery

DCI dichloroisoprenaline; dichloroisoproterenol

DCL diffuse or disseminated cutaneous leishmaniasis

DCLS deoxycholate citrate lactose saccharose

DCM dichloromethane; dilated cardiomyopathy; Doctor of Comparative Medicine; dyssynergia cerebellaris myoclonica

DCMP daunomycin, cytosine arabinoside, 6-mercaptopurine, and prednisolone

dCMP deoxycytidine monophosphate

DCMT Doctor of Clinical Medicine of the Tropics

DCN delayed conditioned necrosis; dorsal column nucleus; dorsal cutaneous nerve

DCNU chlorozotocin

DCO Diploma of the College of Optics

D_{CO} diffusing capacity for carbon monoxide

DCOG Diploma of the College of Obstetricians and Gynaecologists

DCP dicalcium phosphate; Diploma in Clinical Pathology; Diploma in Clinical Psychology; District Community Physician

DCR dacryocystorhinostomy; direct cortical response

DCS dense canalicular system; diffuse cortical sclerosis; dorsal column stimulation, dorsal column stimulator

DCT direct Coombs test; distal convoluted tubule

DCTMA desoxycorticosterone trimethylacetate

dCTP deoxycytidine triphosphate

DCTPA desoxycorticosterone triphenylacetate

DCX double charge exchange

DCx double convex

DD dangerous drug; degenerative disease; developmental disability; differential diagnosis; died of the disease; Di Guglielmo's disease; disc diameter; discharged dead; double diffusion; drug dependence; dry dressing; Dupuytren's disease

dd daily [Lat. *de die*]; let it be given to [Lat. *detur ad*]

D6D delta-6-desaturase

DDA Dangerous Drugs Act; dideoxyadenosine

DDAVP, dDAVP 1-deamino-8-D-arginine vasopressin

DDC dangerous drug cabinet; diethyldithiocarbamate; direct display console; diverticular disease of the colon

DDc double concave

DDD AV universal [pacemaker]; degenerative disc disease; dehydroxydinaphthyl disulfide; dense deposit disease; dichlorodiphenyldichloroethane; dihydroxydinaphthyl disulfide

DDE dichlorodiphenyldichloroethylene

DDG deoxy-D-glucose

DDH Diploma in Dental Health

DDIB Disease Detection Information Bureau

dd in d from day to day [Lat. *de die in diem*]

DDM Diploma in Dermatological Medicine; Doctor in Dental Medicine

DDO Diploma in Dental Orthopaedics

DDP cisplatin; density-dependent phosphoprotein; difficult denture patient; distributed data processing

DDPA Delta Dental Plans Association

DDR diastolic descent rate; Diploma in Diagnostic Radiology

DDRB Doctors' and Dentists' Review Body

DDS damaged disc syndrome; dendrodendritic synaptosome; dental distress syndrome; depressed DNA synthesis; dialysis disequilibrium syndrome; diaminodiphenylsulfone; directional Doppler sonography; Director of Dental Services; Doctor of Dental Surgery; dodecyl sulfate; double decidual sac; dystrophy-dystocia syndrome

DDSc Doctor of Dental Science

DDSO diaminodiphenylsulfoxide

DDST Denver Developmental Screening Test

DDT dichlorodiphenyltrichloroethane; ductus deferens tumor

ddTTP dideoxythymidine triphosphate

DE deprived eye; digestive energy; dose equivalent; dream elements; drug evaluation; duration of ejection

D&E dilatation and evacuation

2DE two-dimensional echocardiography

DEA dehydroepiandrosterone; diethanolamine; Drug Enforcement Agency

DEAE diethylaminoethyl [cellulose]

DEAE-D diethylaminoethyl dextran

DEB diepoxybutane; diethylbutanediol; Division of Environmental Biology

DEBA diethylbarbituric acid

DEBRA Dystrophic Epidermolysis Bullosa Research Association

deb spis of the proper consistency [Lat. *debita spissutudine*]

DEC decrease; deoxycholate citrate; diethylcarbamazine; dynamic environmental conditioning

Dec, dec decant

dec deciduous; decompose, decomposition; decrease, decreased

decd deceased

decoct decoction

decomp decomposition, decompose

decr decrease, decreased

decub lying down [Lat. *decubitus*]
DED date of expected delivery; delayed erythema dose
DEEG depth electroencephalogram, depth electroencephalography
de d in d from day to day [Lat. *de die in diem*]
DEF decayed primary teeth requiring filling, decayed primary teeth requiring extraction, and primary teeth successfully filled
def defecation; deficiency, deficient
defib defibrillation
defic deficiency, deficient
deform deformed, deformity
Deg, deg degeneration, degenerative; degree
degen degeneration, degenerative
deglut let it be swallowed [Lat. *deglutiatur*]
DEH dysplasia epiphysealis hemimelica
DEHP di(2-ethylhexyl)phthalate
DEHS Division of Emergency Health Services
dehyd dehydration, dehydrated
DEJ, dej dentino-enamel junctio
del deletion; delivery; delusion
deliq deliquescence, deliquescent
Δ Greek capital letter *delta*
δ Greek lower case letter *delta*; immunoglobulin D
Dem Demerol
DEN dengue
denat denatured
DENT Dental Exposure Normalization Technique
Dent, dent dentistry, dentist, dental, dentition; let it be given [Lat. *dentur*]
dent tal dos give of such doses [Lat. *dentur tales doses*]
DEP diethylpropanediol; dilution end point
dep dependent; purified [Lat. *depuratus*]
DEPA diethylene phospharamide
depr depression, depressed
DEPS distal effective potassium secretion
DEP ST SEG depressed ST segment
dept department
DER disulfiram-ethanol reaction
DeR degeneration reaction
der derivative chromosome
deriv derivative, derived

Derm, derm dermatology, dermatologist, dermatological
DES dialysis encephalopathy syndrome; diethylstilbestrol; diffuse esophageal spasm; disequilibrium syndrome; doctor's emergency service
desat desaturated
desc descendant
DESI drug efficacy study implementation
DEST dichotic environmental sounds test
dest distill, distilled [Lat. *destilla, destillatus*]
DET diethyltryptamine
det let it be given [Lat. *detur*]
Det-6 detroid-6 [human sternal marrow cells]
determ determination, determined
det in dup, det in 2 plo let twice as much be given [Lat. *detur in duplo*]
detn detention
detox detoxification
d et s let it be given and labeled [Lat. *detur et signetur*]
DEV deviant, deviation; duck embryo vaccine
devel development
DevPd developmental pediatrics
DEX dexamethasone
dex right [Lat. *dexter*]
DF decapacitation factor; decontamination factor; deferoxamine; deficiency factor; defined flora [animal]; degree of freedom; diabetic father; dietary fibers; discriminant function; disseminated foci; distribution factor, dorsiflexion
df degrees of freedom
DFA direct fluorescent antibody
DFB dinitrofluorobenzene
DFC dry-filled capsule
DFD defined formula diets; diisopropyl phosphorofluoridate
DFDT difluoro-diphenyl-trichloroethane
DFE diffuse fasciitis with eosinophilia; distal femoral epiphysis
DFHom Diploma of the Faculty of Homeopathy
DFI disease-free interval
DFMO difluoromethylornithine
DFMR daily fetal movement record
DFO, DFOM deferoxamine
DFP diastolic filling period; diisopropylfluorophosphate

DF³²P radiolabeled diisopropylfluorophosphate
DFR diabetic floor routine
DFSP dermatofibrosarcoma protuberans
DFT defibrillation threshold
DFU dead fetus in utero; dideoxyfluorouridine
DFV diarrhea with fever and vomiting
DG dentate gyrus; deoxyglucose; diagnosis; diastolic gallop; diglyceride; distogingival
dg decigram
DGAVP desglycinamide-9-[Arg-8]-vasopressin
DGBG dimethylglyoxal bisguanylhydrazone
DGI disseminated gonococcal infection
DGLA dihomogamma-linolenic acid
dGMP deoxyguanosine monophosphate
DGMS Division of General Medical Sciences
DGN diffuse glomerulonephritis
DGO Diploma in Gynaecology and Obstetrics
DGP 2,3-diglycerophosphate
DGS diabetic glomerulosclerosis
dGTP deoxyguanosine triphosphate
DGV dextrose-gelatin-Veronal [buffer]
DH day hospital; dehydrogenase; delayed hypersensitivity; dermatitis herpetiformis; developmental history; diaphragmatic hernia; disseminated histoplasmosis; dominant hand; ductal hyperplasia; Dunkin-Hartley [guinea pig]
D/H deuterium/hydrogen [ratio]
DHA dehydroascorbic acid; dehydroepiandrosterone; dihydroacetic acid; dihydroxyacetone; district health authority
DHAD mitoxantrone hydrochloride
DHAP dihydroxyacetone phosphate
DHAS dehydroepiandrosterone sulfate
DHBS dihydrobiopterin synthetase
DHBV duck hepatic B virus
DHC dehydrocholesterol; dehydrocholate
DHCA deep hypothermia and circulatory arrest
DHD district health department
DHE dihydroergotamine
DHEA dehydroepiandrosterone
DHEAS dehydroepiandrosterone sulfate
DHEC dihydroergocryptine
DHES Division of Health Examination Statistics

DHEW Department of Health, Education, and Welfare
DHF dengue hemorrhagic fever
DHFR dihydrofolate reductase
DHg Doctor of Hygiene
DHGG deaggregated human gamma-globulin
DHHS Department of Health and Human Services
DHI Dental Health International; dihydroxyindole
DHIA dehydroisoandrosterol
DHL diffuse histiocytic lymphoma
DHM dihydromorphine
DHMA 3,4-dihydroxymandelic acid
DHP dehydrogenated polymer; dihydroprogesterone
DHPG dihydroxyphenylglycol; dihydroxyproproxymethylguanine
DHPR dihydropteridine reductase
DHR delayed hypersensitivity reaction
DHS delayed hypersensitivity; duration of hospital stay
D-5-HS 5% dextrose in Harman's solution
DHSM dihydrostreptomycin
DHSS Department of Health and Social Security; dihydrostreptomycin sulfate
DHT dehydrotestosterone; dihydroergotoxine; dihydrotachysterol; dihydrotestosterone; dihydrothymine
5,7-DHT 5,7-dihydroxytryptamine
DHTP dihydrotestosterone propionate
DHy, DHyg Doctor of Hygiene
DHZ dihydralazine
DI dentinogenesis imperfecta; deoxyribonucleic acid index; deterioration index; diabetes insipidus; diagnostic imaging; disto-incisal; double indemnity; drug information; drug interactions; dyskaryosis index
DIA diabetes; Drug Information Association
dia diathermy
diab diabetes, diabetic
diag diagnosis; diagram
diam diameter
dias diastole, diastolic
diath diathermy
DIB dot immunobinding
DIC dicarbazine; differential interference contrast microscopy; diffuse intravascular

coagulation; disseminated intravascular coagulation

dic dicentric

DICD dispersion-induced circular dichroism

DID dead of intercurrent disease; double immunodiffusion

DIDD dense intramembranous deposit disease

DIDMOAD diabetes insipidus, diabetes mellitus, optic atrophy, deafness [syndrome]

DIE died in emergency department

dieb alt on alternate days [Lat. *diebus alternis*]

dieb tert every third day [Lat. *diebus tertiis*]

DIF diffuse interstitial fibrosis; dose increase factor

DIFF, diff difference, differential; diffusion

DIFP diisopropyl fluorophosphonate

DIG digoxin

dig let it be digested [Lat. *digeretur*]

DIH Diploma in Industrial Health

DIHPPA di-iodohydroxyphenylpyruvic acid

dil dilute, dilution, diluted

dilat dilatation

DILD diffuse infiltrative lung disease

Diluc at daybreak [Lat. *diluculo*]

dilut dilute, dilution, diluted

DIM divalent ion metabolism

dim diminished; one half [Lat. *dimidius*]

DIMIT 3,5-dimethyl-3'-isopropyl-L-thyronine

DIMOAD diabetes insipidus, diabetes mellitus, optic atrophy and deafness

DIMS disorders of initiating and maintaining sleep

d in p aeq divide into equal parts [Lat. *dividetur in partes aequales*]

DIP desquamative interstitial pneumonitis; diisopropyl phosphate; distal interphalangeal; drip infusion pyelogram; dual-in-line package

Dip diplomate

dip diploid

DIPA diisopropylamine

DipBact Diploma in Bacteriology

DIPC diffuse interstitial pulmonary calcification

DipChem Diploma in Chemistry

DipClinPath Diploma in Clinical Pathology

diph diphtheria

diph-tox AP alum precipitated diphtheria toxoid

DIPJ distal interphalangeal joint

DipMicrobiol Diploma in Microbiology

DipSocMed Diploma in Social Medicine

DIR double isomorphous replacement

Dir, dir director; direction, directions [Lat. *directione*]

DIRD drug-induced renal disease

dir prop with proper direction [Lat. *directione propria*]

DIS Diagnostic Interview Schedule

DI-S debris index, simplified

dis disability, disabled; disease; dislocation; distance

disc discontinue

disch discharge, discharged

DISH diffuse idiopathic skeletal hyperostosis

disinfect disinfection

disloc dislocation, dislocated

disod disodium

disp dispensary, dispense

diss dissolve, dissolved

dissem disseminated, dissemination

dist distal; distill, distillation, distilled; distance

DIT diiodotyrosine

dITP deoxyinosine triphosphate

div divergence, divergent; divide, divided, division

DIVBC disseminated intravascular blood coagulation

DIVC disseminated intravascular coagulation

div in par aeq divide into equal parts [Lat. *dividetur in partes aequales*]

DJD degenerative joint disease

DK dark; decay; diabetic ketoacidosis; diseased kidney; dog kidney [cells]

dk deka

DKA diabetic ketoacidosis

dkg dekagram

dkm dekameter

DKTC dog kidney tissue culture

DKV deer kidney virus

DL danger list; developmental level; difference limen; disabled list; distolingual; equimolecular mixture of the dextrorotatory and levorotatory enantiomorphs

DL, D-L Donath-Landsteiner [antibody]

D_L diffusing capacity of the lungs

dl deciliter

DLa distolabial

DLaI distolabioincisal

DLaP distolabiopulpal

DLC Dental Laboratory Conference

DLCO single breath diffusing capacity

D_{LCO} carbon monoxide diffusion in the lungs

D_{LCO2} carbon dioxide diffusion in the lungs

D_{LCO}^{SB} single-breath carbon monoxide diffusing capacity of the lungs

D_{LCO}^{SS} steady state carbon monoxide diffusing capacity of the lungs

DLE discoid lupus erythematosus; disseminated lupus erythematosus

D_1LE diagonal 1 lower extremity

D_2LE diagonal 2 lower extremity

DLF Disabled Living Foundation; dorsolateral funiculus

DLG distolingual groove

DLI distolinguoincisal; double label index

DLIS digoxin-like immunoreactive substance

DLL dihomo-gammalinoleic acid

DLLI dulcitol lysine lactose iron

DLMP date of last menstrual period

DLNMP date of last normal menstrual period

DLO Diploma in Laryngology and Otology; distolinguo-occlusal

D_{LO2} diffusing capacity of the lungs for oxygen

DLP distolinguopulpal; dysharmonic luteal phase

D_5LR dextrose in 5% lactated Ringer's solution

DLT dihydroepiandrosterone loading test

DLV defective leukemia virus

DM dextromaltose; dextromorphan; diabetes mellitus; diabetic mother; diastolic murmur; dopamine; double minute [chromosome]

D_M membrane component of diffusion

dm decimeter

dm^2 square decimeter

dm^3 cubic decimeter

DMA dimethylamine; dimethylaniline; dimethylarginine; direct memory access

DMAB dimethylaminobenzaldehyde

DMAC N,N-dimethylacetamide

DMAE dimethylaminoethanol

DMBA 7,12-dimethylbenz[a]anthracene

DMC demeclocycline; di(p-chlorophenyl)methylcarbinol; direct microscopic count

DMCC direct microscopic clump count

DMCT, DMCTC dimethylchlortetracycline

DMD Doctor of Dental Medicine; Duchenne's muscular dystrophy

DMDT dimethoxydiphenyl trichloroethane

DMDZ desmethyldiazepam

DME degenerative myoclonus epilepsy; dimethyl diester; dimethyl ether; diphasic meningoencephalitis; director of medical education; dropping mercury electrode; Dulbecco's modified Eagle's [medium]

DMEM Dulbecco's modified Eagle's medium

DMF decayed, missing, and filled [teeth]; N,N-dimethylformamide; diphasic milk fever

DMGBL dimethyl-gammabutyrolactone

DMH diffuse mesangial hypercellularity

DMI diaphragmatic myocardial infarction; direct migration inhibition

DMJ Diploma in Medical Jurisprudence

DMKA diabetes mellitus ketoacidosis

DMM dimethylmyleran

DMN dimethylnitrosamine; dorsal motor nucleus

DMNA dimethylnitrosamine

DMO 5,5-dimethyl-2,4-oxazolidinedione (dimethadone)

DMOOC diabetes mellitus out of control

DMP diffuse mesangial proliferation; dimethylphthalate

DMPA depot medroxyprogesterone acetate

DMPE, DMPEA 3,4-dimethoxyphenylethylamine

DMPP dimethylphenylpiperazinium

DMPS dysmyelopoietic syndrome

DMR Diploma in Medical Radiology
DMRD Diploma in Medical Radio-Diagnosis
DMRE Diploma in Medical Radiology and Electrology
DMRT Diploma in Medical Radio-Therapy
DMS delayed microembolism syndrome; demarcation membrane system; department of medicine and surgery; dermatomyositis; dimethylsulfate; dimethylsulfoxide; District Management Team; Doctor of Medical Science; dysmyelopoietic syndrome
DMSA dimercaptosuccinic acid
DMSO dimethylsulfoxide
DMT dermatophytosis; N,N-dimethyltryptamine; Doctor of Medical Technology
DMU dimethanolurea
DMV Doctor of Veterinary Medicine
DN diabetic neuropathy; dibucaine number; dicrotic notch; Diploma in Nursing; Diploma in Nutrition; District Nurse; Doctor of Nursing
D/N dextrose/nitrogen ratio
Dn dekanem
dn decinem
DNA deoxyribonucleic acid
DNAse, DNase deoxyribonuclease
DNB dinitrobenzene; Diplomate of the National Board [of Medical Examiners]
DNBP dinitrobutylphenol
DNC did not come; dinitrocarbanilide; Disaster Nursing Chairman
DNCB dinitrochlorobenzene
DND died a natural death
DNE Director of Nursing Education; Doctor of Nursing Education
DNFB dinitrofluorobenzene
DNMS Director of Naval Medical Services
DNO District Nursing Officer
DNOC dinitroorthocresol
DNP deoxyribonucleoprotein; dinitrophenol
DNPH dinitrophenylhydrazine
DNPM dinitrophenol-morphine
DNR daunorubicin; do not resuscitate
DNS diaphragmatic nerve stimulation; Doctor of Nursing Services; dysplastic nevus syndrome
D$_5$NSS 5% destrose in normal saline solution

DNT did not test
DO diamine oxidase; digoxin; Diploma in Ophthalmology; Diploma in Osteopathy; dissolved oxygen; disto-occlusal; Doctor of Ophthalmology; Doctor of Optometry; Doctor of Osteopathy; doctor's orders; drugs only
D$_O$ oxygen diffusion
do the same, as before [Lat. *dictum*]
DOA date of admission; dead on arrival; Department of Agriculture
DOAC Dubois oleic albumin complex
DOB date of birth; doctor's order book
DObstRCOG Diploma of the Royal College of Obstetricians and Gynaecologists
DOC deoxycholate; deoxycorticosterone; died of other causes
doc doctor; document
DOCA deoxycorticosterone acetate
DOCG deoxycorticosterone glucoside
DOCLINE Documents On-Line
DOcSc Doctor of Ocular Science
DOD date of death; died of disease; dissolved oxygen deficit
DOE desoxyephedrine; direct observation evaluation; dyspnea on exertion
DOES disorders of excessive sleepiness
DOFOS disturbance of function occlusion syndrome
DOH department of health
DOHyg Diploma in Occupational Hygiene
DOI died of injuries
DOM deaminated O-methyl metabolite; department of medicine; dimethoxymethylamphetamine; dissolved organic matter; dominance, dominant
DOMA dihydromandelic acid
DOMF 2'7'-dibromo-4'-(hydroxymercuri)fluorescein
DOMS Diploma in Ophthalmic Medicine and Surgery
DON Director of Nursing; diazooxonorleucine
don until [Lat. *donec*]
donec alv sol fuerit until the bowels are opened (until a bowel movement takes place) [Lat. *donec alvus soluta fuerit*]
DOOR deafness, onycho-osteodystrophy, mental retardation [syndrome]
DOPA, dopa dihydroxyphenylalanine

DOPAC dihydrophenylacetic acid

dopase dihydroxyphenylalanine oxidase

DOph Doctor of Ophthalmology

DOPP dihydroxyphenylpyruvate

DOPS diffuse obstructive pulmonary syndrome; dihydroxyphenylserine

Dors dorsal

DOrth Diploma in Orthodontics; Diploma in Orthoptics

DOS deoxystreptamine; disk operating system; Doctor of Ocular Science; Doctor of Optical Science

dos dosage, dose

DOSC Dubois oleic serum complex

DOSS distal over-shoulder strap; docusate sodium

DOT Dictionary of Occupational Titles

DOTC Dameshek's oval target cell

Dox doxorubicin

DP data processing; deep pulse; degradation product; degree of polymerization; dementia praecox; dental prosthodontics, dental prosthesis; dexamethasone pretreatment; diastolic pressure; diffusion pressure; digestible protein; diphosgene; diphosphate; dipropionate; directional preponderance; disability pension; distal pit; distopulpal; Doctor of Pharmacy; Doctor of Podiatry; donor's plasma; dorsalis pedis; with proper direction [Lat. *directione propria*]

DPA Department of Public Assistance; diphenylalanine; dipicolinic acid; dipropylacetic acid

DPC delayed primary closure; desaturated phosphatidylcholine; direct patient care; discharge planning coordinator; distal palmar crease

DPD Department of Public Dispensary; depression pure disease; diffuse pulmonary disease; diphenamid; Diploma in Public Dentistry

DPDL diffuse poorly differentiated lymphocytic lymphoma

dpdt double-pole double-throw [switch]

DPE dipiperidinoethane

DPF Dental Practitioners' Formulary

DPG 2,3-diphosphoglycerate; displacement placentogram

2,3-DPG 2,3-diphosphoglycerate

2,3-DPGM 2,3-diphosphoglycerate mutase

DPGP diphosphoglycerate phosphatase

DPH Department of Public Health; diphenhydramine; diphenylhexatriene; diphenylhydantoin; Diploma in Public Health Doctor of Public Health; Doctor of Public Hygiene

DPhC Doctor of Pharmaceutical Chemistry

DPhc Doctor of Pharmacology

DPHN Doctor of Public Health Nursing

DPhys Diploma in Physiotherapy

DPhysMed Diploma in Physical Medicine

DPI days post inoculation; disposable personal income

DPJ dementia paralytica juvenilis

DPL dipalmitoyl lecithin; distopulpolingual

DPLa distopulpolabial

DPM Diploma in Psychological Medicine; discontinue previous medication; Doctor of Physical Medicine; Doctor of Podiatric Medicine; Doctor of Preventive Medicine; Doctor of Psychiatric Medicine; dopamine

dpm disintegrations per minute

DPN diabetic polyneuropathy; diphosphopyridine nucleotide; disabling pansclerotic morphea

DPNH reduced diphosphopyridine nucleotide

DPO dimethoxyphenyl penicillin

DPP differential pulse polarography

DPPC dipalmitoylphosphatidylcholine

DPS dimethylpolysiloxane

dps disintegrations per second

dpst double-pole single-throw [switch]

DPT Demerol, Phenergan, and Thorazine; dichotic pitch discrimination test; diphtheria–pertussis–tetanus [vaccine]; diphtheritic pseudotabes; dipropyltryptamine

DPTA diethylenetriamine penta-acetic acid

DPTI diastolic pressure time index

DQ deterioration quotient; developmental quotient

DQE detective quantum efficiency

DR degeneration reaction; delivery room; diabetic retinopathy; diagnostic radiology; doctor; dorsal root; dose ratio

Dr doctor

dr dorsal root; dram; dressing
DRACOG Diploma of Royal Australian College of Obstetricians and Gynaecologists
DRACR Diploma of Royal Australasian College of Radiologists
DRAM dynamic random access memory
dr ap dram, apothecary
DRAT differential rheumatoid agglutination test
DRBC denaturated red blood cell; donkey red blood cell
DRCOG Diploma of Royal College of Obstetricians and Gynaecologists
DRCPath Diploma of Royal College of Pathologists
DREZ dorsal root entry zone
DRF daily replacement factor; Deafness Research Foundation; dose reduction factor
DRG diagnosis related groups; dorsal respiratory group; dorsal root ganglion
DrHyg Doctor of Hygiene
DRI discharge readiness inventory
dRib deoxyribose
DRID double radial immunodiffusion
DRME Division of Research in Medical Education
Dr Med Doctor of Medicine
DrMT Doctor of Mechanotherapy
DRNDP diribonucleoside-3',3'-diphosphate
DRnt diagnostic roentgenology
DRO differential reinforcement of other behavior; Disablement Resettlement Officer
DRP dorsal root potential
DrPH Doctor of Public Health; Doctor of Public Hygiene
DRQ discomfort relief quotient
DRS drowsiness; Duane retraction syndrome; dynamic renal scintigraphy
drsg dressing
DS dead air space; dead space; defined substrate; dehydroepiandrosterone sulfate; delayed sensitivity; density standard; dental surgery; dermatan sulfate; dermatology and syphilology; desynchronized sleep; dextran sulfate; dextrose-saline; diastolic murmur; dilute strength; dioptric strength; disaster services; disoriented; disseminated

sclerosis; dissolved solids; Doctor of Science; donor's serum; double-stranded; double strength; Down's syndrome; drug store; dry swallow
D/S dextrose/saline
D&S dermatology and syphilology
D-5-S 5% dextrose in saline solution
ds double-stranded
DSA digital subtraction angiography
DSACT, D-SACT direct sinoatrial conduction time
DSAP disseminated superficial actinic porokeratosis
DSAS discrete subaortic stenosis
DSBL disabled
DSC disodium chromoglycate; Doctor of Surgical Chiropody; Down's syndrome child
DSc Doctor of Science
DSCF Doppler-shifted constant frequency
DSCG disodium chromoglycate
DSD depression spectrum disease; discharge summary dictated; dry sterile dressing
dsDNA double-stranded deoxyribonucleic acid
DSE Doctor of Sanitary Engineering
DSH deliberate self harm; dexamethasone suppressible hyperaldosteronism
DSI deep shock insulin; Depression Status Inventory; Down Syndrome International
DSIM Doctor of Science in Industrial Medicine
DSIP delta sleep-inducing peptide
dslv dissolve
DSM Diagnostic and Statistical Manual [of Mental Disorders]; Diploma in Social Medicine; drink skim milk
DSP delayed sleep phase; dibasic sodium phosphate; digital subtraction phlebography
DSPC disaturated phosphatidylcholine
DSS decusate sodium; dengue shock syndrome; dioctyl sodium sulfosuccinate
DSSc Diploma in Sanitary Science
DSSEP dermatomal somatosensory evoked potential
DST desensitization test; dexamethasone suppression test; dihydrostreptomycin
DSUH directed suggestion under hypnosis

DSur Doctor of Surgery
DT delirium tremens; dental technician; digitoxin; diphtheria-tetanus [toxoid]; discharge tomorrow; dispensing tablet; distance test; duration of tetany; dye test
D/T total ratio of deaths
dT deoxythymidine
DTA differential thermal analysis
DTB dedicated time block
DTBC d-tubocurarine
DTBN di-t-butyl nitroxide
dTc d-tubocurarine
DTCD Diploma in Tuberculosis and Chest Diseases
DTCH Diploma in Tropical Child Health
DTD give such a dose [Lat. *datur talis dosis*]
dTDP deoxythymidine diphosphate
DTF detector transfer function
DTH delayed-type hypersensitivity; Diploma in Tropical Hygiene
DTIC dacarbazine; dimethyltriazeno-imidazole carboxamide
D time dream time
DTLA Detroit Test of Learning Aptitudes
DTM dermatophyte test medium; Diploma in Tropical Medicine
DTM&H Diplomate of Tropical Medicine and Hygiene
dTMP deoxythymidine monophosphate
DTN diphtheria toxin, normal
DTNB 5,5'-dithiobis-(2-nitrobenzoic) acid
DTP diphtheria-tetanus-pertussis [vaccine]; distal tingling on percussion; Tinel's sign
DTPA diethylenetriaminepentaacetic acid
DTPH Diploma in Tropical Public Health
DTR deep tendon reflex
DTS dense tubular system; donor transfusion, specific
DT's delirium tremens
DTT diphtheria tetanus toxoid
dTTP deoxythymidine triphosphate
DT-VAC diphtheria-tetanus vaccine
DTVM Diploma in Tropical Veterinary Medicine
DTVP developmental test of visual perception
DTZ diatrizoate
DU decubitus ulcer; density unknown; deoxyuridine; diagnosis undetermined;

dog unit; duodenal ulcer; duroxide uptake; Dutch [rabbit]
dU deoxyuridine
du dial unit
DUB dysfunctional uterine bleeding
D_1UE diagonal 1 upper extremity
D_2UE diagonal 2 upper extremity
DUI driving under the influence
dulc sweet [Lat. *dulcis*]
dUMP deoxyuridine monophosphate
duod duodenum, duodenal
dup duplication
dur hard [Lat. *duris*]
dur dolor while pain lasts [Lat. *durante dolore*]
DV dependent variable; dilute volume; distemper virus; domiciliary visit; double vibration; double vision
D&V diarrhea and vomiting
dv double vibrations
DVA distance visual acuity; duration of voluntary apnea; vindesine
DVB divinylbenzene
DVCC Disease Vector Control Center
DV&D Diploma in Venereology and Dermatology
dVDAVP 1-deamine-4-valine-D-arginine vasopressin
DVE duck virus enteritis
DVH Diploma in Veterinary Hygiene; Division for the Visually Handicapped
DVI AV sequential [pacemaker]
DVIU direct vision internal urethrotomy
DVL deep vastus lateralis
DVM digital voltmeter; Doctor of Veterinary Medicine
DVMS Doctor of Veterinary Medicine and Surgery
DVN dorsal vagal nucleus
DVR digital vascular reactivity; Doctor of Veterinary Radiology; double valve replacement
DVS Doctor of Veterinary Science; Doctor of Veterinary Surgery
DVSc Doctor of Veterinary Science
DVT deep venous thrombosis
DW deionized water; dextrose in water; distilled water; dry weight
D/W dextrose in water
D_5W 5% aqueous dextrose solution
dw dwarf [mouse]

DWA died from wounds by the action of the enemy
DWD died with disease
DWDL diffuse well-differentiated lymphocytic lymphoma
DWI driving while impaired
DWS disaster warning system
DWT dichotic word test
dwt pennyweight
DX dextran
Dx diagnosis
DXD discontinued
DXM dexamethasone
DXR deep x-ray
DXRT deep x-ray therapy
DXT deep x-ray therapy; dextrose
dXTP deoxyxanthine triphosphate
DY dense parenchyma
Dy dysprosium
dy dystrophia muscularis [mouse]
dyn dyne
DZ dizygotic; dizziness
dz disease; dozen

–E–

E air dose; cortisone [compound E]; edema; elastance; electric field vector; electrode potential; electromotive force; electron; embyro; emmetropia; encephalitis; endangered [animal]; endoplasm; energy; *Entamoeba*; enzyme; epinephrine; erythrocyte; erythroid; *Escherichia*; esophagus; estradiol; ethyl; expectancy [wave]; expected frequency in a cell of a contingency table; experiment, experimenter; expired air; extralymphatic; extraction fraction; eye; glutamic acid; internal energy; mathematical expectation; redox potential; stereodescriptor to indicate the configuration at a double bond [Ger. *entgegen* opposite]
E* lesion on the erythrocyte cell membrane at the site of complement fixation
E_0 electric affinity
E_1 estrone
E_2 17ß-estradiol
E_3 estriol

E_4 estetrol
4E four plus edema
E° standard electrode potential
e base of natural logarithms, approximately 2,7182818285; egg transfer; electric charge; electron; elementary charge
e⁻ negative electron
e⁺ positron
ε see *epsilon*
η see *eta*
EA early antigen; educational age; egg albumin; electric affinity; electrophysiological abnormality; embryonic antibody; endocardiographic amplifier; Endometriosis Association; epiandrosterone; erythrocyte antibody; esophageal atresia; estivo-autumnal; ethacrynic acid
ea each
EAA Epilepsy Association of America; essential amino acid; extrinsic allergic alveolitis
EAB Ethics Advisory Board
EAC Ehrlich ascites carcinoma; erythrocyte, antibody, complement; external auditory canal
EACA epsilon-aminocaproic acid
EACD eczematous allergic contact dermatitis
ead the same [Lat. *eadem*]
E-ADD epileptic attentional deficit disorder
EAE experimental allergic encephalomyelitis
EAHF eczema, asthma, and hay fever
EAHLG equine antihuman lymphoblast globulin
EAHLS equine antihuman lymphoblast serum
EAI Emphysema Anonymous, Inc.
EAM external acoustic meatus
EAMG experimental autoimmune myasthenia gravis
EAN experimental allergic neuritis
EAP electric acupuncture; epiallopregnanolone
EAQ eudismic affinity quotient
Ea R reaction of degeneration [Ger. *Entartungs-Reaktion*]
EAST external rotation, abduction stress test
EAT Ehrlich ascites tumor; electroaerosol therapy; experimental autoimmune thymitis

EATC Ehrlich ascites tumor cell

EAV equine abortion virus

EAVC enhanced atrioventricular conduction

EB elementary body; endometrial biopsy; epidermolysis bullosa; Epstein-Barr [virus]; estradiol benzoate; Evans blue

EBA epidermolysis bullosa acquisita; orthoethoxybenzoic acid

EBCDIC Extended Binary Coded Decimal Interchange Code

EBD epidermolysis bullosa dystrophica

EBF erythroblastosis fetalis

EBG electroblepharogram, electroblepharography

EBI emetine bismuth iodide; estradiol binding index

EBK embryonic bovine kidney

EBL estimated blood loss

EBM electrophysiologic behavior modification; expressed breast milk

EBNA Epstein-Barr virus-associated nuclear antigen

E/BOD electrolyte biochemical oxygen demand

EBP estradiol-binding protein

EBS electric brain stimulation; Emergency Bed Service; epidermolysis bullosa simplex

EBSS Earle's balanced salt solution

EBV effective blood volume; Epstein-Barr virus

EC electrochemical; electron capture; embryonal carcinoma; endothelial cell; enteric coating; entering complaint; enterochromaffin; Enzyme Commission; epidermal cell; *Escherichia coli*; excitation-contraction; experimental control; expiratory center; extracellular; extracranial; eyes closed

E-C ether-chloroform [mixture]

E/C estrogen/creatinine ratio

Ec ectochonchion

ECA electrocardioanalyzer; epidemiological catchment area; ethacrynic acid; ethylcarboxylate adenosine

ECBD exploration of common bile duct

ECBO enteric cytopathogenic bovine orphan [virus]

ECBV effective circulating blood volume

ECC embryonal cell carcinoma; emergency cardiac care; extracorporeal circulation

ECCLS European Committee for Clinical Laboratory Standards

ECCO₂R extracorporeal carbon dioxide removal

ECD electrochemical detector; electron capture detector; endocardial cushion defect

ECDO enteric cytopathic dog orphan [virus]

ECF effective capillary flow; eosinophilic chemotactic factor; erythroid colony formation; extended care facility; extracellular fluid

ECFA eosinophilic chemotactic factor of anaphylaxis

ECFMG Educational Commission on Foreign Medical Graduates; Educational Council for Foreign Medical Graduates

ECFMS Educational Council for Foreign Medical Students

ECFV extracellular fluid volume

ECG electrocardiogram, electrocardiography

ECGF endothelial cell growth factor

ECGS endothelial cell growth supplement

ECHO echocardiography; enteric cytopathic human orphan [virus]; Etoposide, cyclophosphamide, Adriamycin, and vincristine

ECHSCP Exeter Community Health Services Computer Project

ECI electrocerebral inactivity; eosinophilic cytoplasmic inclusions; extracorporeal irradiation

ECIB extracorporeal irradiation of blood

EC-IC extracranial-intracranial

ECIL extracorporeal irradiation of lymph

ECL emitter-coupled logic; enterochromaffin-like [type]

ECLT euglobulin clot lysis time

ECM embryonic chick muscle; erythema chronicum migrans; extracellular matrix

ECMO enteric cytopathic monkey orphan [virus]; extracorporeal membrane oxygenation

E co *Escherichia coli*

ECOG Eastern Cooperative Oncology Group

ECoG electrocorticogram, electrocorticography

ECP effector cell precursor; endocardial

potential; eosinophil cationic protein; *Escherichia coli* polypeptide; estradiol cyclopentane propionate; external cardiac pressure; external counterpulsation; free cytoporphyrin of erythrocytes

ECPO enteric cytopathic porcine orphan [virus]

ECPOG electrochemical potential gradient

ECR emergency chemical restraint

ECRB extensor carpi radialis brevis

ECRL extensor carpi radialis longus

ECS elective cosmetic surgery; electro-cerebral silence; electroconvulsive shock, electroshock

ECSO enteric cytopathic swine orphan [virus]

ECT electroconvulsive therapy; enteric coated tablet; euglobulin clot test

ECTA Everyman's Contingency Table Analysis

ECU extended care unit; extensor carpi ulnaris

ECV extracellular volume

ECW extracellular water

ED ectopic depolarization; effective dose; Ehlers-Danlos [syndrome]; electrodialysis; electron diffraction; emergency department; emotional disorder, emotionally disturbed; Entner-Doudoroff [pathway]; enzyme deficiency; epidural; epileptiform discharge; equine dermis [cells]; erythema dose; ethyl dichlorarsine; ethynodiol; extensive disease; extra-low dispersion

E-D ego-defense

ED$_{50}$ median effective dose

E$_d$ depth dose

EDA electrodermal activity; electrodermal audiometry; electron donor acceptor

EDAM electron-dense amorphous material

EDAX energy dispersive x-ray analysis

EDB early dry breakfast; extensor digitorum brevis

EDC emergency decontamination center; estimated date of conception; expected date of confinement; extensor digitorum communis

EDCI energetic dynamic cardiac insufficiency

EDCS end-diastolic chamber stiffness; end-diastolic circumferential stress

EDD effective drug duration; expected date of delivery

EDDA expanded duty dental auxiliary

edent edentia, edentulous

EDIM epizootic diarrhea of infant mice

E-diol estradiol

EDL end-diastolic length; end-diastolic load; estimated date of labor; extensor digitorum longus

ED/LD emotionally disturbed and learning disabled

EDM early diastolic murmur

EDN electrodesiccation; eosinophil-derived neurotoxin

EDNA Emergency Department Nurses Association

EDP electron dense particle; electronic data processing; end-diastolic pressure

EDR effective direct radiation; electrodermal response

EDS edema disease of swine; egg drop syndrome; Ehlers-Danlos syndrome; excessive daytime sleepiness

EDTA ethylenediamine tetraacetic acid

Educ education

EDV end-diastolic volume

EDVI end-diastolic volume index

EDWTH end-diastolic wall thickness

EDX, EDx electrodiagnosis

EDXA energy-dispersive x-ray analysis

EE embryo extract; end-to-end; *Enterobacteriaceae* enrichment [broth]; ethinyl estradiol; equine encephalitis; eye and ear

E-E erythema-edema [reaction]

EEA electroencephalic audiometry

EEC enteropathogenic *Escherichia coli*; ectrodactyly-ectodermal dysplasia-clefting [syndrome]

EECD endothelial-epithelial corneal dystrophy

EEE eastern equine encephalitis; eastern equine encephalomyelitis; experimental enterococcal endocarditis

EEEV eastern equine encephalomyelitis virus

EEG electroencephalogram, electroencephalography

EEGA electroencephalographic audiometry

EELS elecron energy loss spectroscopy

EEM ectodermal dysplasia, ectro-dactyly, macular dystrophy [syndrome]
EEME, EE3ME ethinylestradiol-3-methyl ether
EEMG evoked electromyogram
EENT eye, ear, nose, and throat
EEP end-expiratory pressure; equivalent effective photon
EEPI extraretinal eye position information
EER electroencephalographic response
EES erythromycin ethylsuccinate; ethyl ethanesulfate
EESG evoked electrospinogram
EF ectopic focus; edema factor; ejection fraction; elastic fibril; electric field; elongation factor; embryo fibroblasts; emergency facility; encephalitogenic factor; endurance factor; eosinophilic fasciitis; epithelial focus; equivalent focus; erythroblastosis fetalis; extrafine; extended field [radiotherapy]; extrinsic factor
EFA Epilepsy Foundation of America; essential fatty acid; extrafamily adoptee
EFAD essential fatty acid deficiency
EFC endogenous fecal calcium; ephemeral fever of cattle
EFDA expanded function dental assistant
EFE endocardial fibroelastosis
eff effect; efferent
effect effective
effer efferent
EFFU epithelial focus-forming unit
EFL effective focal length
EFM electronic fetal monitoring
EFP effective filtration pressure; endoneural fluid pressure
EFR effective filtration rate
EFV extracellular fluid volume
EFVC expiratory flow-volume curve
EFW estimated fetal weight
EG esophagogastrectomy
eg for example [Lat. *exempli gratia*]
EGA estimated gestational age
EGBUS external genitalia, Bartholin, urethral, Skene's glands
EGC epithelioid-globoid cell
EGD esophagogastroduodenoscopy
EGDF embryonic growth and development factor
EGF epidermal growth factor

EGG electrogastrogram
EGH equine growth hormone
EGL eosinophilic granuloma of the lung
EGM electrogram
EGOT erythrocytic glutamic oxaloacetic transaminase
E-GR erythrocyte glutathione reductase
EGRA equilibrium-gated radionuclide angiography
EGT ethanol gelation test
EGTA esophageal gastric tube airway; ethyleneglycol-bis-(ß-aminoethylether)-N,N,N',N'-tetraacetic acid
EH enlarged heart; epoxide hydratase; essential hypertension
E&H environment and heredity
E$_h$ redox potential
EHA Emotional Health Anonymous; Environmental Health Agency
EHAA epidemic hepatitis-associated antigen
EHB elevate head of bed
EHBA extrahepatic biliary atresia
EHBF estimated hepatic blood flow; exercise hyperemia blood flow; extrahepatic blood flow
EHC enterohepatic circulation; enterohepatic clearance; essential hypercholesterolemia; extended health care
EHD epizootic hemorrhagic disease
EHDP ethane-1-hydroxy-1,1-diphosphate
EHDV epizootic hemorrhagic disease virus
EHF epidemic hemorrhagic fever; exophthalmos-hyperthyroid factor; extreme high frequency
EHH esophageal hiatal hernia
EHL effective half-life; endogenous hyperlipidemia; Environmental Health Laboratory; extensor hallucis longus
EHME employee health maintenance examination
EHNA 9-erythro-2-(hydroxy-3-nonyl) adenine
EHO extrahepatic obstruction
EHP di-(20-ethylhexyl) hydrogen phosphate; Environmental Health Perspectives; excessive heat production; extrahigh potency
EHPAC Emergency Health Preparedness Advisory Committee

EHPT Eddy hot plate test
EHSDS experimental health services delivery system
EHV equine herpes virus
EI electrolyte imbalance; enzyme inhibitor; eosinophilic index
E/I expiration/inspiration [ratio]
EIA electroimmunoassay; enzyme immunoassay; equine infectious anemia; exercise-induced asthma; an interface between a computer and a system for transmitting digital information
EIAB extra-intracranial arterial bypass
EIB exercise-induced bronchospasm
EIC elastase inhibition capacity; enzyme inhibition complex
EID egg infectious dose; electro-immunodiffusion
EIEC enteroinvasive *Escherichia coli*
EIEE early infantile epileptic encephalopathy
EIF erythrocyte initiation factor; eukaryotic initiation factor
eIF erythrocyte initiation factor
EIMS electron ionization mass spectrometry
EIP extensor indicis proprius
EIPS endogenous inhibitor of prostaglandin synthase
EIRnv extra incidence rate of non-vaccinated groups
EIRP effective isotropic radiated power
EIRv extra incidence rate of vaccinated groups
EIS Environmental Impact Statement; Epidemic Intelligence Service
EIT erythroid iron turnover
EJ elbow jerk; external jugular
EJP excitation junction potential
ejusd of the same [Lat. *ejusdem*]
EK erythrokinase
EKC epidemic keratoconjunctivitis
EKG electrocardiogram, electrocardiography
EKY electrokymogram, electrokymography
EL early latent; erythroleukemia; exercise limit; external lamina
el elixir
ELA endotoxin-like activity
ELAS extended lymphadenopathy syndrome

ELB early light breakfast; elbow
ELD egg lethal dose
elec electricity, electric
elect electuary
elem elementary
elev elevation, elevated, elevator
ELH egg-laying hormone
ELIA enzyme-linked immunoassay
ELICT enzyme-linked immunocytochemical technique
ELIEDA enzyme-linked immunoelectron diffusion assay
ELISA enzyme-linked immunosorbent assay
elix elixir
ELM external limiting membrane; extravascular lung mass
ELOP estimated length of program
ELP endogenous limbic potential
ELS Eaton-Lambert syndrome; electron loss spectroscopy
ELSS emergency life support system
ELT euglobulin lysis time
ELV erythroid leukemia virus
EM ejection murmur; electron micrograph; electron microscopy, electron microscope; electrophoretic mobility; Embden-Meyerhof [pathway] emergency medicine; emotional disorder, emotionally disturbed; erythema multiforme; erythrocyte mass; erythromycin
E/M electron microscope, electron microscopy
E&M endocrine and metabolic
Em emmetropia
EMA electronic microanalyzer; emergency assistance, emergency assistant
EMAP evoked muscle action potential
EMB embryology; engineering in medicine and biology; eosin-methylene blue; ethambutol; explosive mental behavior
EMBASE Excerpta Medica Database
EMBL European Molecular Biology Laboratory
embryol embryology
EMC electron microscopy; emergency medical care; encephalomyocarditis; essential mixed cryoglobulinemia
EMC&R emergency medical care and rescue
EMCRO Experimental Medical Care Review Organization

EMCV encephalomyocarditis virus
EMD esophageal mobility disorder
EMEM Eagle's minimal essential medium
EMER electromagnetic molecular electron resonance
emer emergency
EMF electromagnetic flowmeter; electromotive force; Emergency Medicine Foundation; endomyocardial fibrosis; erythrocyte maturation factor; evaporated milk formula
emf electromotive force
EMG electromyogram, electromyography; eye movement gauge; exomphalos-macroglossia-gigantism [syndrome]
EMGN extramembranous glomerulonephritis
EMI electromagnetic interference; emergency medical information
EMIC emergency maternal and infant care
EMIT enzyme multiplication immunoassay technique
EMJH Ellinghausen-McCullough-Johnson-Harris [medium]
EMMA eye movement measuring apparatus
EMO Epstein-Macintosh-Oxford [inhaler]; exophthalmos, myxedema circumscriptum praetibiale, and osteoarthropathia hypertrophicans [syndrome]
emot emotion, emotional
EMP electric membrane property; Embden-Meyerhof pathway
emp as directed [Lat. *ex modo prescripto*]; plaster [Lat. *emplastrum*]
emp vesic blistering plaster [Lat. *emplastrum vesicatorium*]
EMR educable mentally retarded; electromagnetic radiation; emergency mechanical restraint; essential metabolism ratio
EMRA Emergency Medicine Residents Association
EMRC European Medical Research Council
EMS early morning specimen; Electronic Medical Service; Emergency Medical Service; endometriosis; ethyl methane-sulfonate
EMT emergency medical tag; emergency medical technician; emergency medical treatment

EMT-A emergency medical technician-ambulance
EMT-I emergency medical technician-intermediate
EMT-P emergency medical technician-paramedic
emu electromagnetic unit
emul emulsion
EMV eye, motor, voice [Glasgow coma scale]
EN enrolled nurse; erythema nodosum
En, en enema
ENA extractable nuclear antigen
END early neonatal death; endocrinology; endorphin
end endoreduplication
Endo endodontics; endotracheal
Endocrin endocrine, endocrinology
ENDOR electron nuclear double resonance
ENeG electroneurography
enem enema
ENG electronystagmogram, electronystagmography
Eng English
ENL erythema nodosum leproticum
Eno enolase
ENP ethyl-p-nitrophenylthiobenzene phosphate; extractable nucleoprotein
ENR eosinophilic nonallergic rhinitis; extrathyroid neck radioactivity
ENS enteral nutritional support
ENT ear, nose, and throat; extranodular tissue
Entom entomology
ENU N-ethyl-N-nitrosourea
env, environ environment, environmental
enz enzymatic
EO eosinophil; ethylene oxide; eyes open
E_0 skin dose
EOA esophageal obturator airway; examination, opinion, and advice
EOD entry on duty; every other day
EOF end of file
E of M error of measurement
EOG electro-oculogram, electro-oculography; electro-olfactogram, electro-olfactography
EOL end of life
EOM equal ocular movement; external otitis media; extraocular movement; extraocular muscle

EOMA emergency oxygen mask assembly
EOMI extraocular muscles intact
EOR exclusive OR
EOS eosinophil; European Orthodontic Society
eos, eosin eosinophil
EOT effective oxygen transport
EOU epidemic observation unit
EP ectopic pregnancy; edible portion; electrophoresis; electroprecipitin; emergency procedure; endogenous pyrogen; endorphin; end point; environmental protection; enzyme product; eosinophilic pneumonia; epicardial electrogram; epithelium, epithelial; epoxide; erythrocyte protoporphyrin; erythrophagocytosis; erythropoietic porphyria; erythropoietin; evoked potential; extreme pressure
EPA eicosapentaenoic acid; Environmental Protection Agency; erect posterior-anterior
EPAP expiratory positive airway pressure
EPA/RCRA Environmental Protection Agency Resource Conservation and Recovery Act
EPB extensor pollicis brevis
EPC end-plate current; epilepsia partialis continua; external pneumatic compression
EPDML epidemiology, epidemiologic
EPEC enteropathogenic *Escherichia coli*
EPEG etoposide
EPF early pregnancy factor; endocarditis parietalis fibroplastica; endothelial proliferating factor; exophthalmos-producing factor
EPG eggs per gram [count]; electropneumography, electropneumogram; ethanolamine phosphoglyceride
EPH edema-proteinuria-hypertension
EPI epinephrine; epithelium, epithelial; evoked potential index
epid epidemic
epil epilepsy, epileptic
epineph epinephrine
epis episiotomy
epith epithelium
EPL extensor pollicis longus
EPM electron probe microanalysis; electrophoretic mobility; energy-protein malnutrition
EPN O-ethyl O-p-nitrophenylphosphonothionate

EPO erythropoietin
EPP end-plate potential; equal pressure point; erythropoietic protoporphyria
EPPS Edwards Personal Preference Schedule
EPR electron paramagnetic resonance; electrophrenic respiration; emergency physical restraint; estradiol production rate
EPROM erasable programmable read-only memory
EPS elastosis perforans serpiginosa; electrophysiologic study; exophthalmos-producing substance; extrapyramidal symptom, extrapyramidal syndrome
ep's epithelial cells
EPSDT Early and Periodic Screening, Diagnosis and Treatment Program
EPSEM equal probability of selection method
ε Greek letter *epsilon*; heavy chain of IgE; permittivity; specific absorptivity
EPSP excitatory postsynaptic potential
EPT early pregnancy test
EPTE existed prior to enlistment
EPTFE expanded polytetrafluoroethylene
EPTS existed prior to service
EPXMA electron probe x-ray microanalyzer
EQ educational quotient; encephalization quotient; equal to
Eq, eq equation, equivalent
equip equipment
equiv equivalency, equivalent
ER ejection rate; emergency room; endoplasmic reticulum; enhanced reactivation; enhancement ratio; environmental resistance; equine rhinopneumonia; equivalent roentgen [unit]; estrogen receptor; evoked response; extended release; extended resistance; external resistance
ER⁻ decreased estrogen receptor
ER⁺ increased estrogen receptor
Er erbium; erythrocyte
er endoplasmic reticulum
ERA electrical response activity; electroencephalic response audiometry; Electroshock Research Association; estrogen receptor assay; evoked response audiometry
ERBF effective renal blood flow
ERC endoscopic retrograde cholangiography; enteric cytopathic human orphan-

rhino-coryza [virus]; erythropoietin-responsive cell

ERCP endoscopic retrograde cholangiopancreatography

ERD evoked response detector

ERDA Energy Research and Development Administration

ERF Education and Research Foundation; Eye Research Foundation

E-RFC e-rosette forming cell

ERG electron radiography; electroretinography, electroretinogram

ERIA electroradioimmunoassay

ERM electrochemical relaxation method

ERP early receptor potential; effective refractory period; elodoisin-related peptide; endoscopic retrograde pancreatography; equine rhinopneumonitis; estrogen receptor protein; event-related potential

ERPF effective renal plasma flow

ERSP event-related slow potential

ERT estrogen replacement therapy

ERV equine rhinopneumonitis virus; expiratory reserve volume

ERY erysipelas

Ery *Erysipelothrix*

ES ejection sound; electrical stimulus, electrical stimulation; electroshock; emergency service; emission spectrometry; endometritis-salpingitis; endoscopic sphincterotomy; end-to-side; enzyme substrate; epileptic syndrome; esterase; exfoliation syndrome; Expectation Score; exterior surface

Es einsteinium

es soap enema [Lat.*enema saponis*]

ESA Electrolysis Society of America

ESB electrical stimulation of the brain

ESC electromechanical slope computer; erythropoietin-sensitive stem cell

ESCA electron spectroscopy for chemical analysis

Esch *Escherichia*

ESCN electrolyte and steroid cardiopathy with necrosis

ESD electronic summation device; esterase-D

ESE electrostatic unit [Ger. *electrostatische Einheit*]

ESF erythropoietic stimulating factor

ESFL end-systolic force-length relationship

ESL end-systolic length

ESM ejection systolic murmur; ethosuximide

ESMIS Emergency Medical Services Management Infomation System

ESN educationally subnormal; estrogen-stimulated neurophysin

ESN(M) educationally subnormal–moderate

ESN(S) educationally subnormal–severe

eso esophagoscopy; esophagus

ESP effective systolic pressure; endometritis-salpingitis-peritonitis; end-systolic pressure; eosinophil stimulation promoter; especially; evoked synaptic potential; extrasensory perception

ESPA electrical stimulation produced analgesia

ESR Einstein stoke radius; electron spin resonance; erythrocyte sedimentation rate

ESRD end-stage renal disease

ESS empty sella syndrome; endostreptosin; erythrocyte-sensitizing substance; euthyroid sick syndrome

ess essential

EST electric shock theshold; electroshock therapy; esterase

est ester; estimation, estimated

esth esthetics, esthetic

ESU electrosurgical unit; electrostatic unit

E-sub excitor substance

ESV end-systolic volume; esophageal valve

ESVI end-systolic volume index

ESWL extracorporeal shock-wave lithotripsy

ET educational therapy; effective temperature; ejection time; endotoxin; endotracheal; endotracheal tube; essential thrombocythemia; essential tremor; ethanol; etiocholanolone test; etiology; eustachian tube; exchange transfusion; exercise test

ET$_3$ erythrocyte triiodothyronine

ET$_4$ effective thyroxine [test]

Et ethyl

et and

ETA electron transfer agent; ethionamide

η Greek letter *eta*; absolute viscosity

ETC estimated time of conception

ET$_c$ corrected ejection time
ETEC enterotoxin of *Escherichia coli*, enterotoxic *Escherichia coli*
ETF electron-transferring flavoprotein; eustachian tube function
ETH elixir terpin hydrate; ethanol
eth ether
ETHC elixir terpin hydrate with codeine
ETIO etiocholandone
etiol etiology
ETK erythrocyte transketolase
ETKM every test known to man
ETM erythromycin
ETO estimated time of ovulation
ETOH, EtOH alcohol, alcoholic
ETOX ethylene oxide
ETP electron transport particle; entire treatment period; eustachian tube pressure
ETR effective thyroxine ratio
ETT exercise tolerance test; extra-pyramidal thyroxine
ETU emergency and trauma unit; emergency treatment unit
ETV extravascular thermal volume
EU Ehrlich unit; entropy unit; enzyme unit
Eu europium; euryon
EUA examination under anesthesia
EUL expected upper limit
EURONET European On-Line Network
EUROTOX European Committee on Chronic Toxicity Hazards
EUS external urethral sphincter
EUV extreme ultraviolet laser
EV emergency vehicle; enterovirus; epidermodysplasia verruciformis; estradiol valerate; evoked potential [response]; expected value; extravascular
eV, ev electron volt
ev eversion
EVA ethyl violet azide; ethylene vinyl acetate
evac evacuation, evacuated, evacuate
eval evaluation, evaluate, evaluated
evap evaporation, evaporated
EVCI expected value of clinical information
ever eversion, everted
EVLW extravascular lung water
EVM electronic voltmeter
EVP evoked visual potential
EVR evoked response

EW emergency ward
EWB estrogen withdrawal bleeding
EWL egg-white lysozyme; evaporation water loss
E(X) expected value of the random variable X
ex examination, examined; example; excision; exercise; exophthalmos
EXAFS extended x-ray absorption fine structure
exam examination, examined, examine
EXBF exercise hyperemia blood flow
exc excision
ExEF ejection fraction during exercise
EXELFS extended electron-loss line fine structure
exer exercise
exhib let it be given [Lat. *exhibeatur*]
exp experiment, experimental; exponential function; exposure
exp lap exploratory laparotomy
expect expectorant
exper experiment, experimental
ExPGN extracapillary proliferative glomerulonephritis
expir expiration, expiratory, expired
exptl experimental
Ext extraction, extract
ext extension; extensor; exterior; external; extract; extremity
ext rot external rotation
EXU excretory urogram
EY egg yolk
EYA egg yolk agar
Ez eczema

–F–

F bioavailability; a cell that donates F factor in bacterial conjugation; a conjugative plasmid in F^+ bacterial cells; degree of fineness of abrasive particles; facies; factor; Fahrenheit; family; farad; Faraday constant; fasting; fat; father; feces; fellow; female; fertility; fetal; fiat; fibroblast; fibrous; field of vision; filament; *Filaria*; fine; finger; flow; fluorine; focus; foil; foramen; force; form, forma; formula; fraction, fractional; fracture; free; French [catheter]; frontal; frontal electrode placement in electroencephalography; function; *Fusiformis*; gilbert; Helmholz free energy; hydrocortisone [compound F]; inbreeding coefficient; phenylalanine; variance ratio

F_1 first filial generation

F_2 second filial generation

F344 Fischer 344 [rat]

°**F** degree on the Fahrenheit scale

F' a hybrid F plasmid

F^- a bacterial cell lacking an F plasmid

F^+ a bacterial cell having an F plasmid

f atomic orbital with angular momentum quantum number 3; farad; femto; fluid; focal; form, forma; fostered [experimental animal]; frequency; make [Lat. *fiat*]; numerical expression of the relative aperture of a camera lens

FA Families Anonymous; Fanconi's anemia; far advanced; fatty acid; febrile antigen; femoral artery; fibroadenoma; fibrosing alveolitis; field ambulance; filterable agent; first aid; fluorescent antibody; fluorescent assay; folic acid; follicular area; forearm; fortified aqueous [solution]; free acid; Freund's adjuvant; Friedreich's ataxia

fa fatty [rat]

FAA formaldehyde, acetic acid, alcohol

FAB formalin ammonium bromide; fragment, antigen-binding [of immunoglobulins]; French-American-British Co-Operative Group [classification]; functional arm brace

Fab fragment, antigen-binding [of immunoglobulins]

$F(ab')_2$ fragment, antigen-binding [of immunoglobulins]

Fabc fragment, antigen and complement binding [of immunoglobulins]

FABP fatty acid-binding protein; folate-binding protein

FAC femoral arterial cannulation; ferric ammonium citrate; 5-fluorouracil, Adriamycin, and cyclophosphamide; free available chlorine

Fac factor

FACA Fellow of the American College of Anesthetists; Fellow of the American College of Angiology; Fellow of the American College of Apothecaries

FACAI Fellow of the American College of Allergists

Facb fragment, antigen, and complement binding

FACC Fellow of the American College of Cardiologists

FACCP Fellow of the American College of Chest Physicians

FACD Fellow of the American College of Dentists

FACEP Fellow of the American College of Family Physicians

FACES unique facies, anorexia, cachexia, and eye and skin lesions [syndrome]

FACFS Fellow of the American College of Foot Surgeons

FACG Fellow of the American College of Gastroenterology

FACH forceps to after-coming head

FACHA Fellow of the American College of Health Administrators

FACMTA Federal Advisory Council on Medical Training Aids

FACNHA Foundation of American College of Nursing Home Administrators

FACO Fellow of the American College of Otolaryngology

FACOG Fellow of the American College of Obstetricians and Gynecologists

FACOSH Federal Advisory Committee on Occupational Safety and Health

FACP Fellow of the American College of Physicians

FACPM Fellow of the American College of Preventive Medicine

FACS Fellow of the American College of Surgeons; fluorescence-activated cell sorter

FACSM Fellow of the American College of Sports Medicine

FACT Flannagan Aptitude Classification Test

FAD familial Alzheimer dementia; familial autonomic dysfunction; fetal activity-acceleration determination; flavin adenine dinucleotide

FADF fluorescent antibody dark-field

$FADH_2$ reduced form of flavin adenine dinucleotide

FADN flavin adenine dinucleotide
FAE fetal alcohol effect
FAF fatty acid free
FAH Federation of American Hospitals
Fahr Fahrenheit
FAI first aid instruction; functional aerobic impairment
FALG fowl antimouse lymphocyte globulin
FAM 5-fluorouracil, Adriamycin, and mitomycin C
Fam, fam family, familial
FAMA Fellow of the American Medical Association; fluorescent antibody to membrane antigen
FAME fatty acid methyl ester
FAMMM familial atypical multiple mole-melanoma [syndrome]
FAN fuchsin, amido black, and naphthol yellow
FANA fluorescent antinuclear antibody
F and R force and rhythm [of pulse]
FANPT Freeman Anxiety Neurosis and Psychosomatic Test
FANY first aid nursing yeomanry
FAP fibrillating action potential; frozen animal procedure
FAPA Fellow of the American Psychiatric Association; Fellow of the American Psychoanalytical Association
FAPHA Fellow of the American Public Health Association
far faradic
FARE Federation of Alcoholic Rehabilitation Establishments
FAS fatty acid synthetase; Federation of American Scientists; fetal alcohol syndrome
FASC free-standing ambulatory surgical center
fasc fasciculus, fascicular
FASEB Federation of American Societies for Experimental Biology
FAST fluorescent antibody staining technique; fluoro-allergo sorbent test
FAT family attitudes test; fluorescent antibody technique; fluoroescent antibody test
FAV feline ataxia virus; floppy aortic valve; fowl adenovirus
FB fasting blood sugar; feedback; fiberoptic bronchoscopy; finger breadth; foreign body; *Fusobacterium*

FBCOD foreign body of the cornea, oculus dexter (right eye)
FBCOS foreign body of the cornea, oculus sinister (left eye)
FBCP familial benign chronic pemphigus
FBE full blood examination
FBEC fetal bovine endothelial cell
FBF forearm blood flow
FBG fasting blood glucose
FBG, fbg fibrinogen
FBH familial benign hypocalciuric hypercalcemia
FBI flossing, brushing, and irrigation
FBL follicular basal lamina
FBM fetal breathing movements
FBN Federal Bureau of Narcotics
FBP femoral blood pressure; fibrinogen breakdown product
FBPsS Fellow of the British Psychological Society
FBS fasting blood sugar; feedback system; fetal bovine serum
FBSS failed back surgery syndrome
FC fasciculus cuneatus; fast component [of a neuron]; febrile convulsions; feline conjunctivitis; ferric citrate; fibrocyte; finger clubbing; finger counting; Foley catheter; frontal cortex
5-FC 5-fluorocytosine
Fc centroid frequency; fragment, crystallizable [of immunoglobulin]
Fc' a fragment of an immunoglobulin molecule produced by papain digestion
fc foot candles
F + C flare + cells
FCA ferritin-conjugated antibodies; Freund's complete adjuvant
FCAP Fellow of the College of American Pathologists
F cath Foley catheter
FCC follicular center cells
fcc face-centered-cubic
FCD feces collection device; fibrocystic disease; fibrocystic dysplasia
FCHL familial combined hyperlipidemia
FChS Fellow of the Society of Chiropodists
FCL fibroblast cell line
fcly face lying
FCM flow cytometry
FCMC family centered maternity care

FCMD Fukuyama type congenital muscular dystrophy
FCMS Fellow of the College of Medicine and Surgery
FCMW Foundation for Child Mental Welfare
FCO Fellow of the College of Osteopathy
FCP final common pathway
FCPS Fellow of the College of Physicians and Surgeons
FCR flexor carpi radialis; fractional catabolic rate
FcR Fc receptor
FCRA fecal collection receptacle assembly; Fellow of the College of Radiologists of Australasia
FCRC Frederick Cancer Research Center
FCS fecal containment system; feedback control system; fetal calf serum
FCSP Fellow of the Chartered Society of Physiotherapy
FCST Fellow of the College of Speech Therapists
FCU flexor carpi ulnaris
FD familial dysautonomia; fan douche; fatal dose; fetal danger; focal distance; Folin-Denis [assay]; follicular diameter; foot drape; forceps delivery; freeze drying
Fd the animo-terminal portion of the heavy chain of an immunoglobulin molecule
FD$_{50}$ median fatal dose
FDA Food and Drug Administration; right frontoanterior [position of the fetus]
FD&C Food, Drug and Cosmetic Act; food, drugs, and cosmetics
FDCPA Food, Drug, and Consumer Product Agency
FDD Food and Drugs Directorate
FDDC ferric dimethyldithiocarbonate
FDE female day-equivalent; final drug evaluation
FDF fast death factor
FDG fluorodeoxyglucose
fdg feeding
FDGF fibroblast-derived growth factor
FDH familial dysalbuminemic hyperthyroxinemia; focal dermal hypoplasia
FDI International Dental Federation [Fédération Dentaire Internationale]

FDIU fetal death in utero
FDLV fer de lance virus
FDN eosinophil-derived neurotoxin
FDNB 1-fluoro-2,4-dinitrobenzene
FDO Fleet Dental Officer
FDP fibrin degradation product; fibrinogen degradation product; flexor digitorum profundus; fructose-1,6-diphosphate
FDPase fructose-1,6-diphosphatase
FDS Fellow in Dental Surgery; flexor digitorum superficialis
FDSRCSEng Fellow in Dental Surgery of the Royal College of Surgeons of England
FDV Friend disease virus
FDZ fetal danger zone
FE fatty ester; fetal erythroblastosis; fetal erythrocyte; fluid extract
Fe female; ferret; iron [Lat. *ferrum*]
fe female
feb fever [Lat. *febris*]
feb dur while the fever lasts [Lat. *febre durante*]
FEBP fetal estrogen-binding protein
FEBS Federation of European Biochemical Societies
FEC forced expiratory capacity; free erythrocyte coproporphyrin; Friend erythroleukemia cell
FECG fetal electrocardiogram
F$_{ECO2}$ fractional concentration of carbon dioxide in expired gas
FECP free erythrocyte coproporphyrin
FECT fibroelastic connective tissue
FECVC functional extracellular fluid volume
FeD iron deficiency
Fed federal
FEE forced equilibrating expiration
FEF forced expiratory flow
FEF$_{50}$ forced expiratory flow at 50%
FEF$_{50}$/FIF$_{50}$ ratio of expiratory flow to inspiratory flow at 50% of forced vital capacity
FEGO International Federation of Gynecology and Obstetrics
FEHBP Federal Employee Health Benefits Program
FEKG fetal electrocardiogram
FeLV feline leukemia virus
fem female; femur, femoral

fem intern at inner side of the thighs [Lat. *femoribus internus*]

FENa, FE$_{Na}$ fractional excretion of sodium

F$_{EO2}$ fractional concentration of oxygen in expired gas

FEP fluorinated ethylene-propylene; free erythrocyte protoporphyrin

FEPP free erythrocyte protoporphyrin

FEPB functional electronic peroneal brace

fert fertility, fertilized

ferv boiling [Lat. *fervens*]

FES fat embolism syndrome; flame emission spectroscopy; forced expiratory spirogram

FeSV feline sarcoma virus

FET field-effect transistor; forced expiratory time

FETs forced expiratory time in seconds

FETE Far Eastern tick-borne encephalitis

FEUO for external use only

FEV familial exudative vitreoretinopathy; forced expiratory volume

fev fever

FEV1, FEV$_1$ forced expiratory volume in one second

FEVB frequency ectopic ventricular beat

FF degree of fineness of abrasive particles; fat-free; father factor; fecal frequency; fertility factor; filtration fraction; finger-to-finger; fixation fluid; flat feet; flip-flop; fluorescent focus; force fluids; forearm flow; foster father; fresh frozen; fundus firm

FFA Fellow of the Faculty of Anaesthetists; free fatty acid

FFAP free fatty acid phase

FFARCS Fellow of the Faculty of Anaesthetists of the Royal College of Surgeons

FFC free from chlorine

FFCM Fellow of the Faculty of Community Medicine

FFD Fellow in the Faculty of Dentistry; focus-film distance

FFDCA Federal Food, Drug, and Cosmetic Act

FFDSRCS Fellow of the Faculty of Dental Surgery Royal College of Surgeons

FFDW fat-free dry weight

FFF degree of fineness of abrasive particles; field-flow fractionation; flicker fusion frequency

FFG free fat graft

FFHom Fellow of the Faculty of Homeopathy

FFI free from infection; fundamental frequency indicator

FFIT fluorescent focus inhibition test

FFM fat-free mass

FFOM Fellow of the Faculty of Occupational Medicine

FFP fresh frozen plasma

FFR Fellow of the Faculty of Radiologists

FFS fat-free solids

FFT flicker fusion threshold

FFU focal forming unit

FFW fat-free weight

FFWW fat-free wet weight

FG fast-glycolytic [fiber]; Feeley-Gorman [agar]; fibrinogen; Flemish giant [rabbit]

FGD fatal granulomatous disease

FGDS fibrogastroduodenoscopy

FGF father's grandfather; fibroblast growth factor; fresh gas flow

FGG focal global glomerulosclerosis; fowl gamma-globulin

FGM father's grandmother

FGN fibrinogen; focal glomerulo-nephritis

FGS fibrogastroscopy; focal glomer-ular sclerosis

FGT fluorescent gonorrhea test

FH familial hypercholesterolemia; family history; fasting hyperbilirubinemia; femoral hypoplasia; fetal head; fetal heart; fibromuscular hyperplasia; Frankfort horizontal [plane]

FH$_4$ tetrahydrofolic acid

fh fostered by hand [experimental animal]; let a draught be made [Lat. *fiat haustus*]

FHA familial hypoplastic anemia; Fellow of the Institute of Hospital Administrators

FHC Ficoll-Hypaque centrifugation; Fuchs' heterochromic cyclitis

FHF fulminant hepatic failure

FHH familial hypocalciuric hypercalce-mia; fetal heart heard

FHIP family health insurance plan

FHM fathead minnow [cells]

FHNH fetal heart not heard

FHR familial hypophosphatemic rickets; fetal heart rate

FHS fetal heart sound; fetal hydantoin syndrome

FHT fetal heart; fetal heart tone

FHTG familial hypertriglyceridemia

FH-UFS femoral hypoplasia–unusual facies syndrome

FHV falcon herpesvirus

FI fever caused by infection; fibrinogen; fixed interval; flame ionization; forced inspiration

FIA fluorescent immunoassay; Freund's incomplete adjuvant

FIB Fellow of the Institute of Biology; fibrin; fibrinogen; fibrositis; fibula

fib, fibrill fibrillation

FIC Fogarty International Center

FICA Federal Insurance Contributions Act

FICD Fellow of the Institute of Canadian Dentists; Fellow of the International College of Dentists

F_{ICO_2} fractional concentration of carbon dioxide in inspired gas

FICS Fellow of the International College of Surgeons

FID flame ionization detector; free induction decay

FIF feedback inhibition factor; fibroblast interferon; forced inspiratory flow; formaldehyde-induced fluorescence

FIFO first in, first out

FIGD familial idiopathic gonadotropin deficiency

FIGLU formiminoglutamic acid

FIH fat-induced hyperglycemia

fil filament

filt filter, filtration

FIM field ion microscopy

FIMLT Fellow of the Institute of Medical Laboratory Technology

FIN fine intestinal needle

FI_{O_2} forced inspiratory oxygen; fraction of inspired oxygen

FiO_2 fraction of inspired oxygen

FIP feline infectious peritonitis

FIR far infrared; fold increase in resistance

FIRDA frontal, intermittent delta activity

fist fistula

FIT fusion inferred threshold

FITC fluorescein isothiocyanate

FIUO for internal use only

FJN familial juvenile nephrophthisis

FJRM full joint range of movement

FK feline kidney

FL fatty liver; feline leukemia; filtration leukapheresis; focal length; Friend leukemia; frontal lobe

FL-2 feline lung [cells]

Fl fluid; fluorescence

fl femtoliter; flexion, flexible; fluid

FLA left frontoanterior [position of the fetus] [Lat. *fronto-laeva anterior*]

Fla let it be done according to rule [Lat. *fiat lege artis*]

flac flaccidity, flaccid

flav yellow [Lat. *flavus*]

fld fluid

fl dr fluid dram

FLEX Federation Licensing Examination

flex flexor, flexion

FLK funny looking kid

FLKS fatty liver and kidney syndrome

FLM fasciculus longitudinalis medialis

floc flocculation

fl oz fluid ounce

FLP left frontoposterior [position of the fetus] [Lat. *fronto-laeva posterior*]

FLS fatty liver syndrome; Fellow of the Linnean Society; fibrous long-spacing [collagen]

FLSP fluorescein-labeled serum protein

FLT left frontotransverse [position of the fetus] [Lat. *fronto-laeva transversa*]

fluor fluorescence; fluorescent; fluorometry; fluoroscopy

FLV feline leukemia virus; Friend leukemia virus

FM facilities management; feedback mechanism; fibromuscular; flavin mononucleotide; flowmeter; foramen magnum; forensic medicine; foster mother; frequency modulation; make a mixture [Lat. *fiat mistura*]

Fm fermium

fm femtometer

FMA Frankfort-mandibular plane angle

FMC family medicine center; flight medicine clinic; focal macular choroidopathy

FMD family medical doctor; fibromuscular dysplasia; foot and mouth disease

FMDV foot and mouth disease virus

FME full mouth extraction

F-met, fMet formyl methionine

FMF familial Mediterranean fever; fetal movement felt; flow microfluorometry

FMG foreign medical graduate

FMGEMS Foreign Medical Graduate Examination in Medical Sciences

FMH fat-mobilizing hormone; fibromuscular hyperplasia

FML flail mitral leaflet; fluorometholone

FMLP, f-MLP N-formyl-methionyl-leucyl-phenylalanine

FMN flavin mononucleotide; frontomaxillo-nasal [suture]

FMNH, FMNH$_2$ reduced form of flavin mononucleotide

FMO Fleet Medical Officer; Flight Medical Officer

fmol femtomole

FMP first menstrual period

FMR Friend-Moloney-Rauscher [antigen]

FMS fat-mobilizing substance; Fellow of the Medical Society; full mouth series

FMU first morning urine

FMX full mouth x-ray

FN false negative; fluoride number

F-N finger to nose

FNA fine needle aspiration

FNAB fine needle aspiration biopsy

FNC fatty nutritional cirrhosis

FNCJ fine needle catheter jejunostomy

FND febrile neutrophilic dermatosis; frontonasal dysplasia

Fneg false negative

FNP family nurse practitioner

FNS functional neuromuscular stimulation

FNT false neurochemical transmitter

FO foramen ovale; fronto-occipital

Fo fomentation, fomenting

FOA Federation of Orthodontic Associations

FOAVF failure of all vital forces

FOB fecal occult blood; feet out of bed; fiberoptic bronchoscopy; foot of bed

FOCAL formula calculation

FOD free of disease

FOG fast oxidative glycolytic [fiber]

fol leaf [Lat. *folium*]

FOMi 5-fluorouracil, vincristine, and mitomycin C

FOOB fell out of bed

FOP fibrodysplasia ossificans progressiva

FOPR full outpatient rate

For forensic

for foreign; formula

form formula

fort strong [Lat. *fortis*]

FORTRAN formula translation

FP false positive; family planning; family practice; family practitioner; fibrinopeptide; filter paper; fixation protein; flavin phosphate; flavoprotein; fluorescence polarization; food poisoning; freezing point; frontoparietal; frozen plasma

F-6-P fructose-6-phosphate

Fp frontal polar electrode placement in electroencephalography

fp foot-pound; forearm pronated; freezing point; let a potion be made [Lat. *fiat potio*]

FPA Family Planning Association; fibrinopeptide A; filter paper activity; fluorophenylalanine

FPB femoral popliteal bypass; fibrinopeptide B

FPC familial polyposis coli; family planning clinic; fish protein concentrate

FpCA 1-fluoromethyl-2-p-chlorophenylethylamine

FPD feto-pelvic disproportion; flame photometric detector

FPG fasting plasma glucose; fluorescence plus Giemsa; focal proliferative glomerulonephritis

FPH$_2$ reduced form of flavin phosphate

FPHE formaldehyde-treated pyruvaldehyde-stabilized human erythrocytes

FPI formula protein intolerance

f pil let pills be made [Lat. *fiat pilulae*]

FPM filter paper microscopic [test]

fpm feet per minute

FPN ferric chloride, perchloric acid, and nitric acid [solution]

FPO Federation of Prosthodontic Organizations; freezing point osmometer

FPR fluorescence photobleaching recovery; fractional proximal resorption

FPRA first pass radionuclide angiogram

FPS Fellow of the Pathological Society; Fellow of the Pharmaceutical Society; fetal PCB (q.v.) syndrome

fps feet per second; frames per second

FPV fowl plague virus

FPVB femoral popliteal vein bypass

FR failure rate; feedback regulation; Fischer-Race [notation]; fixed ratio; flocculation reaction; flow rate; free radical; frequent relapses

F&R force and rhythm

Fr fracture; francium; French

FRA fibrinogen-related antigen; fluorescent rabies antibody

frac fracture

FRACDS Fellow of the Royal Australasian College of Dental Surgery

FRACGP Fellow of the Royal Australasian College of General Practitioners

FRACO Fellow of the Royal Australasian College of Ophthalmologists

FRACP Fellow of the Royal Australasian College of Physicians

FRACR Fellow of the Royal Australasian College of Radiologists

fract fracture

fract dos in divided doses [Lat. *fracta dosi*]

FRAI Fellow of the Royal Anthropological Institute

FRANZCP Fellow of the Royal Australian and New Zealand College of Psychiatrists

FRAP fluorescence recovery after photo-bleaching

FRAT free radical assay technique

fra(X) fragile X chromosome, fragile X syndrome

Fr BB fracture of both bones

FRC Federal Radiation Council; frozen red cells; functional reserve capacity; functional residual capacity

FRCD Fellow of the Royal College of Dentists

FRCGP Fellow of the Royal College of General Practitioners

FRCOG Fellow of the Royal College of Obstetricians and Gynaecologists

FRCP Fellow of the Royal College of Physicians

FRCPA Fellow of the Royal College of Pathologists of Australia

FRCPath Fellow of the Royal College of Pathologists

FRCP(C) Fellow of the Royal College of Physicians of Canada

FRCPE Fellow of the Royal College of Physicians of Edinburgh

FRCPI Fellow of the Royal College of Physicians of Ireland

FRCPsych Fellow of the Royal College of Psychiatrists

FRCS Fellow of the Royal College of Surgeons

FRCS(C) Fellow of the Royal College of Surgeons of Canada

FRCSEd Fellow of the Royal College of Surgeons of Edinburgh

FRCSEng Fellow of the Royal College of Surgeons of England

FRCSI Fellow of the Royal College of Surgeons of Ireland

FRCVS Fellow of the Royal College of Veterinary Surgeons

FRE Fischer rat embryo

FREIR Federal Research on Biological and Health Effects of Ionizing Radiation

frem fremitus

freq frequency

FRES Fellow of the Royal Entomological Society

FRF Fertility Research Foundation; follicle-stimulating hormone-releasing factor

FRH follicle-stimulating hormone-releasing hormone

FRh fetal rhesus monkey kidney [cell]

FRHS fast-repeating high sequence

frict friction

frig cold [Lat. *frigidus*]

FRIPHH Fellow of the Royal Institute of Public Health and Hygiene

FRJM full range joint movement

FRMedSoc Fellow of the Royal Medical Society

FRMS Fellow of the Royal Microscopical Society

FROM full range of movements

FRP functional refractory period

FRS Fellow of the Royal Society; ferredoxin-reducing substance; first rank symptom; furosemide

FRSH Fellow of the Royal Society of Health

FRT Family Relations Test; full recovery time

Fru fructose

frust in small pieces [Lat. *frustillatim*]

Frx fracture

FS factor of safety; Fanconi syndrome; Felty syndrome; Fisher syndrome; food service; forearm supination; fragile site; Friesinger score; frozen section; full scale [IQ]; full soft [diet]; function study; human foreskin cells; simple fracture

F/S female, spayed [animal]

fsa let it be made skillfully [Lat. *fiat secundum artem*]

fsar let it be made according to the rules [Lat. *fiat secundum artem reglas*]

FSBT Fowler single breath test

FSC Food Standards Committee

FSD focus-skin distance

FSF fibrin stabilizing factor

FSG fasting serum glucose; focal segmental sclerosis

FSGHS focal segmental glomerular hyalinosis and sclerosis

FSGN focal sclerosing glomerulonephritis

FSGS focal segmental glomerulosclerosis

FSH fascioscapulohumeral; focal and segmental hyalinosis; follicle-stimulating hormone

FSH/LR-RH follicle-stimulating hormone and luteinizing hormone releasing hormone

FSH-RF follicle-stimulating hormone-releasing factor

FSH-RH follicle-stimulating hormone-releasing hormone

FSI foam stability index; Food Sanitation Institute

FSMB Federation of State Medical Boards

FSP familial spastic paraplegia; fibrin split products; fibrinogen split products

F-SP special form [Lat. *forma specialis*]

FSR Fellow of the Society of Radiographers; fragmented sarcoplasmic reticulum; fusiform skin revision

FSS focal segmental sclerosis; Freeman-Sheldon syndrome; French steel sound

FST foam stability test

FSU family service unit

FSV feline fibrosarcoma virus

FSW field service worker

FT false transmitter; family therapy; fast twitch; fibrous tissue; free thyroxine; full term; function test

FT$_3$ free triiodothyronine

FT$_4$ free thyroxine

ft foot, feet; let there be made [Lat. *fiat or fiant*]

FTA fluorescent titer antibody; fluorescent treponemal antibody

FTA-ABS, FTA-Abs fluorescent treponemal antibody, absorbed [test]

FTAT fluorescent treponemal antibody test

FTBD fit to be detained; full term born dead

FTBE focal tick-borne encephalitis

FTBS Family Therapist Behavioral Scale

FTC Federal Trade Commission

ftc foot candle

ft cataplasm let a poultice be made [Lat. *fiat cataplasma*]

ft cerat let a cerate be made [Lat. *fiat ceratum*]

ft collyr let an eyewash be made [Lat. *fiat collyrium*]

FTD femoral total density

ft emuls let an emulsion be made [Lat. *fiat emulsio*]

ft enem let an enema be made [Lat. *fiat enema*]

ft garg let a gargle be made [Lat. *fiat gargarisma*]

FTI free thyroxine index

FT$_3$I free triiodothyronine index

ft infus let an injection be made [Lat. *fiat infusum*]

FTIR functional terminal innervation ratio

ftL foot lambert

FTLB full-term live birth

ft lb foot pound

ft linim let a liniment be made [Lat. *fiat linimentum*]

FTM fluid thioglycolate medium; fractional test meal

ft mas let a mass be made [Lat. *fiat massa*]

ft mas div in pil let a mass be made and divided into pills [Lat. *fiat massa dividenda in pilulae*]

ft mist let a mixture be made [Lat. *fiat mistura*]

FTN finger to nose

FTND full-term normal delivery

FTO fructose-terminated oligosaccharide

ft pil let pills be made [Lat. *fiat pilulae*]

ft pulv let a powder be made [Lat. *fiat pulvis*]

FTS feminizing testis syndrome; flexor-tenosynovitis; thymulin [Fr. *facteur thymique sérique*]

FTSG full thickness skin graft

ft solut let a solution be made [Lat. *fiat solutio*]

ft suppos let a suppository be made [Lat. *fiat suppositorium*]

FTT failure to thrive

FTU fluorescence thiourea

ft ung let an ointment be made [Lat. *fiat unguentum*]

FU fecal urobilinogen; fetal urobilinogen; fluorouracil; follow-up; fractional urinalysis

F/U follow-up, fundus of umbilicus

F&U flanks and upper quadrants

5-FU 5-fluorouracil

Fu Finsen unit

FUB functional uterine bleeding

Fuc fucose

FUDR, FUdR 2-fluoro-2'-deoxyuridine

FUFA free volatile fatty acid

FUM 5-fluorouracil and methotrexate; fumarate; fumigation

FUN follow-up note

funct function, functional

FUO fever of unknown origin

FUR fluorouracil riboside

FUS feline urologic syndrome

FUT fibrinogen uptake test

FV fluid volume; Friend virus

FVA Friend virus anemia

FVC forced vital capacity

FVIC forced inspiratory vital capacity

FVL femoral vein ligation; flow volume loop

FVP Friend virus polycythemia

FVR feline viral rhinotracheitis; forearm vascular resistance

FW Felix-Weil [reaction]; Folin-Wu [reaction]; fragment wound

Fw F wave

fw fresh water

FWA Family Welfare Association

FWB full weight bearing

FWHM full width at half maximum

FWPCA Federal Water Pollution Control Administration

FWR Felix-Weil reaction; Folin-Wu reaction

Fx fracture

Fx-dis fracture-dislocation

FXN function

FY fiscal year

FYI for your information

FZ focal zone; furazolidone

Fz frontal midline placement of electrodes in electroencephalography

FZS Fellow of the Zoological Society

–G–

G acceleration [force];conductance; free energy; gallop; gap; gas; gastrin; gauge; gauss; geometric efficiency; giga; gingiva, gingival; glabella; globular; globulin; glucose; glycine; glycogen; goat; gold inlay; gonidial; good; goose; grade; Grafenberg spot; gram; gravida; gravitation constant; Greek; green; guanidine; guanine; guanosine; gynecology; unit of force of acceleration

G_1 presynthetic gap [phase of cells prior to DNA synthesis]

G_2 postsynthetic gap [phase of cells following DNA synthesis]

GI primigravida

GII secundigravida

GIII tertigravida

G° standard free energy

g force [pull of gravity]; gender; gram; gravity; group; ratio of magnetic moment of a particle to the Bohr magneton; standard acceleration due to gravity, 9.80665 m/s^2

g relative centrifugal force

γ see *gamma*

GA Gamblers Anonymous; gastric analysis; general anesthesia; general appearance; gentisic acid; gestational age; gingivoaxial; glucoamylase; glucose; glucose/acetone; glucuronic acid; Golgi apparatus; gramicidin A; granulocyte adherence; guessed average; gut-associated

Ga gallium; granulocyte agglutination

ga gauge

GAA gossypol acetic acid

GABA, gaba gamma-aminobutyric acid

GABA-T gamma-aminobutyric acid transaminase

GABOB gamma-amino-beta-hydroxybutyric acid

GAD glutamic acid decarboxylase

GADH gastric alcohol dehydrogenase

GAG glycosaminoglycan

GAIPAS General Audit Inpatient Psychiatric Assessment Scale

GAL galactosyl; glucuronic acid lactone

Gal galactose

gal galactose; gallon

GalN galactosamine

GALT galactose-1-p-uridyltransferase; gut-associated lymphoid tissue

GALV gibbon ape leukemia virus

Galv, galv galvanic

γ Greek letter *gamma*; a carbon separated from the carboxyl group by two other carbon atoms; a constituent of the gamma protein plasma fraction; heavy chain of immunogammaglobulin; a monomer in fetal hemoglobin; photon

γG immunoglobulin G

G and D growth and development

gang, gangl ganglion, ganglionic

GAP D-glyceraldehyde-3-phosphate

GAPD, GAPDH glyceraldehyde-phosphate dehydrogenase

GAPO growth retardation, alopecia, pseudo-anodontia, and optic atrophy [syndrome]

Garg, garg gargle

GAS gastric acid secretion; gastroenterology; general adaptation syndrome; generalized arteriosclerosis

GASA growth-adjusted sonographic age

gastroc gastrocnemius [muscle]

GAT group adjustment therapy

GB gallbladder; glial bundle; goof balls; Guillain-Barré [syndrome]

GBA ganglionic blocking agent; gingivobuccoaxial

GBD gender behavior disorder; glass blower's disease

GBG glycine-rich beta-glycoprotein; gonadal steroid-binding globulin

GBH gamma-benzene hexachloride; graphite benzalkonium-heparin

GBHA glyoxal-bis-(2-hydroxyanil)

GBIA Guthrie bacterial inhibition assay

GBL glomerular basal lamina

GBM glomerular basement membrane

GBP galactose-binding protein; gated blood pool

GBS gallbladder series; group B *Streptococcus*; Guillain-Barré syndrome

GBSS Gey's balanced saline solution; Guillain-Barré-Strohl syndrome

GC ganglion cell; gas chromatography; geriatric care; glucocorticoid; gonococcus; gonorrhea; granular casts; granulomatous colitis; granulosa cell; guanine cytosine; guanylcyclase

Gc group-specific component

GCA giant cell arteritis

g-cal gram calorie

GCB gonococcal base

GCFT gonorrhea complement fixation test

GCI General Cognitive Index

GCIIS glucose controlled insulin infusion system

g-cm gram-centimeter

GC-MS gas chromatography-mass spectrometry

GCN giant cerebral neuron

GCR Group Conformity Rating

GCS Glasgow Coma Score; glucocorticosteroid; glutamylcysteine synthetase

GCSA Gross cell surface antigen

GCT giant cell thyroiditis

GCV great cardiac vein

GCVF great cardiac vein flow

GCW glomerular capillary wall

GCWM General Conference on Weights and Measures

GD General Diagnostics; general dispensary; gestational day; gonadal dysgenesis; Graves' disease

Gd gadolinium

G&D growth and development
GDA germine diacetate
GDB gas density balance; guide dogs for the blind
GDC giant dopamine-containing cell; General Dental Council
GDF gel diffusion precipitin
GDH glutamate dehydrogenase; glycerophosphate dehydrogenase; glycol dehydrogenase; growth and differentiation hormone
g/dl grams per deciliter
GDM gestational diabetes mellitus
GDMO General Duties Medical Officer
GDP guanosine diphosphate
GDS Global Deterioration Scale; gradual dosage schedule
GDW glass-distilled water
GE gastric emptying; gastroemotional; gastroenterology; gastroenterostomy; gel electrophoresis; generalized epilepsy; generator of excitation; gentamicin
Ge germanium
G/E granulocyte/erythroid [ratio]
GEC galactose elimination capacity; glomerular epithelial cell
GECC Government Employees' Clinic Centre
GEF gonadotropin enhancing factor
GEH glycerol ester hydrolase
gel gelatin
gel quav in any kind of jelly [Lat. *gelatina quavis*]
GEN gender; generation
Gen genetics, genetic; genus
gen general; genital
genet genetic, genetics
gen et sp nov new genus and species [Lat. *genus et species nova*]
genit genitalia, genital
gen nov new genus [Lat. *genus novum*]
GENPS genital neoplasm-papilloma syndrome
GENT gentamicin
GEP gastroenteropancreatic
GER gastroesophageal reflux; geriatrics; granular endoplasmic reticulum
Ger German
GERD gastroesophageal reflux disease
geriat geriatrics, geriatric
GERL Golgi-associated endoplasmic reticulum lysosome

Geront gerontology, gerontologist, gerontologic
GES glucose-electrolyte solution
GEST gestation
GET gastric emptying time; graded treadmill exercise test
Gev giga electron volt
GEX gas exchange
GF gastric fluid; germ-free; glass factor; glomerular filtration; gluten-free; grandfather; growth factor
gf gram-force
GFA glial fibrillary acidic [protein]
GFAP glial fibrillary acidic protein
GFD gluten-free diet
GFFS glycogen and fat-free solid
GFH glucose-free Hanks [solution]
GFI glucagon-free insulin; ground-fault interrupter
GFL giant follicular lymphoma
GFP gamma-fetoprotein; gel-filtered platelet
GFR glomerular filtration rate
GFS global focal sclerosis; guafenesin
GG gamma globulin; glycylglycine
GGA general gonadotropic activity
GGE generalized glandular enlargement
GGG gamboge [Lat. *gummi guttae gambiae*]; glycine-rich gamma-glycoprotein
GG or S glands, goiter, or stiffness [of neck]
GGPNA gamma-glutamyl-p-nitroanilide
GGT gamma-glutamyltranspeptidase; gamma-glutamyltransferase
GGVB gelatin, glucose, and veronal buffer
GH general hospital; genetic hypertension; genetically hypertensive [rat]; growth hormone
GHA Group Health Association
GHAA Group Health Association of America
GHBA gamma-hydroxybutyric acid
GHD growth hormone deficiency
GHQ General Health Questionnaire
GHR granulomatous hypersensitivity reaction
GHRF growth hormone-releasing factor
GH-RH growth hormone-releasing hormone
GH-RIF growth hormone-release inhibiting factor

GHV goose hepatitis virus
GHz gigahertz
GI gastrointestinal; gelatin infusion [medium]; gingival index; globin insulin; glomerular index; granuloma inguinale; growth inhibition
gi gill
GIB gastrointestinal bleeding
GID gender identity disorder
GIF growth hormone-inhibiting factor
GIGO garbage in, garbage out
GIH gastrointestinal hemorrhage; growth-inhibiting hormone
GII gastrointestinal infection
GIK glucose-insulin-potassium [solution]
GIM gonadotropin-inhibiting material
Ging, ging gingiva, gingival
g-ion gram-ion
GIP gastric inhibitory polypeptide; giant cell interstitial pneumonia; gonorrheal invasive peritonitis
GIS gas in stomach; gastrointestinal series
GIT gastrointestinal tract
GITT glucose insulin tolerance test
GJ gap junction; gastric juice; gastro-jejunostomy
GK glomerulocystic kidney; glycerol kinase
GL glycolipid; glycosphingolipid; greatest length; gustatory lacrimation
Gl beryllium [Lat. *glucinium*]; glabella
gl gill; gland, glandular
g/l grams per liter
GLA gamma-linolenic acid; gingivo-linguoaxial
glac glacial
GLAD gold-labelled antigen detection
gland glandular
GLC gas-liquid chromatography
Glc glucose
glc glaucoma
GlcA gluconic acid
GlcN glucosamine
GlcUA D-glucuronic acid
GLD globoid leukodystrophy
GLH giant lymph node hyperplasia
GLI glicentin; glucagon-like immuno-reactivity
GLIM generalized linear interactive model
GLM general linear model

Gln glucagon; glutamine
GLNH giant lymph node hyperplasia
Glo glyoxylase
GLO1 glyoxylase 1
glob globular; globulin
GLP glucose-L-phosphate; glycolipo-protein; good laboratory practice; group living program
GLR graphic level recorder
GLS generalized lymphadenopathy syndrome
GLTN glomerulotubulonephritis
GLU glucuronidase; glutamic acid, glutamine
Glu glucuronidase; glutamic acid, glutamine
glu glucose
GLU-5 five-hour glucose tolerance test
GLUC glucosidase
gluc glucose
GLV Gross leukemia virus
GLY, gly glycine; glycocoll
glyc glyceride
GM gastric mucosa; Geiger-Müller [counter]; general medicine; genetic manipulation; geometric mean; giant melanosome; gram; grand mal [epilepsy]; grandmother; grand multiparity; growth medium
G-M Geiger-Müller [counter]
Gm an allotype marker on the heavy chains of immunoglobins
gm gram
GMA glyceral methacrylate
GMB gastric mucosal barrier; granulo-membranous body
GMC general medical clinic; general medical council; grivet monkey cell
GM-CFU granulocyte-macrophage colony forming unit
GMD geometric mean diameter; glyco-peptide moiety modified derivative
GMENAC Graduate Medical Education National Advisory Committee
GMK green monkey kidney [cells]
g/ml grams per milliliter
gm/l grams per liter
gm-m gram-meter
g-mol gram-molecule
GMP guanosine monophosphate
3':5'-GMP guanosine 3':5'-cyclic phosphate

GMS General Medical Service; Gomori methenamine silver stain
GM&S general medicine and surgery
GMSC General Medical Services Committee
GMT geometric mean titer; gingival margin trimmer
GMW gram molecular weight
GN glomerulonephritis; glucose nitrogen [ratio]; gnotobiote; graduate nurse; gram-negative
G/N glucose/nitrogen ratio
Gn gnathion; gonadotropin
GNB gram-negative bacillus
GNBM gram-negative bacillary meningitis
GNC general nursing care; General Nursing Council
GND Gram-negative diplococci
GNID gram-negative intracellular diplococci
GNP gerontologic nurse practitioner
GnRF gonadotropin-releasing factor
GnRH gonadotropin-releasing hormone
GNTP Graduate Nurse Transition Program
GO glucose oxidase
G&O gas and oxygen
Go gonion
G$_0$ quiescent phase of cells leaving the mitotic cycle
GOAT Galveston Orientation and Amnesia Test
GOBAB gamma-hydroxy-beta-amino-butyric acid
GOE gas, oxygen, and ether
GOG Gynecologic Oncology Group
GOH geroderma osteodysplastica hereditaria
G Ω gigohm
GOR general operating room
GOT aspartate aminotransferase; glucose oxidase test; glutamate oxaloacetate transaminase
GOTM glutamic-oxaloacetic trans-aminase, mitochondrial
GP general paralysis, general paresis; general practice, general practitioner; genetic prediabetes; geometric progression; globus pallidus; glucose phosphate; glycopeptide; glycoprotein; gram-positive; guinea pig

G/P gravida/para
GPI glycoprotein I
G3P, G-3-P glycerol-3-phosphate
G6P, G-6-P glucose-6-phosphate
gp glycoprotein; group
GPA grade point average; Group Practice Association; guinea pig albumin
GPAIS guinea pig anti-insulin serum
G6Pase, G-6-Pase glucose-6-phos-phatase
GPB glossopharyngeal breathing
GPC gastric parietal cell; gel permeation chromatography; granular progenitor cell; guinea pig complement
GPD glucose-6-phosphate dehydrog-enase
G6PD, G-6-PD glucose-6-phosphate dehydrogenase
G-6-PDA glucose-6-phosphate dehy-drogenase enzyme variant A
G6PDH, G-6-PDH glucose-6-phos-phate dehydrogenase
GPE guinea pig embryo
GPF granulocytosis-promoting factor
GPGG guinea pig gamma-globulin
GPh Graduate in Pharmacy
GPHLV guinea pig herpes-like virus
GPI general paralysis of the insane; glucosephosphate isomerase
GPIMH guinea pig intestinal mucosal homogenate
GPIPID guinea pig intraperitoneal infectious dose
GPK guinea pig kidney [antigen]
GPKA guinea pig kidney absorption [test]
Gply gingivoplasty
GPM general preventive medicine; giant pigment melanosome
GPMAL gravida, para, multiple births, abortions, and live births
GPN graduate practical nurse
GPPQ General Purpose Psychiatric Questionnaire
GPRBC guinea pig red blood cell
GPS gray platelet syndrome; guinea pig serum; guinea pig spleen
GPT glutamic-pyruvic transaminase
GpTh group therapy
GPU guinea pig unit
GPUT galactose phosphate uridyl transferase
GQAP general question asking program

GR gamma-rays; gastric resection; general research; glucocorticoid receptor; glutathione reductase

gr grain; gram; gravity; gray

gr⁻ gram-negative

gr⁺ gram-positive

GRA gated radionuclide angiography; gonadotropin-releasing agent

Grad by degrees [Lat. *gradatim*]

grad gradient; gradually; graduate

GRAE generally regarded as effective

gran granule, granulated

GRAS generally recognized as safe

grav gravid

grav I pregnancy one; primigravida

GRD gastroesophageal reflux disease

grd ground

GRF gonadotropin-releasing factor; growth hormone-releasing factor

GRG glycine-rich glycoprotein

GRH growth hormone-releasing hormone

GRIF growth hormone release-inhibiting factor

GRN granules

GrN gram-negative

Grn green

GRP gastrin-releasing peptide

GrP gram-positive

$Gr_1P_0AB_1$ one pregnancy, no births, one abortion

GRPS glucose-Ringer-phosphate solution

GRW giant ragweed [test]

GS gallstone; Gardner syndrome; gastric shield; general surgery; Gilbert syndrome; glomerular sclerosis; glutamine synthetase; goat serum; Goldenhar syndrome; grip strength; group section

gs group specific

G/S glucose and saline

g/s gallons per second

GSA general somatic afferent; group-specific antigen; Gross virus antigen; guanidinosuccinic acid

GSBG gonadal steroid-binding globulin

GSC gas-solid chromatography; gravity settling culture

GSCN giant serotonin-containing neuron

GSD genetically significant dose; glycogen storage disease

GSE general somatic efferent; gluten-sensitive enteropathy

GSF galactosemic fibroblast; genital skin fibroblast

GSH glomerulus-stimulating hormone; golden Syrian hamster; reduced glutathione

GSN giant serotonin-containing neuron

GSoA Gerontological Society of America

GSP galvanic skin potential

GSR galvanic skin response; generalized Shwartzman reaction

GSS gamete-shedding substance; Gerstmann-Sträussler-Scheinker [disease]

GSSG oxidized glutathione

GSSR generalized Sanarelli-Shwartzman reaction

GST glutathione-S-transferase; gold sodium thiomalate; graphic stress telethermometry; group striction

GSW gunshot wound

GSWA gunshot wound, abdominal

GT generation time; genetic therapy; gingiva treatment; Glanzmann's thrombasthenia; glucose tolerance; glycityrosine; glutamyl transpeptidase; granulation tissue; greater trochanter; group tensions; group therapy

GT1–GT10 glycogen storage disease, types 1 to 10

gt drop [Lat. *gutta*]

g/t granulation time

G&T gowns and towels

GTB gastrointestinal tract bleeding

GTF glucose tolerance factor; glucosyltransferase

GTH gonadotropic hormone

GTN gestational trophoblastic neoplasia; glomerulotubulonephritis; glyceryl trinitrate

GTO Golgi tendon organ

GTP glutamyl transpeptidase; guanosine triphosphate

GTR granulocyte turnover rate

GTS Gilles de la Tourette syndrome

GTT gelatin-tellurite-taurocholate [agar]; glucose tolerance test

gtt drops [Lat. *guttae*]

GU gastric ulcer; genitourinary; glycogenic unit; gonococcal urethritis; gravitational ulcer

GUA group of units of analysis

Gua guanine

GULHEMP general physique, upper

extremity, lower extremity, hearing, eyesight, mentality, and personality
Guo guanosine
GUS genitourinary sphincter; genitourinary system
gutt to the throat [Lat. *gutturi*]
guttat drop by drop [Lat. *guttatim*]
gutt quibusd with a few drops [Lat. *guttis quibusdam*]
GV gentian violet; germinal vesicle; Gross virus
GVBD germinal vesicle breakdown
GVF good visual fields
GVG gamma-vinyl-gamma-aminobutyric acid
GVH, GvH graft-versus-host
GVHD, GvHD graft-versus-host disease
GVHR, GvHR graft-versus-host reaction
GVTY gingivectomy
GW germ warfare; glycerin in water; gradual withdrawal; group work
GX glycinexylidide
GXT graded exercise test
Gy gray
GYN gynecologic, gynecologist, gynecology
GZ Guilford-Zimmerman [test]

–H–

H bacterial antigen in serologic classification of bacteria [Ger. *Hauch* film]; deflection in the His bundle in electrogram [spike]; draft [Lat. *haustus*]; electrically induced spinal reflex; enthalpy; fucosal transferase producing gene; heart; heavy; height; hemagglutination; hemolysis; *Hemophilus;* henry; heroin; high; histidine; Holzknecht unit; homosexual; horizontal; hormone; horse; hospital; Hounsfield unit; hour; human; hydrogen; hydrolysis; hygiene; hyoscine; hypermetropia; hyperopia; hypodermic; hypothalamus; magnetic field strength; magnetization; mustard gas; oersted; the region of a sarcomere containing only myosin filaments [Ger. *heller* lighter] [band]

H^+ hydrogen ion
$[H^+]$ hydrogen ion concentration
H_0 null hypothesis
H1, ^{1}H, H^1 protium
H_1 alternative hypothesis
H2, ^{2}H, H^2 deuterium
H3, ^{3}H, H^3 tritium
h coefficient of heat transfer; hand-rearing [of experimental animals]; hecto; height; henry; human; hour [Lat. *hora*]; negatively staining region of a chromosome; Planck's constant; specific enthalpy
HA H antigen; Hartley [guinea pig]; headache; hearing aid; height age; hemadsorption; hemagglutinating antibody; hemagglutination; hemagglutinin; hemolytic anemia; hemophiliac with adenopathy; hepatic artery; hepatitis A; hepatitis-associated; Heyden antibiotic; high anxiety; histamine; histocompatibility antigen; hospital administration; hospital admission; hospital apprentice; Hounsfield unit; hyaluronic acid; hydroxyapatite; hyperalimentation; hyperandrogenism; hypersensitivity alveolitis
HA2 hemadsorption virus 2
Ha absolution hypermetropia; hafnium; hamster
ha hectare
HAA hearing aid amplifier; hemolytic anemia antigen; hepatitis-associated antigen; hospital activity analysis
HA Ag hepatitis A antigen
HABA 2(4'-hydroxyazobenzene) benzoic acid
HAChT high affinity choline transport
HACR hereditary adenomatosis of the colon and rectum
HACS hyperactive child syndrome
HAD hemadsorption; hospital administration, hospital administrator
HAd hemadsorption
HAd-I hemadsorption-inhibition
HAE hereditary angioneurotic edema
HAG heat-aggregated globulin
HAGG hyperimmune antivariola gammaglobulin
HAHTG horse antihuman thymus globulin
HAI hemagglutination inhibition; hepatic arterial infusion
H&A Ins health and accident insurance

HAIR-AN hyperandrogenism, insulin resistance, and acanthosis nigricans [syndrome]
HaK hamster kidney
HAL hepatic artery ligation
hal halothane
halluc hallucinations
HALP hyperalphalipoproteinemia
HaLV hamster leukemia virus
HAM hearing aid microphone; hypoparathyroidism, Addison's disease, and mucocutaneous candidiasis [syndrome]
HAm human amnion
HAMA Hamilton anxiety [scale]
HAMD Hamilton depression [scale]
HAN heroin-associated nephropathy; hyperplastic alveolar nodule
H and E hematoxylin and eosin [stain]
Handicp handicapped
HANE hereditary angioneurotic edema
HANES health and nutrition examination survey
HAP Handicapped Aid Program; heredopathia atactica polyneuritiformis; histamine phosphate acid; humoral antibody production; hydrolyzed animal protein; hydroxyapatite
HAPA hemagglutinating anti-penicillin antibody
HAPC hospital-acquired penetration contact
HAPE high-altitude pulmonary edema
HAPO high altitude pulmonary [o]edema
HAPS hepatic arterial perfusion scintigraphy
HAREM heparin assay rapid easy method
HAS Hamilton anxiety scale; health advisory service; highest asymptomatic [dose]; hospital administrative service; hospital advisory service; hypertensive arteriosclerotic
HASHD hypertensive arteriosclerotic heart disease
HASP Hospital Admissions and Surveillance Program
HAsP health aspects of pesticides
HAT heterophil antibody titer; hypoxanthine, aminopterin, and thymidine; hypoxanthine, azaserine, and thymidine
HATG horse antihuman thymocyte globulin
HATH Heterosexual Attitudes Toward Homosexuality [scale]

HATTS hemagglutination treponemal test for syphilis
HAU hemagglutinating unit
haust a draft [Lat. *haustus*]
HAV hemadsorption virus; hepatitis A virus
HB health board; heart block; hepatitis B; His bundle; housebound; hybridoma bank
Hb hemoglobin
HbA hemoglobin A, adult hemoglobin
HBAb hepatitis B antibody
HBABA hydroxybenzeneazobenzoic acid
HBAg hepatitis B antigen
HBB hospital blood bank; hydroxybenzyl benzimidazole
HbBC hemoglobin binding capacity
HBBW hold breakfast blood work
HB$_c$ hepatitis B core [antigen]
HbC hemoglobin C
HB$_c$Ag, HBcAg, HBCAG hepatitis B core antigen
HBCG heat-aggregated BCG [q.v.]
HbCO carboxyhemoglobin
HBD has been drinking; hydroxybutyric dehydrogenase
HbD hemoglobin D
HBDH hydroxybutyrate dehydrogenase
HBDT human basophil degranulation test
HBE His bundle electrogram
HbE hemoglobin E
HB$_e$Ag, HBeAg, HBEAG hepatitis B early antigen
HBF hemispheric blood flow; hemoglobinuric bilious fever; hepatic blood flow
HbF fetal hemoglobin, hemoglobin F
HBGM home blood glucose monitoring
HbH hemoglobin H
Hb-Hp hemoglobin-haptoglobin [complex]
HBI high serum-bound iron
HBIg hepatitis B immunoglobulin
HBL hepatoblastoma
HBLA human B-lymphocyte antigen
HBM Health Belief Model
HbM hemoglobin M
HbMet methemoglobin
HBO hyperbaric oxygenation, hyperbaric oxygen
HbO$_2$ oxyhemoglobin

HBP hepatic binding protein; high blood pressure

HB$_s$ hepatitis B surface [antigen]

HbS hemoglobin S, sickle-cell hemoglobin

HB$_s$Ag, HBsAg, HBSAG hepatitis B surface antigen

HBsAg/adr hepatitis B surface antigen manifesting group-specific determinant *a*, and subtype specific determinants, *d* and *r*

HBSS Hank's balanced salt solution

HbSS hemoglobin SS

HBT human brain thromboplastin; human breast tumor

HBV hepatitis B vaccine; hepatitis B virus

HBW high birth weight

HbZ hemoglobin Z, hemoglobin Zürich

HC hair cell; hairy cell; handicapped; head circumference; head compression; healthy control; hepatic catalase; hereditary coproporphyria; hippocampus; home care; Hospital Corps; house call; Huntington's chorea; hyaline casts; hydraulic concussion; hydrocarbon; hydrocortisone; hydroxycorticoid; hypertrophic cardiomyopathy

H&C hot and cold

Hc hydrocolloid

HCA heart cell aggregate; hepatocellular adenoma; home care aide; Hospital Corporation of America

HCAP handicapped

HCB hexachlorobenzene

HCC hepatitis contagiosa canis; hepatocellular carcinoma; hydroxycholecalciferol

25-HCC 25-hydroxycholecalciferol

HCD heavy-chain disease; high carbohydrate diet; homologous canine distemper

HCF hereditary capillary fragility; hypocaloric carbohydrate feeding

HCFA Health Care Financing Administration

HCG, hCG human chorionic gonadotropin

HCH 1,2,3,4,5,6-hexachlorocyclohexane

HcImp hydrocolloid impression

HCIS Health Care Information System

HCL hairy-cell leukemia; human cultured lymphoblasts

HCLF high carbohydrate, low fiber [diet]

HCM health care management; hypertrophic cardiomyopathy

HCMM hereditary cutaneous malignant melanoma

HCN hereditary chronic nephritis

HCO$_3$- bicarbonate

HCP handicapped; hepatocatalase peroxidase; hereditary coproporphyria; hexachlorophene; high cell passage

H&CP hospital and community psychiatry

HCR heme-controlled repressor; host-cell reactivation

HCRE Homeopathic Council for Research and Education

HCS Hajdu-Cheney syndrome; health care support; hourglass contraction of the stomach; human chorionic somatotropin; human cord serum

hCS, hCSM human chorionic somatomammotropin

HCSD Health Care Studies Division

HCT hematocrit; historic control trial; homocytotrophic; hydrochlorothiazide; hydroxycortisone

Hct hematocrit

hCT human chorionic thyrotropin

HCTC Health Care Technology Center

HCTZ hydrochlorothiazide

HCU homocystinuria; hyperplasia cystica uteri

HCVD hypertensive cardiovascular disease

Hcy homocysteine

HD Hajna-Damon [broth]; Hansen's disease; hearing distance; heart disease; hemodialysis; hemolyzing dose; herniated disc; high density; high dose; hip disarticulation; Hirschsprung's disease; Hodgkin's disease; hormone-dependent; house dust; human diploid [cells]; Huntington's disease; hydatid disease; hydroxydopamine

H&D Hunter and Driffield [curve]

HD$_{50}$ hemolyzing dose of complement that lyses 50% of sensitized erythrocytes

hd at bedtime [Lat. *hora decubitus*]; head

HDA Huntington's Disease Association; hydroxydopamine

HDARAC high dose cytarabine (ARA C)
HDBH hydroxybutyric dehydrogenase
HDC histidine decarboxylase
HDCS human diploid cell strain
HDCV human diploid cell rabies vaccine
HDD Higher Dental Diploma
HDF human diploid fibroblast
HDFP Hypertension Detection and Follow-up Program
HDH heart disease history
HDI hemorrhagic disease of infants
HDL high density lipoprotein
HDL-C high density lipoprotein–cholesterol
HDL-c high density lipoprotein–cell surface
HDLP high density lipoprotein
HDLS hereditary diffuse leukoencephalopathy with spheroids
HDLW distance from which a watch ticking is heard by left ear
HDMTX high dose methotrexate
HDN hemolytic disease of the newborn
HDP hexose diphosphate; hydroxydimethylpyrimidine
HDPAA heparin-dependent platelet-associated antibody
HDRF Heart Disease Research Foundation
HDRW distance from which a watch ticking is heard by right ear
HDS Healthcare Data Systems; Health Data Services; herniated disc syndrome; Hospital Discharge Survey
HDU hemodialysis unit
HE hektoen enteric [agar]; hemagglutinating encephalomyelitis; hepatic encephalopathy; hereditary eliptocytosis; hollow enzyme; human enteric; hypogonadotropic eunuchoidism
H&E hematoxylin and eosin [stain]; hemorrhage and exudate; heredity and environment
He heart; helium
HEAL Health Education Assistance Loan
HEAT human erythrocyte agglutination test
hebdom a week [Lat. *hebdomada*]
HEC Health Education Council; human endothelial cell; hydroxyergocalciferol

HED hydrotropic electron-donor; unit skin dose [of x-rays] [Ger. *Haut-Einheits-Dosis*]
HEENT head, ear, eyes, nose, and throat
HEEP health effects of environmental pollutants
HEF hamster embryo fibroblast
HEG hemorrhagic erosive gastritis
HEHR highest equivalent heart rate
HEI high-energy intermediate; human embryonic intestine [cells]
HEIS high-energy ion scattering
HEK human embryonic kidney
HEL hen egg white lysozyme; human embryonic lung; human erythroleukemia
HeLa Helen Lake [human cervical carcinoma cells]
HELF human embryo lung fibroblast
HELLP hemolysis, elevated liver enzymes, and low platelet count [syndrome]
HELP Health Education Library Program; Health Emergency Loan Program; Health Evaluation and Learning Program; heat escape lessening posture; Heroin Emergency Life Project; Hospital Equipment Loan Project
HEM hematology
HEMA Health Education Media Association
hemat hematology, hematologist
hemi hemiparesis, hemiparalysis; hemiplegia
HEMPAS hereditary erythrocytic multinuclearity with positive acidified serum
HEMRI hereditary multifocal relapsing inflammation
HEP high egg passage [virus]; high energy phosphate; human epithelial cell
hEP human endorphin
HEp-1 human cervical carcinoma cells
HEp-2 human laryngeal tumor cells
HEPA high efficiency particulate air [filter]
HEPES N-2-hydroxyethylpiperazine-N-2-ethanesulfonic [acid]
HEPM human embryonic palatal mesenchymal [cell]
HER hemorrhagic encephalopathy of rats
hered heredity, hereditary
hern hernia, herniated
HERS Health Evaluation and Referral

Service; hemorrhagic fever with renal syndrome

HES health examination survey; human embryonic skin; human embryonic spleen; hydroxyethyl starch; hypereosinophilic syndrome

HESCA Health Sciences Communications Association

HET Health Education Telecommunications; helium equilibration time

het heterozygous

HETE hydroxy-eicosatetraenoic [acid]

HETP height equivalent to a theoretical plate; hexaethyltetraphosphate

HEV hemagglutinating encephalomyelitis virus; hepato-encephalomyelitis virus; high endothelial venule

HEW [Department of] Health, Education, and Welfare

HEX hexosaminidase

Hex hexamethylmelamine

HEX A hexosaminidase A

HF Hageman factor; hard filled [capsule]; hay fever; heart failure; helper factor; hemorrhagic factor; hemorrhagic fever; high fat [diet]; high flow; high frequency; human fibroblast

Hf hafnium

hf half; high frequency

HFC hard filled capsule; high frequency current; histamine-forming capacity

HFD hemorrhagic fever of deer; high forceps delivery; hospital field director

HFDK human fetal dipolid kidney

HFF human foreskin fibroblast

HFI hereditary fructose intolerance

HFIF human fibroblast interferon

HFJV high-frequency jet ventilation

HFL human fetal lung

HFM hemifacial microsomia

HFMA Healthcare Financial Management Association

HFO high-frequency oscillatory [ventilation]

HFOV high-frequency oscillatory ventilation

HFP hexafluoropropylene; hypofibrinogenic plasma

HFPPV high frequency positive pressure ventilation

HFR high frequency recombination

Hfr high frequency of recombination

HFRS hemorrhagic fever with renal syndrome

HFS Hospital Financial Support

hfs hyperfine structure

hFSH, HFSH human follicle-stimulating hormone

HFST hearing for speech test

HFT high-frequency transduction; high-frequency transfer

Hft high-frequency transfer

HFV high frequency ventilation

HG hand grip; herpes gestationis; Heschl's gyrus; human gonadotropin; hypoglycemia

Hg mercury [Lat. *hydrargyrum*]

hg hectogram; hemoglobin

HGA homogentisic acid, homogentisate

Hgb hemoglobin

HGF hyperglycemic-glucogenolytic factor

Hg-F fetal hemoglobin

HGG herpetic geniculate ganglionitis; human gammaglobulin

HGH, hGH human growth hormone

HGMCR human genetic mutant cell repository

HGO hepatic glucose output; human glucose output

HGP hepatic glucose production; hyperglobulinemic purpura

HGPRT hypoxanthine guanine phosphoribosyl transferase

HH hard-of-hearing; healthy hemophiliac; hiatal hernia; holistic health; home help; hydroxyhexamide; hypergastrinemic hyperchlorhydria; hyperhidrosis; hypogonadotropic hypogonadism; hyporeninemic hypoaldosteronism

H&H hematocrit and hemoglobin

HHA Health Hazard Appraisal; Home Health Agency; hereditary hemolytic anemia; hypothalamo-hypophyseo-adrenal [system]

HHb hypohemoglobinemia; un-ionized hemoglobin

HHCS high-altitude hypertrophic cardiomyopathy syndrome

HHD hypertensive heart disease

HHE hemiconvulsion-hemiplegia-epilepsy [syndrome]

HHG hypertrophic hypersecretory gastropathy

HHH hyperornithinemia, hyperammonemia, homocitrillinuria [syndrome]

HHHO hypotonia, hypomentia, hypogonadism, obesity [syndrome]

HHM humoral hypercalcemia of malignancy

H+Hm compound hypermetropic astigmatism

HHRH hereditary hypophosphatemic rickets with hypercalciuria; hypothalamic hypophysiotropic releasing hormone

HHS [Department of] Health and Human Services; hereditary hemolytic syndrome; human hypopituitary serum; hyperkinetic heart syndrome

HHSSA Home Health Services and Staffing Association

HHT hereditary hemorrhagic telangiectasia; homoharringtonine; hydroxyheptadecatrienoic acid

HI head injury; health insurance; hemagglutination inhibition; hepatobiliary imaging; high impulsiveness; histidine; hormone-dependent; hospital insurance; humoral immunity; hydroxyindole; hypomelanosis of Ito; hypothermic ischemia

H-I hemagglutination-inhibition

Hi histamine

HIA Hearing Industries Association; heat infusion agar; hemagglutination inhibition antibody; hemagglutination inhibition assay

HIAA Health Insurance Association of America

5-HIAA 5-hydroxyindoleacetic acid

HIB heart infusion broth; hemolytic immune body

HIBAC Health Insurance Benefits Advisory Council

HIC Heart Information Center

HiCn cyanomethemoglobin

HID headache, insomnia, depression [syndrome]; human infectious dose

HIDA Health Industry Distributors Association; hepato-iminodiacetic acid (lidofenin)

HIE human intestinal epithelium; hyper-IgE [syndrome]

HIES hyper-IgE syndrome

HIF higher integrative functions

HIFBS heat-inactivated fetal bovine serum

HIFC hog instrinsic factor concentrate

HIFCS heat-inactivated fetal calf serum

HIG, hIG human immunoglobulin

HIH hypertensive intracerebral hemorrhage

HIHA high impulsiveness, high anxiety

HiHb hemiglobin (methemoglobin)

HII Health Industries Institute; Health Insurance Institute

HILA high impulsiveness, low anxiety

HIM hepatitis-infectious mononucleosis

HIMA Health Industries Manufacturers Association

HIMC hepatic intramitochondrial crystalloid

HIMT hemagglutination inhibition morphine test

Hint Hinton [test]

HIO hypoiodism

HIOMT hydroxyindole-O-methyl transferase

HIOS high index of suspicion

HIP health illness profile; health insurance plan; hospital insurance program

HIPE Hospital Inpatient Enquiry

HiPIP high potential iron protein

HIPO hemihypertrophy, intestinal web, preauricular skin tag, and congenital corneal opacity [syndrome]; Hospital Indicator for Physicians Orders

HIR head injury routine

HIS health information system; Health Interview Survey; histidine; hospital information system; hyperimmune serum

His histidine

HISSG Hospital Information Systems Sharing Group

HIST hospital in-service training

hist histamine, history

HISTLINE History of Medicine On-Line

Histo histoplasmin skin test

histol histological, histologist, histology

HIT hemagglutination inhibition test; heparin-induced thrombocytopenia; hypertrophic infiltrative tendonitis

HITB, HiTb *Hemophilus influenzae* type B

HITTS heparin-induced thrombosis-thrombocytopenia syndrome

HIU hyperplasia interstitialis uteri

HIV human immunodeficiency virus

HJ Howell-Jolly [bodies]

HJR hepatojugular reflex

HK heat-killed; heel-to-knee; hexokinase; human kidney

H-K hands to knee

HKC human kidney cell

HKLM heat-killed*Listeria monocytogenes*

HKS hyperkinesis syndrome

HL hairline; half life; hearing level; hearing loss; heparin lock; histocompatibility locus; Hodgkin's lymphoma; hypertrichosis lanuginosa; latent hypermetropia

H&L heart and lungs [machine]

H/L hydrophile/lipophile [ratio]

Hl hypermetropic, latent

hl hectoliter

HLA histocompatibility leukocyte antigen; histocompatibility locus antigen; homologous leukocyte antibody; human leukocyte antigen; human lymphocyte antigen

HL-A human leukocyte antigen

HLA-LD human lymphocyte antigen-lymphocyte defined

HLA-SD human lymphocyte antigen-serologically defined

HLB hydrophilic-lipophilic balance; hypotonic lysis buffer

HLBI human lymphoblastoid interferon

HLCL human lymphoblastoid cell line

HLD hypersensitivity lung disease

HLDH heat-stable lactic dehydrogenase

HLEG hydrolysate lactalbumin Earle's glucose

HLF heat-labile factor

hLH human luteinizing hormone

HLHS hypoplastic left heart syndrome

HLI human leukocyte interferon

H-L-K heart, liver, and kidneys

HLN hyperplastic liver nodules

HLP hepatic lipoperoxidation; hind leg paralysis; hyperlipoproteinemia

HLR heart-lung resuscitation

HLS Health Learning System; Hippel-Lindau syndrome

HLT human lipotropin; human lymphocyte transformation

HLV herpes-like virus

HM hand movements; health maintenance; hemifacial microsomia; Holter monitoring; hospital management; human milk; hydatidiform mole; hyperimmune mouse

Hm manifest hypermetropia

hm hectometer

HMAC Health Manpower Advisory Council

HMAS hyperimmune mouse ascites

HMB homatropine methobromide

HMBA hexamethylene bisacetamide

HMC hand-mirror cell; heroin, morphine, and cocaine; hospital management committee; major histocompatibility complex

HMCCMP human mammary carcinoma cell membrane proteinase

HMD hyaline membrane disease

HME Health Media Education; heat and moisture exchanger; heat, massage, and exercise

HMF hydroxymethylfurfural

HMG high mobility group; human menopausal gonadotropin; 3-hydroxy-3-methyl-glutaryl

hMG human menopausal gonadotropin

HMG CoA 3-hydroxy-3-methylglutaryl coenzyme A

HMIS hospital medical information system

HML human milk lysosome

HMM heavy meromyosin; hexamethylmelamine

HMMA 4-hydroxy-3-methoxymandelic acid

HMO health maintenance organization; heart minute output

HMP hexose monophosphate pathway; hot moist packs

HMPA hexamethylphosphoramide

HMPG hydroxymethoxyphenylglycol

HMPS hexose monophosphate shunt

HMPT hexamethylphosphorotriamide

HMR histiocytic medullary reticulosis

H-mRNA H-chain messenger ribonucleic acid

HMRTE human milk reverse transcriptase enzyme

HMSAS hypertrophic muscular subaortic stenosis

HMSN hereditary motor and sensory neuropathy

HMSS Hospital Management Systems Society

HMT histamine-N-methyltransferase; hospital management team

HMTA hexamethylenetetramine

HMW high-molecular-weight

HMWGP high molecular weight glycoprotein

HMX heat, massage, and exercise

HN head nurse; hemagglutinin neuraminidase; hematemesis neonatorum; hemorrhage of newborn; hereditary nephritis; hilar node; histamine-containing neuron; home nursing; hospitalman; human nutrition; hypertrophic neuropathy

H&N head and neck

hn tonight [Lat. *hoc nocte*]

HNA heparin neutralizing activity

HNB human neuroblastoma

HNC hypernephroma cell; hyperosmolar nonketotic coma; hypothalamoneurohypophyseal complex

HNP hereditary nephritic protein; herniated nucleus pulposus; human neurophysin

hnRNA heterogeneous nuclear ribonucleic acid

hnRNP heterogeneous nuclear ribonucleoprotein

HNS head and neck surgery; home nursing supervisor

HNSHA hereditary nonspherocytic hemolytic anemia

HNV has not voided

HO high oxygen; house officer; hyperbaric oxygen

H/O history of

Ho holmium; horse

HoaRhLG horse anti-rhesus lymphocyte globulin

HoaTTG horse anti-tetanus toxoid globulin

HOB head of bed

HOC human ovarian cancer; hydroxycorticoid

HOCM hypertrophic obstructive cardiomyopathy

hoc vesp this evening [Lat. *hoc vespere*]

HOD hyperbaric oxygen drenching

HofF height of fundus

HOGA hyperornithinemia with gyrate atrophy

HOH hard of hearing

HoIg horse immunoglobulin

HOME Home Observation for Measurement of the Environment

Homeop homeopathy

HOMO highest occupied molecular orbital

HOOD hereditary onycho-osteodysplasia

HOODS hereditary onycho-osteodysplasia syndrome

HOP high oxygen pressure

HOPE health-oriented physical education; holistic orthogonal parameter estimation

hor horizontal

hor decub at bedtime [Lat. *hora decubitus*]

hor interm at the intermediate hours [Lat. *horis intermediis*]

hor som at bedtime [Lat. *hori somni*]

hor un spatio at the end of one hour [Lat. *horae unius spatio*]

HOS human osteosarcoma

HoS horse serum

Hosp, hosp hospital

HOST hypo-osmotic shock treatment

HOT human old tuberculin

HP halogen phosphorus; handicapped person; haptoglobin; hemiplegia; *Hemophilus pleuropneumoniae*; high potency; high power; high pressure; high protein; highly purified; horizontal plane; horsepower; hospital participation; hot pack; house physician; human pituitary; hydrophilic petrolatum; hydrostatic pressure; hydroxypyruvate; hyperparathyroidism; hypophoria

H&P history and physical examination

Hp haptoglobin

HPA *Helix pomatia* agglutinin; hemagglutinating penicillin antibody; hypothalamo-pituitary-adrenocortical [system]

HPAA hydroperoxyarachidonic acid; hydroxyphenylacetic acid; hypothalamo-pituitary-adrenal axis

HPAC hypothalamo-pituitary-adrenocortical

HPBC hyperpolarizing bipolar cell

HPBF hepatotrophic portal blood factor

HPC hippocampal pyramidal cell; hydroxypropylcellulose

HPD high protein diet

HPE history and physical examination

HPF heparin-precipitable fraction; hepatic plasma flow; high-power field [microscope]; hypocaloric protein feeding

HPFH hereditary persistence of fetal hemoglobin

hPFSH, HPFSH human pituitary follicle stimulating hormone

hPG, HPG human pituitary gonadotropin

HPI history of present illness

HPL human parotid lysozyme; human

peripheral lymphocyte; human placental lactogen

hPL human placental lactogen; human platelet lactogen

HPLAC high pressure liquid affinity chromatography

HPLC high-performance liquid chromatography; high-power liquid chromatography; high-pressure liquid chromatography

HPN home parenteral nutrition; hypertension

HPNS high pressure neurological syndrome

HPO high-presure oxygen; hydroperoxide; hydrophilic ointment; hypertrophic pulmonary osteoarthropathy

HPP hereditary pyropoikilocytosis

HPP, hPP hydroxypyrozolopyrimidine; human pancreatic polypeptide

HPPA hydroxyphenylpyruvic acid

HPPH 5-(4-hydroxyphenyl)-5-phenylhydantoin

HPPO high partial pressure of oxygen; hydroxyphenyl pyruvate oxidase

HPr human prolactin

hPRL human prolactin

HPRT hypoxanthine-guanine phosphoribosyltransferase

HPS hematoxylin, phloxin, and saffron; high protein supplement; His-Purkinje system; hypertrophic pyloric stenosis; hypothalamic pubertal syndrome

HPSL Health Professions Student Loan

HPT human placental thyrotropin; hyperparathyroidism

HPTIN human pancreatic trypsin inhibitor

HPV *Hemophilus pertussis* vaccine; hepatic portal vein; human papillomavirus

HPVD hypertensive pulmonary vascular disease

HPV-DE high-passage virus-duck embryo

HPV-DK high-passage virus-dog kidney

HPVG hepatic portal venous gas

HPZ high pressure zone

[3H]QNB (-)[3H]quinuclidinyl benzilate

HR heart rate; hemorrhagic retinopathy; higher rate; hormonal response; hospital record; hospital report; hyperimmune reaction

hr hairless [mouse]; hour

H&R hysterectomy and radiation

HRA Human Resources Administration; health risk appraisal; heart rate audiometry

HRBC horse red blood cell

HRC high resolution chromatography; horse red cell; human rights committee

HRE high resolution electrocardiography; hormone receptor enzyme

HREM high resolution electron microscopy

HRIG, HRIg human rabies immunoglobulin

HRL head rotation to the left

HRLA human reovirus-like agent

hRNA heterogeneous ribonucleic acid

HRP histidine-rich protein; horseradish peroxidase

HRPD Hamburg Rating Scale for Psychiatric Disorders

HRR head rotation to the right

HRRI heart rate retardation index

HRS Hamilton Rating Scale; hepatorenal syndrome; hormone receptor site

HRSA Health Resources and Services Administration

HRS-D Hamilton Rating Scale for Depression

HRT heart rate

HRTE human reverse transcriptase enzyme

HRTEM high resolution transmission electron microscopy

HRV heart rate variability; human rotavirus

HS half strength; hand surgery; Hartmann's solution; head sling; heart sounds; heat-stable; Hegglin syndrome; heme synthetase; heparin sulfate; hereditary spherocytosis; herpes simplex; homologous serum; horizontally selective; Horner syndrome; horse serum; hospital ship; hospital staff; hour of sleep; house surgeon; Hurler's syndrome; hypereosinophilic syndrome

hs at bedtime [Lat. *hora somni*]

H/S helper-suppressor [ratio]

HSA Health Services Administration; Health Systems Agency; horse serum albumin; human serum albumin; hypersomnia-sleep apnea

HSAG N-2-hydroxyethylpiperazine-N-2-ethanesulfonate-saline-albumin- gelatin

HSAP heat-stable alkaline phosphatase

HSAS hypertrophic subaortic stenosis

HSC Health and Safety Commission; human skin collagenase

HS-CoA reduced coenzyme A

HSD hydroxysteroid dehydrogenase

H(SD) Holtzman Sprague-Dawley [rat]

HSE herpes simplex encephalitis

HSF histamine sensitizing factor; hypothalamic secretory factor

HSG herpes simplex genitalis; hysterosalpingogram, hysterosalpingography

hSGF human skeletal growth factor

HSGP human sialoglycoprotein

HSI human seminal plasma inhibitor

HSK herpes simplex keratitis

HSL herpes simplex labialis

HSLC high speed liquid chromatography

HSM hepatosplenomegaly; holosystolic murmur

HSMHA Health Services and Mental Health Administration

HSN hereditary sensory neuropathy

HSP Health Systems Plan; hemostatic screening profile; Hospital Service Plan; human serum prealbumin; human serum protein

HSQB Health Standards and Quality Bureau

HSR Harleco synthetic resin; heated serum reagin; homogeneously staining region

HSRC Health Services Research Center; Human Subjects Review Committee

HSRD hypertension secondary to renal disease

HSRI Health Systems Research Institute

HSS high speed supernatant; hypertrophic subaortic stenosis

HSTF human serum thymus factor

HSV herpes simplex virus

HSV-1 herpes simplex virus type 1

HSV-2 herpes simplex virus type 2

HSVE herpes simplex virus encephalitis

HSVtk herpes simplex virus thymidine kinase

HSyn heme synthase

HT Hashimoto's thyroiditis; heart; heart transplantation, heart transplant; hemagglutination titer; high temperature; histologic technician; home treatment; Hubbard tank; human thrombin; hydro-

cortisone test; hydrotherapy; hydroxytryptamine; hypermetropia, total; hypertension; hypertransfusion; hypodermic tablet; hypothalamus

H&T hospitalization and treatment

5-HT 5-hydroxytryptamine

Ht height of heart; heterozygote; hyperopia, total; hypothalamus

ht a draught [Lat. *haustus*]; heart; heart tones; height; high tension

HTA heterophil transplantation antigen; hydroxytryptamine; hypophysiotropic area

HTACS human thyroid adenyl-cyclase stimulator

ht aer heated aerosol

HT(ASCP) Histologic Technician certified by the Board of Registry of the American Society of Clinical Pathologists

HTB house tube feeding; human tumor bank

HTC hepatoma cell; hepatoma tissue culture; homozygous typing cell

HTD human therapeutic dose

HTDW heterosexual development of women

HTF heterothyrotropic factor

HTG hypertriglyceridemia

HTH homeostatic thymus hormone

HTHD hypertensive heart disease

HTIG homologous tetanus immune globulin

HTL hamster tumor line; histotechnologist; human thymic leukemia

HTLA high-titer, low acidity; human T-lymphocyte antigen

HTL(ASCP) Histotechnologist certified by the Board of Registry of the American Society of Clinical Pathologists

HTLV human T-cell leukemia/lymphoma virus

HTLV-MA cell membrane antigen associated with the human T-cell leukemia virus

HTLV-I-MA human T-cell leukemia virus-I-associated membrane antigen

HTN Hantaan-[like virus]; hypertension; hypertensive nephropathy

HTO hospital transfer order

HTOH hydroxytryptophol

HTP House-Tree-Person [test]; hydroxytryptophan; hypothromboplastinemia

5-HTP 5-hydroxy-L-tryptophan

HTS head traumatic syndrome; human thyroid-stimulating hormone, human thyroid stimulator

HTSH, hTSH human thyroid-stimulating hormone

HTST high temperature, short time

HTV herpes-type virus

HTVD hypertensive vascular disease

HTX histrionicotoxin

HU heat unit; hemagglutinating unit; hemolytic unit; human urine, human urinary; hydroxyurea; hyperemia unit

Hu human

HUC hypouricemia

HU-FSH human urinary follicle-stimulating hormone

HUIFM human leukocyte interferon meloy

HUK human urinary kallikrein

HUP Hospital Utilization Project

HUR hydroxyurea

HURA health in underserved rural areas

HUS hemolytic uremic syndrome; hyaluronidase unit for semen

HuSA human serum albumin

HUTHAS human thymus antiserum

HV Hantaan virus; hepatic vein; herpes virus; hospital visit; hyperventilation

H&V hemigastrectomy and vagotomy

HVA homovanillic acid

HVAC heating, ventilating, and air conditioning

HVC Health Visitor's Certificate

HVD hypertensive vascular disease

HVE high-voltage electrophoresis

HVH herpesvirus hominis

HVJ hemagglutinating virus of Japan

HVL, hvl half-value layer

HVM high-velocity missile

HVPE high voltage paper electrophoresis

HVR hypoxic ventilation response

HVS herpesvirus of Saimiri; hyperventilation syndrome

HVSD hydrogen-detected ventricular septal defect

HVTEM high voltage transmission electron microscopy

HVUS hypocomplementemic vasculitis urticaria syndrome

HWB hot water bottle

HWC Health and Welfare, Canada

HWS hot water-soluble

HX histiocytosis X; hydrogen exchange; hypophysectomized

Hx history; hypoxanthine

HXM hexamethylmelamine

Hy hypermetropia; hyperopia; hypothenar; hysteria

HYD hydration, hydrated; hydroxyurea

hydr hydraulic

hydro hydrotherapy

hyg hygiene, hygienic, hygienist

HYL, Hyl hydroxylysine

HYP hydroxyproline; hypnosis

Hyp hydroxyproline; hyperresonance; hypertrophy; hypothalamus

hyp hypophysis, hypophysectomy

hyper-IgE hyperimmunoglobulinemia E

hypn hypertension

hypno hypnosis

Hypo hypodermic, hypodermic injection

hypox hypophysectomized

HypRF hypothalamic releasing factor

Hypro hydroxyproline

hys, hyst hysterectomy; hysteria, hysterical

HZ herpes zoster

Hz hertz

–I–

I electric current; impression; incisor [permanent]; independent; index; indicated; induction; inhibition, inhibitor; inosine; intensity; internal medicine; intestine; iodine; ionic strength; moment of inertia; region of a sarcomere that contains only actin filaments; Roman numeral one

i incisor [deciduous]; insoluble; isochromosome; optically inactive

ι see *iota*

IA ibotenic acid; immune adherence; impedance angle; indolaminergic accumulation; indulin agar; infantile autism; infected area; inferior angle; internal auditory; intra-amniotic; intra-aortic; intra-arterial; intra-articular; intra-atrial; intra-auricular

Ia immune response gene-associated antigen

IAA imidazoleacetic acid; indoleacetic acid; International Antituberculosis Association; interruption of the aortic arch

IAB Industrial Accident Board; intra-abdominal; intra-aortic balloon

IABA intra-aortic balloon assistance

IABC intra-aortic balloon counterpulsation

IABM idiopathic aplastic bone marrow

IABP intra-aortic balloon pumping

IAC ineffective airway clearance; internal auditory canal; intra-arterial chemotherapy

IACD implantable automatic cardioverter-defibrillator

IACS International Academy of Cosmetic Surgery

IACV International Association of Cancer Victims and Friends

IAD internal absorbed dose

IADH inappropriate antidiuretic hormone

IADHS inappropriate antidiuretic hormone syndrome

IADR International Association for Dental Research

IAds immunoadsorption

IAEA International Atomic Energy Agency

IAFI infantile amaurotic familial idiocy

IAG International Association of Gerontology; International Academy of Gnathology

IAGP International Association of Geographic Pathology

IAGUS International Association of Genito-Urinary Surgeons

IAH implantable artificial heart

IAHA immune adherence hemagglutination

IAHS International Association of Hospital Security

IAL International Association of Laryngectomees

IAM Institute of Aviation Medicine; internal auditory meatus

i am intra-amniotic

IAMM International Association of Medical Museums

IAO immediately after onset; intermittent aortic occlusion; International Association of Orthodontists

IAOM International Association of Oral Myology

IAP immunosuppressive acidic protein; inosinic acid pyrophosphorylase; Institute of Animal Physiology; intermittent acute porphyria; International Academy of Pathology; International Academy of Proctology; islet-activating protein

IAPB International Association for Prevention of Blindness

IAPM International Academy of Preventive Medicine

IAPP International Association for Preventive Pediatrics

IAR iodine-azide reaction

IARC International Agency for Research on Cancer

IARF ischemic acute renal failure

IARSA idiopathic acquired refractory sideroblastic anemia

IAS immunosuppressive acidic substance; infant apnea syndrome; interatrial septum; interatrial shunting; intra-amniotic saline

IASA interatrial septal aneurysm

IASD interatrial septal defect; interauricular septal defect

IASHS Institute for Advanced Study in Human Sexuality

IASL International Association for Study of the Liver

IASP International Association for Study of Pain

IAT iodine azide test; invasive activity test

IAV intra-arterial vasopressin

IB immune body; inclusion body; index of body build; infectious bronchitis; Institute of Biology

ib in the same place [Lat. *ibidem*]

IBAT intravascular broncho-alveolar tumor

IBB intestinal brush border

IBC Institutional Biosafety Committee; iodine-binding capacity; iron-binding capacity

IBCA isobutyl-2-cyanoacrylate

IBD inflammatory bowel disease; irritable bowel disease

IBE International Bureau for Epilepsy

IBED Inter-African Bureau for Epizootic Diseases

iB-EP immunoreactive beta-endomorphin

IBF immature brown fat; immunoglobulin-binding factor

IBG insoluble bone gelatin

IBI intermittent bladder irrigation

ibid in the same place [Lat. *ibidem*]

IBK infectious bovine keratoconjunctivitis

IBMP International Board of Medicine and Psychology

IBMX 3-isobutyl-1-methylxanthine

IBP International Biological Program; intra-aortic balloon pumping; iron-binding protein

IBPMS indirect blood pressure measuring system

IBR infectious bovine rhinotracheitis

IBRO International Brain Research Organization

IBRV infectious bovine rhinotracheitis virus

IBS imidazole buffered saline; irritable bowel syndrome

IBSA iodinated bovine serum albumin

IBU international benzoate unit

i-Bu isobutyl

IBV infectious bronchitis vaccine; infectious bronchitis virus

IBW ideal body weight

IC immune complex; immunocytochemistry; individual counseling; inferior colliculus; inner canthal [distance]; inorganic carbon; inspiratory capacity; inspiratory center; institutional care; integrated circuit; integrated concentration; intensive care; intercostal; intermediate care; intermittent claudication; interstitial cell; intracavitary; intracellular; intracerebral; intracranial; intracutaneous; irritable colon; islet cells; isovolumic contraction

IC$_{50}$ inhibitory concentration of 50%

ic between meals [Lat. *inter cibos*]

ICA Institute of Clinical Analysis; internal carotid artery; intracranial aneurysm; islet cell antibody

ICAA International Council on Alcohol and Addictions; Invalid Children's Aid Association

ICAMI International Committee Against Mental Illness

ICAO internal carotid artery occlusion

ICBF inner cortical blood flow

ICBP intracellular binding protein

ICC immunocompetent cells; immunocytochemistry; Indian childhood cirrhosis; intensive coronary care; internal conversion coefficient

ICCE intracapsular cataract extraction

ICCM idiopathic congestive cardiomyopathy

ICCR International Committee for Contraceptive Research

ICCU intensive coronary care unit; intermediate coronary care unit

ICD immune complex disease; induced circular dichroism; Institute for Crippled and Disabled; International Center for the Disabled; International Classification of Diseases, Injuries, and Causes of Death; intrauterine contraceptive device; ischemic coronary disease; isocitrate dehydrogenase; isolated conduction defect

ICDA International Classification of Diseases, Adapted

ICD-CM International Classification of Diseases–Clinical Modification

ICDH isocitrate dehydrogenase

ICD-O International Classification of Diseases–Oncology

ICE iridocorneal endothelial [syndrome]

ICF indirect centrifugal flotation; intensive care facility; intermediate-care facility; International Cardiology Foundation; intracellular fluid; intravascular coagulation fibrinolysis

ICF(M)A International Cystic Fibrosis (Mucoviscidosis) Association

ICF-MR intermediate-care facility for the mentally retarded

ICG indocyanine green; isotope cisternography

ICGN immune-complex glomerulonephritis

ICH idiopathic cortical hyperostosis; infectious canine hepatitis; intracerebral hematoma; intracranial hemorrhage

ICHD Inter-Society Commission for Heart Disease Resources

ICHPPC International Classification of Health Problems in Primary Care

ICLA International Committee on Laboratory Animals

ICM inner cell mass; intercostal margin; International Confederation of Midwives; ion conductance modulator

ICN intensive care nursery; International Council of Nurses

ICNND Interdepartmental Committee on Nutrition in National Defense

ICO impedance cardiac output

ICP incubation period; infection-control practitioner; intracranial pressure

ICPA International Commission for the Prevention of Alcoholism

ICPEMC International Commission for Protection against Environmental Mutagens and Carcinogens

ICPI Intersociety Committee on Pathology Information

ICR [distance between] iliac crests; Institute for Cancer Research; Institute for Cancer Research [mouse]; International Congress of Radiology; intracardiac catheter recording; intracranial reinforcement; ion cyclotron resonance

ICRC International Committee of the Red Cross

ICRD Index of Codes for Research Drugs

ICRETT International Cancer Research Technology Transfer

ICREW International Cancer Research Workshop

I-CRF immunoreactive corticotropin-releasing factor

ICRF-159 razoxane

ICRP International Commission on Radiological Protection

ICRU International Commission on Radiation Units and Measurements

ICS ileocecal sphincter; immotile cilia syndrome; impulse-conducting system; intensive care, surgical; intercellular space; intercostal space; International College of Surgeons; International Craniopathic Society; intracranial stimulation; irritable colon syndrome

ICSA islet cell surface antibody

ICSC idiopathic central serous choroidopathy

ICSH International Committee for Standardization in Hematology; interstitial cell-stimulating hormone

ICSP International Council of Societies of Pathology

ICSS intracranial self-stimulation

ICSU International Council of Scientific Unions

ICT indirect Coombs test; inflammation of connective tissue; insulin coma therapy; intensive conventional therapy; intracardiac thrombus; isovolumic contraction time

Ict icterus

iCT immunoreactive calcitonin

ICTMM International Congress on Tropical Medicine and Malaria

ICTS idiopathic carpal tunnel syndrome

ICTV International Committee for the Taxonomy of Viruses

ICU intensive care unit

ICV intracerebroventricular

ICVS International Cardiovascular Society

ICW intracellular water

ID identification; iditol dehydrogenase; immunodeficiency; immunodiffusion; inclusion disease; index of discrimination; individual dose; infant death; infectious disease; infective dose; inhibitory dose; initial dose; initial dyskinesia; injected dose; inside diameter; interdigitating; intradermal

I&D incision and drainage

ID$_{50}$ median infective dose

Id infradentale; interdentale

id the same [Lat. *idem*]

i d during the day [Lat. *in diem*]; intradermal

IDA image display and analysis; iminodiacetic acid; iron deficiency anemia

IDAV immunodeficiency-associated virus

IDBS infantile diffuse brain sclerosis

IDC idiopathic dilated cardiomyopathy; interdigitating cell

IDCI intradiplochromatid interchange

IDD insulin-dependent diabetes

IDDM insulin-dependent diabetes mellitus

IDI induction-delivery interval; interdentale inferius

IDIC Internal Dose Information Center

IDL Index to Dental Literature; intermediate density lipoprotein

IDM indirect method; infant of diabetic mother

ID-MS isotope dilution–mass spectrometry

iDNA intercalary deoxyribonucleic acid

idon vehic in a suitable vehicle [Lat. *idoneo vehiculo*]

IDP initial dose period; inosine diphosphate
IDPH idiopathic pulmonary hemosiderosis
IDPN iminodipropionitrile
IDR intradermal reaction
IDS immune deficiency state
IdS interdentale superius
IDSA Infectious Disease Society of America
IDT immune diffusion test
IDU idoxuridine; iododeoxyuridine
IdUA iduronic acid
IDUR idoxuridine
IdUrd idoxuridine
IDV intermittent demand ventilation
IDVC indwelling venous catheter
IE immunizing unit [Ger. *immunitäts Einheit*]; immunoelectrophoresis; infectious endocarditis; intake energy; internal elastica
ie that is [Lat. *id est*]
I/E inspiratory/expiratory [ratio]
IEA immediate early antigen; immunoelectroadsorption; infectious equine anemia; International Epidemiological Association; intravascular erythrocyte aggregation
IEC injection electrode catheter; intraepithelial carcinoma; ion-exchange chromatography
IEE inner enamel epithelium
IEEE Institute of Electrical and Electronic Engineers
IEF International Eye Foundation; isoelectric focusing
IEL internal elastic lamina; intraepithelial lymphocyte
IEM immuno-electron microscopy; inborn error of metabolism
IEMG integrated electromyogram
IEOP immunoelectro-osmophoresis
IEP immunoelectrophoresis; individualized education program; isoelectric point
IF immunofluorescence; indirect fluorescence; infrared; inhibiting factor; initiation factor; interferon; intermediate frequency; interstitial fluid; intrinsic factor; involved field [radiotherapy]
IFA idiopathic fibrosing alveolitis; immunofluorescence assay; immunofluorescent antibody; incomplete Freund's adjuvant; indirect fluorescent antibody; indirect fluorescent assay; International Fertility Association; International Filariasis Association
IFAT indirect fluorescent antibody test
IFC intermittent flow centrifugation; intrinsic factor concentrate
IFCC International Federation of Clinical Chemistry
IFCR International Foundation for Cancer Research
IFCS inactivated fetal calf serum
IFDS isolated follicle-stimulating hormone deficiency syndrome
IFE interfollicular epidermis
IFF inner fracture face
IFFH International Foundation for Family Health
IFGO International Federation of Gynecology and Obstetrics
IFHP International Federation of Health Professionals
IFHPMSM International Federation for Hygiene, Preventive Medicine, and Social Medicine
IFLrA recombinant human leukocyte interferon A
IFMBE International Federation for Medical and Biological Engineering
IFME International Federation for Medical Electronics
IFMP International Federation for Medical Psychotherapy
IFMSA International Federation of Medical Student Associations
IFMSS International Federation of Multiple Sclerosis Societies
IFN interferon
If nec if necessary
IFP inflammatory fibroid polyp; intermediate filament protein
IFPM International Federation of Physical Medicine
IFR infrared; inspiratory flow rate
IFRA indirect fluorescent rabies antibody [test]
IFRP International Fertility Research Program
IFSM International Federation of Sports Medicine
IFT immunofluorescence test
IFU interferon unit
IFV interstitial fluid volume; intracellular fluid volume
IG, Ig immunoglobulin

IG, ig intragastric
IGA infantile genetic agranulocytosis
IgA immunoglobulin A
IgA1, IgA2 subclasses of immuno-globulin A
IGC intragastric cannula
IGD isolated gonadotropin deficiency
IgD immunoglobulin D
IgD1, IgD2 subclasses of immuno-globulin D
IGDM infant of mother with gestational diabetes mellitus
IGE impaired gas exchange
IgE immunoglobulin E
IgE1 subclass of immunoglobulin E
IGF insulin-like growth factor
IGFET insulated gate field effect transistor
IgG immunoglobulin G
IgG1, IgG2, IgG3, IgG4 sub-classes of immunoglobulin G
IGH immunoreactive growth hormone
IGHD isolated growth hormone deficiency
IGIV immune globulin intravenous
IgM immunoglobulin M
IgM1 subclass of immunoglobulin M
IGR immediate generalized reaction
IGS inappropriate gonadotropin secretion
IgSC immunoglobulin-secreting cell
IGT impaired glucose tolerance
IGTT intravenous glucose tolerance test
IGV intrathoracic gas volume
IH idiopathic hirsutism; immediate hypersensitivity; indirect hemagglutin-ation; industrial hygiene; infectious hepatitis; inhibiting hormone; inner half; inpatient hospital; iron hematoxylin
IHA idiopathic hyperaldosteronism; indirect hemagglutination; indirect hemagglutination antibody
IHAC Industrial Health and Advisory Committee
IHBTD incompatible hemolytic blood transfusion disease
IHC idiopathic hemochromatosis; idiopathic hypercalciuria; inner hair cell; intrahepatic cholestasis
IHCP Institute of Hospital and Community Psychiatry
IHD ischemic heart disease
IHF Industrial Health Foundation; Inter-national Hospital Foundation
IHH infectious human hepatitis

IHL International Homeopathic League
IHO idiopathic hypertrophic osteo-arthropathy
IHP idiopathic hypoparathyroidism; idiopathic hypopituitarism; interhospital-ization period; inverted hand position
IHPP Intergovernmental Health Project Policy
IHR intrinsic heart rate
IHRB Industrial Health Research Board
IHS inactivated horse serum; Indian Health Service; International Health Society
IHSA iodinated human serum albumin
IHSC immunoreactive human skin collagenase
IHSS idiopathic hypertrophic subaortic stenosis
IHT insulin hypoglycemia test
I5HT intraplatelet serotonin
Ii incision inferius
II Roman numeral two
II-para secundipara
IIE idiopathic ineffective erythropoiesis
IIF immune interferon; indirect immuno-fluorescence
IIGR ipsilateral instinctive grasp reaction
III Roman numeral three
III-para tertipara
IIME Institute of International Medical Education
IIS International Institute of Stress
IJ internal jugular
IJD inflammatory joint disease
IJP inhibitory junction potential; internal jugular pressure
IK immune body [Ger. *Immunekörper*]; *Infusoria* killing [unit]
IKE ion kinetic energy
IKU *Infusoria* killing unit
IL ileum; incisolingual; interleukin
Il promethium [*illinium*]
ILA insulin-like activity; International Leprosy Association
ILa incisolabial
ILB, ILBW infant, low birth weight
ILC incipient lethal concentration
ILD interstitial lung disease; ischemic leg disease; ischemic limb disease; isolated lactase deficiency
ILE, ILe, Ileu isoleucine
ILL intermediate lymphocytic lymphoma

ILM insulin-like material; internal limiting membrane

ILP inadequate luteal phase; interstitial lymphocytic pneumonia

ILR irreversible loss rate

ILS idiopathic leucine sensitivity; idiopathic lymphadenopathy syndrome; increase in life span; infrared live scanner; intralobal sequestration

ILSI International Life Sciences Institute

ILSS integrated life support system

IM idiopathic myelofibrosis; immunosuppressive method; Index Medicus; industrial medicine; infection medium; infectious mononucleosis; inner membrane; intermediate megaloblast; internal medicine; intramedullary; intramuscular; invasive mole

IMA Industrial Medical Association; inferior mesenteric artery; Interchurch Medical Assistance; internal mammary artery; Irish Medical Association

IMAA iodinated macroaggregated albumin

IMAI internal mammary artery implant

IMB intermenstrual bleeding

IMBC indirect maximum breathing capacity

IMBI Institute of Medical and Biological Illustrators

IMD immunologically mediated disease

ImD$_{50}$ immunizing dose sufficient to protect 50% of the animals in a test group

IMDD idiopathic midline destructive disease

IMDP imidocarb diproprionate

IME independent medical examination

IMEM improved minimum essential medium

IMF intermediate filament

IMG inferior mesenteric ganglion; internal medicine group [practice]

IMH idiopathic myocardial hypertrophy; indirect microhemagglutination [test]

IMHP 1-iodomercuri-2-hydroxypropane

IMI immunologically measurable insulin; inferior myocardial infarction; intramuscular injection

IMIC International Medical Information Center

ImLy immune lysis

IMM inhibitor-containing minimal medium

immat immaturity, immature

IMMC interdigestive migrating motor complex

immobil immobilization, immobilize

immun immune, immunity, immunization

IMP idiopathic myeloid proliferation; impression; individual Medicaid practitioner; inosine 5'-monophosphate; intramembranous particle; intramuscular compartment pressure

IMPA incisal mandibular plane angle

IMPC International Myopia Prevention Center

IMPS Inpatient Multidimensional Psychiatric Scale

Impx impacted

IMR individual medical record; infant mortality rate; Institute for Medical Research

IMS incurred in military service; Indian Medical Service; industrial methylated spirit; integrated medical services

IMSS in-flight medical support system

IMT induced muscular tension; inspiratory muscle training

IMV intermittent mandatory ventilation; isophosphamide, methotrexate, and vincristine

IMViC, imvic indole, methyl red, Voges-Proskauer, citrate [test]

IMVP idiopathic mitral valve prolapse

IMVS Institute of Medical and Veterinary Science

IN icterus neonatorum; infundibular nucleus; insulin; interneuron; intranasal

In indium; inion; inulin

in inch

in^2 square inch

in^3 cubic inch

INA International Neurological Association; Jena Nomina Anatomica

INAA instrumental neutron activation analysis

INAD infantile neuroaxonal dystrophy

INAH isonicotinic acid hydrazide

inbr inbreeding

inc incompatibility; incontinent; increase, increased; incurred

IncB inclusion body

INCD infantile nuclear cerebral degeneration

incr increase, increased; increment

incur incurable
IND industrial medicine; investigational new drug
in d daily [Lat. *in dies*]
indic indication, indicated
INDIV individual
INDM infant of nondiabetic mother
INDO indomethacin
INDOR internuclear double resonance
indust industrial
INE infantile necrotizing encephalomyelopathy
INF infant, infantile; infection, infective, infected; inferior; infirmary; infundibulum; infusion; interferon
inf infant, infantile; pour in [Lat. *infunde*]
infect infection, infected, infective
Inflamm inflammation, inflammatory
ing inguinal
InGP indolglycerophosphate
INH inhalation; isoniazid; isonicotinic acid hydrazide
inhal inhalation
inhib inhibition, inhibiting
INI intranuclear inclusion
inj injection; injury, injured, injurious
inject injection
inj enem let an enema be injected [Lat. *injiciatur enema*]
INN International Nonproprietary Names
innerv innervation, innervated
INO internuclear ophthalmoplegia; inosine
Ino inosine
INOC isonicotinoyloxycarbonyl
inoc inoculation, inoculated
inorg inorganic
Inox inosine, oxidized
INP idiopathic neutropenia
INPH iproniazid phosphate
INPV intermittent negative-pressure ventilation
INREM internal radiation dose
INS idiopathic nephrotic syndrome
ins insertion; insurance, insured
insem insemination
insol insoluble
Insp inspiration
Inst institute
insuf insufflation
insuff insufficient, insufficiency

INT intermediate; intermittent; internal; p-iodonitrotetrazolium
int cib between meals [Lat. *inter cibos*]
INTEG integument
intern internal
Internat international
Intest intestine, intestinal
INTH intrathecal
Intmd intermediate
int noct during the night [Lat. *inter noctem*]
INTOX intoxication
INTR intermittent
inv inversion; involuntary
invest investigation
inv ins inverted insertion
invol involuntary
involv involvement, involved
inv(p+q-) pericentric inversion
inv(p-q+) pericentric inversion
IO inferior oblique; inferior olive; intestinal obstruction; intraocular
I&O, I/O in and out; intake/output
IOA International Osteopathic Association
IOC International Organizing Committee on Medical Librarianship; intern on call
IOD injured on duty; integrated optical density
IOFB intraocular foreign body
IOH idiopathic orthostatic hypotension
IOL intraocular lens
IOM Institute of Medicine
IOMP International Organization for Medical Physics
IOP intraocular pressure
IOR index of response
IOS International Organization for Standardization
IOT intraocular tension; intraocular transfer; ipsilateral optic tectum
IOTA information overload testing aid
ι Greek letter *iota*
IOU intensive care observation unit; international opacity unit
IP icterus praecox; immune precipitate; immunoperoxidase technique; incisoproximal; incisopulpal; incontinentia pigmenti; incubation period; induced potential; induction period; infection prevention; infundibular process; inosine phosphorylase; inpatient; instantaneous pressure; L'Institut Pasteur; International

Pharmacopoeia; interphalangeal; interpupillary; intraperitoneal; ionization potential; isoelectric point

IPA incontinentia pigmenti achromians; independent practice association; individual practice association; International Pediatric Association; International Pharmaceutical Association; International Psychoanalytical Association; isopropyl alcohol

IPAA International Psychoanalytical Association

I-para primipara

IPC International Poliomyelitis Congress; ion pair chromatography; N-phenyl isopropyl carbamate; isopropyl chlorophenyl

IPD inflammatory pelvic disease; intermittent peritoneal dialysis; intermittent pigment darkening; Inventory of Psychosocial Development

IPE infectious porcine encephalomyelitis; interstitial pulmonary emphysema

IPEH intravascular papillary endothelial hyperplasia

IPF idiopathic pulmonary fibrosis; infection-potentiating factor

IPG impedance plethysmography

iPGE immunoreactive prostaglandin E

IPH idiopathic portal hypertension; idiopathic pulmonary hemosiderosis; inflammatory papillary hyperplasia; interphalangeal

IPHR inverted polypoid hamartoma of the rectum

IPI interpulse interval

IPIA immunoperoxidase infectivity assay

IPL inner plexiform layer; intrapleural

IPM impulses per minute; inches per minute

IPN infectious pancreatic necrosis [of trout]

IPP inflatable penile prosthesis; intermittent positive pressure

IPPA inspection, palpation, percussion, and auscultation

IPPB intermittent positive-pressure breathing

IPPB-I intermittent positive-pressure breathing–inspiration

IPPI interruption of pregnancy for psychiatric indication

IPPO intermittent positive-pressure inflation with oxygen

IPPR intermittent positive-pressure respiration

IPPV intermittent positive-pressure ventilation

IPQ intimacy potential quotient

i-Pr isopropyl

IPRL isolated perfused rat liver

IPRT interpersonal reaction test

IPS idiopathic postprandial syndrome; infundibular pulmonary stenosis; initial prognostic score; intraperitoneal shock; ischiopubic synchondrosis

ips inches per second

IPSC inhibitory postsynaptic current

IPSP inhibitory postsynaptic potential

IPT immunoperoxidase technique

iPTH immunoreactive parathyroid hormone

IPU inpatient unit

IPV inactivated poliomyelitis vaccine; infectious pustular vaginitis; infectious pustular vulvovaginitis

IQ intelligence quotient

IQ&S iron, quinine, and strychnine

IR drop of voltage across a resistor produced by a current; immune response; immunization rate; immunoreactive; immunoreagent; index of response; inferior rectus [muscle]; infrared; insoluble residue; insulin resistance; internal resistance

I-R Ito-Reenstierna [reaction]

Ir iridium

ir immunoreactive; intrarectal; intrarenal

IRA immunoregulatory alpha-globulin; inactive renin activity

IR-ACTH immunoreactive adrenocorticotropic hormone

IRBBB incomplete right bundle branch block

IRC inspiratory reserve capacity; International Red Cross

IRCA intravascular red cell aggregation

IRCC International Red Cross Committee

IRDS idiopathic respiratory distress syndrome; infant respiratory distress syndrome

IRF idiopathic retroperitoneal fibrosis

IRG immunoreactive glucagon

IRGH immunoreactive growth hormone

IRGl immunoreactive glucagon

IRH Institute for Research in Hypnosis; Institute of Religion and Health

IRHCS immunoradioassayable human chorionic somatomammotropin
IRhGH immunoreactive human growth hormone
IRI immunoreactive insulin; insulin resistance index
IRIA indirect radioimmunoassay
IRIg insulin-reactive immunoglobulin
IRIS interleukin regulation of immune system; International Research Information Service
IRM innate releasing mechanism; Institute of Rehabilitation Medicine
IRMA immunoradiometric assay; intra-retinal microvascular abnormalities
iRNA immune ribonucleic acid; information ribonucleic acid
IROS ipsilateral routing of signal
IRP immunoreactive plasma; immunoreactive proinsulin
Irr irradiation; irritation
IRRD Institute for Research in Rheumatic Diseases
irreg irregularity, irregular
irrig irrigation, irrigate
IRS infrared spectrophotometry; International Rhinologic Society
IRSA idiopathic refractory sideroblastic anemia
IRT immunoreactive trypsin;
interresponse time
IRTU integrating regulatory transcription unit
IRU industrial rehabilitation unit; interferon reference unit
IRV inspiratory reserve volume; inverse-ratio ventilation
IS immediate sensitivity; immune serum; immunosuppression; incentive spirometer; infant size; information system; insertion sequence; in situ; intercellular space; intercostal space; intracardial shunt; intraspinal; intrasplenic; invalided from service
Is incision superius
is in situ; island; islet
ISA Instrument Society of America; intrinsic simulating activity; intrinsic sympathomimetic activity; iodinated serum albumin
ISADH inappropriate secretion of antidiuretic hormone
ISBI International Society for Burn Injuries

ISBP International Society for Biochemical Pharmacology
ISBT International Society for Blood Transfusion
ISC immunoglobulin-secreting cells; insoluble collagen; International Society of Cardiology; International Society of Chemotherapy; inter-shift coordination; interstitial cell; irreversibly sickled cell
ISCLT International Society for Clinical Laboratory Technology
ISCM International Society of Cybernetic Medicine
ISCN International System for Human Cytogenetic Nomenclature
ISCP International Society of Comparative Pathology
ISD immunosuppressive drug; Information Services Division; inhibited sexual desire; isosorbide dinitrate
ISDN isosorbide dinitrate
ISE inhibited sexual excitement; International Society of Endocrinology; International Society of Endoscopy; ion-selective electrode
ISEK International Society of Electromyographic Kinesiology
ISF interstitial fluid
ISFV interstitial fluid volume
ISG immune serum globulin
ISGE International Society of Gastroenterology
ISH icteric serum hepatitis; International Society of Hematology
ISI infarct size index; injury severity index; Institute for Scientific Information; interstimulus interval
ISKDC International Study of Kidney Diseases in Childhood
ISL interspinous ligament
ISM International Society of Microbiologists
ISMED International Society on Metabolic Eye Disorders
ISMH International Society of Medical Hydrology
ISMHC International Society of Medical Hydrology and Climatology
ISN International Society of Nephrology; International Society of Neurochemistry
ISO International Standards Organization
iso isoproterenol
isol isolation, isolated
isom isometric

ISP distance between iliac spines; intraspinal; isoproterenol
ISPO International Society for Prosthetics and Orthotics
ISPT interspecies ovum penetration test
isq unchanged [Lat. *in status quo*]
ISR information storage and retrieval; Institute for Sex Research; Institute of Surgical Research
ISRM International Society of Reproductive Medicine
ISS Index-Injury Severity Score; International Society of Surgery; ion-scattering spectroscopy; ion surface scattering
ISSN International Standard Serial Number
IST insulin sensitivity test; insulin shock therapy; International Society on Toxicology
ISTD International Society of Tropical Dermatology
ISU International Society of Urology
I-sub inhibitor substance
ISW interstitial water
ISY intrasynovial
IT immunological test; implantation test; inhalation test; inhalation therapy; intentional tremor; intradermal test; intratesticular; intrathecal; intratracheal; intratracheal tube; intratumoral; isomeric transition
I/T intensity/duration
ITA International Tuberculosis Association
ITC imidazolyl-thioguanine chemotherapy; Interagency Testing Committee
ITc International Table calorie
ITE insufficient therapeutic effect; in the ear; intrapulmonary interstitial emphysema
ITFS iliotibial tract friction syndrome
ITh intrathecal
ITI intertrial interval
ITLC instant thin-layer chromatography
ITM improved Thayer-Martin [medium]; Israel turkey meningoencephalitis
ITP idiopathic thrombocytopenic purpura; immunogenic thrombocytopenic purpura; inosine triphosphate; islet-cell tumor of the pancreas; isotachophoresis
ITPA Illinois Test of Psycholinguistic Abilities
ITR intraocular tension recorder; intratracheal

ITT insulin tolerance test
ITU intensive therapy unit
IU immunizing unit; international unit; intrauterine; in utero
iu infectious unit
IUA intrauterine adhesions
IUB International Union of Biochemistry
IUBS International Union of Biological Sciences
IUC idiopathic ulcerative colitis
IUCD intrauterine contraceptive device
IUD intrauterine death; intrauterine device
IUDR idoxuridine
IUFB intrauterine foreign body
IUGR intrauterine growth rate; intrauterine growth retardation
IU/l international units per liter
IUM intrauterine [fetus] malnourished; intrauterine membrane
IU/min international units per minute
IUP intrauterine pregnancy; intrauterine pressure
IUPAC International Union of Pure and Applied Chemistry
IUPD intrauterine pregnancy delivered
IUPHAR International Union of Pharmacology
IUPS International Union of Physiological Sciences
IURES International Union of Reticuloendothelial Societies
IUT intrauterine transfusion
IUVDD International Union against Venereal Diseases and the Treponematoses
IV interventricular; intervertebral; intravascular; intravenous; intraventricular; invasive; iodine value; Roman numeral four; symbol for class 4 controlled substances
IVAP in-vivo adhesive platelet
IVB intraventricular block
IVBC intravascular blood coagulation
IVC inferior vena cava; inspiratory vital capacity; intravascular coagulation; intravenous cholangiogram, intravenous cholangiography; intraventricular catheter
IVCC intravascular consumption coagulopathy
IVCD intraventricular conduction defect
IVCP inferior vena cava pressure

IVCT inferior vena cava thrombosis; intravenously enhanced computed tomography

IVCV inferior vena cavography

IVD intervertebral disk

IVF interventricular foramen; intravascular fluid; in vitro fertiliztion

IVGTT intravenous glucose tolerance test

IVH intravenous hyperalimentation; intraventricular hemorrhage

IVJC intervertebral joint complex

IVM intravascular mass

IVN intravenous nutrition

IVP intravenous push; intravenous pyelogram, intravenous pyelography

IVPB intravenous piggyback

IVPF isovolume pressure flow curve

IVR idioventricular rhythm; intravaginal ring

IVS inappropriate vasopressin secretion; intervening sequence; interventricular septum

IVSA International Veterinary Students Association

IVSD interventricular septal defect

IVSS intravenous soluset

IVT intravenous transfusion; intraventricular; isovolumetric time

IVTTT intravenous tolbutamide tolerance test

IVU intravenous urography

IVV intravenous vasopressin

IWGMT International Working Group on Mycobacterial Taxonomy

IWL insensible water loss

IWMI inferior wall myocardial infarct

i (Xq) long arm isochromosome

IZS insulin zinc suspension

–J–

J dynamic movement of inertia; electric current density; joint; joule; journal; juvenile; juxtapulmonary-capillary receptor; magnetic polarization; a polypeptide chain in polymeric immunoglobulins; a reference point following the QRS complex, at the beginning of the ST segment, in electrocardiography; sound intensity

j jaundice [rat]

JA juxta-articular

JAI juvenile amaurotic idiocy

JAS Jenkins Activity Survey

jaund jaundice

JBE Japanese B encephalitis

J/C joules per coulomb

JCA juvenile chronic arthritis

JCAE Joint Committee on Atomic Energy

JCAH Joint Commission on Accreditation of Hospitals

JCAI Joint Council of Allergy and Immunology

JCC Joint Committee on Contraception

JCF juvenile calcaneal fracture

JCML juvenile chronic myelogenous leukemia

JCP juvenile chronic polyarthritis

jct junction

JCV Jamestown Canyon virus

JD juvenile diabetes

JDF Juvenile Diabetes Foundation

JDM juvenile diabetes mellitus

JE Japanese encephalitis

JEE Japanese equine encephalitis

JEMBEC agar plates for transporting cultures of gonococci

jej jejunum

jentac breakfast [Lat. *jentaculum*]

JF joint fluid

JFET junction field effect transistor

JG juxtaglomerular

JGA juxtaglomerular apparatus

JGC juxtaglomerular cell

JGI juxtaglomerular granulation index

JH juvenile hormone

JHA juvenile hormone analog

JHMO Junior Hospital Medical Officer

JJ jaw jerk

J/kg joules per kilogram

JMS junior medical student

JNA Jena Nomina Anatomica

JND just noticeable difference

jnt joint

JOD juvenile-onset diabetes

JODM juvenile-onset diabetes mellitus

JPS joint position sense

JRA juvenile rheumatoid arthritis

J/s joules per second

JSV Jerry-Slough virus

J/T joules per tesla
jt joint
Ju jugale
JUA joint underwriting association
juv juvenile
JV jugular vein
JVD jugular venous distention
JVP jugular vein pulse; jugular venous pressure
juxt near [Lat. *juxta*]

–K–

K absolute zero; capsular antigen [Ger. *Kapsel*, capsule]; cathode; coefficient of heat transfer; in electroencephalography, a burst of diphasic slow waves in response to stimuli during sleep; electrostatic capacity; equilibrium constant; ionization constant; kanamycin; Kell factor; kelvin; kerma; kidney; killer [cell]; kilo-; kinetic energy; lysine; modulus of compression; the number 1024 in computer core memory; potassium [Lat. *kalium*]; vitamin K

°K degree on the Kelvin scale
K_1 phytonadione
17-K 17-ketosteroid
k Boltzmann constant; constant; kilo; kilohm
κ see *kappa*
KA alkaline phosphatase; kainic acid; keto acid; ketoacidosis; King-Armstrong [unit]
K/A ketogenic/antiketogenic ratio
Ka cathode
K_a acid ionization constant
kA kiloampere
ka cathode
KAAD kerosene, alcohol, acetic acid, and dioxane
KAF conglutinogen-activating factor; killer-assisting factor
KAFO knee-ankle-foot orthosis
KAP knowledge, aptitude, and practice
κ Greek letter *kappa*; magnetic susceptibility
kappa a light chain of human immunoglobulins [chain]

KAT kanamycin acetyltransferase
kat katal
kat/l katals per liter
KAU King-Armstrong unit
KB human oral epidermoid carcinoma cells; Kashin-Bek [disease]; ketone body; knee brace
K_b base ionization constant
kb kilobase
KBG syndrome of multiple abnormalities designated with the original patient's initials
kbp kilobase pair
kBq kilobecquerel
KBS Klüver-Bucy syndrome
KC cathodal closing
kC kilocoulomb
kc kilocycle
K Cal, Kcal, kcal kilocalorie
KCC cathodal closing contraction; Kulchitzky cell carcinoma
KCG kinetocardiogram
kCi kilocurie
kcps kilocycles per second
KCS keratoconjunctivitis sicca
kc/s kilocycles per second
KCT cathodal closing tetanus
KD cathodal duration; Kawasaki disease; killed
K_d dissociation constant; partition coefficient
kd, kDa kilodalton
KDA known drug allergies
KDO ketodeoxyoctonate
KDT cathodal duration tetanus
kdyn kilodyne
KE Kendall compound E; kinetic energy
K_e exchangeable body potassium
KERV Kentucky equine respiratory virus
keV kiloelectron volt
KF Kenner-fecal medium; kidney function
kf flocculation rate in antigen-antibody reaction
KFAB kidney-fixing antibody
KFD Kyasanur forest disease
KFS Klippel-Feil syndrome
kg kilogram
kg-cal kilocalorie
kg/cm² kilogram per square centimeter
KG-1 Koeffler Golde-1 cell line

kgf kilogram-force
kg/l kilograms per liter
kg-m kilogram-meter
kg/m kilograms per meter
kg·m/s² kilogram-meter per second squared
Kgn kininogen
kgps kilograms per second
KGS ketogenic steroid
17-KGS 17-ketogenic steroid
KH Krebs-Henseleit [buffer]
K24H potassium, urinary 24-hour
KHB Krebs-Henseleit buffer
KHb potassium hemoglobinate
KHD kinky hair disease
KHF Korean hemorrhagic fever
KHM keratoderma hereditaria mutilans
KHN Knoop hardness number
KHP King's Honorary Physician
KHS King's Honorary Surgeon; kinky hair syndrome; Krebs-Henseleit solution
kHz kilohertz
KI karyopyknotic index; Krönig's isthmus
KIA Kligler iron agar
KIC ketoisocaproate
KICB killed intracellular bacteria
KID keratitis, ichthyosis, and deafness [syndrome]
kilo kilogram
KIMSV, Ki-MSV Kirsten murine sarcoma virus
KISS saturated solution of potassium iodide
KIU kallikrein inactivation unit
KJ knee jerk
kJ kilojoule
kj knee jerk
KK knee kick
kkat kilokatal
KL kidney lobe; Klebs-Loeffler [bacillus]
kl kiloliter
Klebs *Klebsiella*
KLH keyhole limpet hemocyanin
KLS kidneys, liver, and spleen; Kreuzbein's lipomatous syndrome
KM kanamycin
km kilometer
km² square kilometer
K$_m$ Michaelis-Menten constant
kMc kilomegacycle
kMc/s kilomegacycles per second

KMEF keratin, myosin, epidermin, and fibrin
kmps kilometers per second
KMV killed measles virus vaccine
kN kilonewton
kn knee
KNRK Kirsten sarcoma virus in normal rat kidney
KO keep open; killed organism; knock out
KOC cathodal opening contraction
k Ω kilohm
KP Kaufmann-Peterson [base]; keratitic precipitate; keratitis punctata; killed parenteral [vaccine]
K-P Kaiser-Permanente [diet]
kPa kilopascal
kPa·s/l kilopascal seconds per liter
KPI karyopyknotic index
KPR key pulse rate
KPTT kaolin partial thromboplastin time
KR key-ridge; Kopper Reppart [medium]
Kr krypton
kR kiloroentgen
KRB Krebs-Ringer buffer
KRBG Krebs-Ringer bicarbonate buffer with glucose
KRP Kolmer test with Reiter protein [antigen]; Krebs-Ringer phosphate
KRRS kinetic resonance Raman spectroscopy
KS Kaposi's sarcoma; Kawasaki syndrome; keratan sulfate; ketosteroid; Klinefelter syndrome; Korsakoff syndrome; Kveim-Siltzbach [test]
17-KS 17-ketosteroid
ks kilosecond
KSC cathodal closing contraction
K$_{sp}$ solubility product
KST cathodal closing tetanus
KT kidney transplantation, kidney transplant
KTI kallikrein-trypsin inhibitor
KTSA Kahn test of symbol arrangement
KTW, KTWS Klippel-Trenaunay-Weber [syndrome]
KU kallikrein unit; Karmen unit
Ku kurchatovium; Peltz factor
KUB kidneys and upper bladder; [x-ray examination of the] kidneys, ureter, and bladder
KV killed vaccine
kV, kv kilovolt

kVA kilovolt-ampere
kvar kilovar
KVBA kanamycin-vancomycin blood agar
kVcp, kvcp kilovolt constant potential
KVE Kaposi's varicelliform eruption
KVLBA kanamycin-vancomycin laked blood agar
KVO keep vein open
kVp, kvp kilovolt peak
KW Keith-Wagener [ophthalmoscopic finding]; Kimmelstiel-Wilson
kW, kw kilowatt
KWB Keith-Wagener-Barker [classification]
kW·h, kW-hr, kw-hr kilowatt-hour
K wire Kirschner wire

–L–

L angular momentum; Avogadro's constant; boundary [Lat. *limes*]; coefficient of induction; diffusion length; inductance; *Lactobacillus*; lambda; lambert; latent heat; latex; Latin; left; *Leishmania*; length; lente insulin; lethal; leucine; levo-; ligament; light; light sense; lingual; liter; liver; low; lower; lumbar; luminance; the outer membrane layer of the cell wall of gram-negative bacteria [layer]; radiance; self-inductance; threshold [Lat. *limen*]
L-variant a defective bacterial variant that can multiply on hypertonic medium
L_0 limes zero [*limes nul*]
L_+ *limes tod*
L1, L2, L3, L4, L5 first, second, third, fourth, and fifth lumbar vertebrae
L/3 lower third
l azimuthal quantum number; left; length; lethal; levorotatory; liter; long; longitudinal; specific latent heat
Λ see *lambda*
λ see *lambda*
LA lactic acid; late abortion; late antigen; latex agglutination; left angle; left arm; left atrium; left auricle; leucine aminopeptidase; leukemia antigen; linguo-axial; lobuloalveolar; local anesthesia; long-

acting [drug]; low anxiety; lupus anticoagulant; lymphocyte antibody
L&A light and accommodation
LA50 total body surface area of burn that will kill 50% of patients (lethal area)
La labial; lambda; lambert; lanthanum
la according to the art [Lat. *lege artis*]
LAA leukemia-associated antigen; leukocyte ascorbic acid
LAAO L-amino acid oxidase
lab laboratory
LAC La Crosse [virus]; linguoaxiocervical; lung adenocarcinoma cells
LaC labiocervical
lac laceration
LACN local area communications network
lacr lacrimal
lact lactate; lactating, lactation; lactic
lact hyd lactalbumin hydrolysate
LAD lactic acid dehydrogenase; left anterior descending [artery]; left axis deviation; lipoamide dehydrogenase
LADA left acromio-dorso-anterior [position]
LADD lacrimoauriculodentodigital [syndrome]
LADH lactic acid dehydrogenase; liver alcohol dehydrogenase
LAD-MIN left axis deviation, minimal
LADP left acromio-dorso-posterior [position]
LAE left atrial enlargement
LAEDV left atrial volume in end diastole
LAEI left atrial emptying index
LAESV left atrial volume in end systole
laev left [Lat. *laevus*]
LAF laminar air flow; Latin American female; lymphocyte-activating factor
LAG linguo-axiogingival; lymphangiogram
LaG labiogingival
lag flask [Lat. *lagena*]
LAH lactalbumin hydrolysate; left anterior hemiblock; left atrial hypertrophy; Licentiate of Apothecaries Hall
LAHV leukocyte-associated herpesvirus
LAI latex particle agglutination inhibition; leukocyte adherence inhibition
LaI labioincisal
LAIT latex agglutination inhibition test
LAL left axillary line; *Limulus* amebocyte lysate

LaL labiolingual

LALI lymphocyte antibody-lymphocytolytic interaction

LAM Latin American male; lymphangioleiomyomatosis

lam laminectomy

λ Greek lower case letter *lambda*; craniometric point; decay constant; an immunoglobulin light chain; mean free path; microliter; thermal conductivity; wavelength

LAMMA laser microprobe mass analyzer

LANV left atrial neovascularization

LAO left anterior oblique; Licentiate of the Art of Obstetrics

LAP laparotomy; left atrial pressure; leucine aminopeptidase; leukocyte alkaline phosphatase; low atmospheric pressure; lyophilized anterior pituitary

lap laparotomy

lapid of stone [Lat. *lapideus*]

LAR laryngology; left arm recumbent

lar left arm reclining

LARC leukocyte automatic recognition computer

Laryngol laryngology

LAS laboratory automation system; lateral amyotrophic sclerosis; left anterior-superior; leucine acetylsalicylate; linear alkylsulfonate; local adaptation syndrome; lymphadenopathy syndrome

LASER light amplification by stimulated emission of radiation

L-ASP L-asparaginase

LASS labile aggregation stimulating substance

LAT lateral; latex agglutination test

Lat Latin

lat lateral

lat admov let it be applied to the side [Lat. *lateri admoveatum*]

LATCH literature attached to charts

lat dol to the painful side [Lat. *lateri dolenti*]

l•atm liter atmosphere

LATS long-acting thyroid stimulator

LATS-P long-acting thyroid stimulator-protector

LATu lobulo-alveolar tumor

LAV lymphadenopathy-associated virus

lav lavoratory

LB left breast; left bundle; leiomyoblastoma; lipid body; live birth; loose body; low back [pain]

L&B left and below

Lb pound force

lb pound [Lat. *libra*]

LBB left bundle branch

LBBB left bundle branch block

LBBsB left bundle branch system block

LBCD left border of cardiac dullness

LBCF Laboratory Branch complement fixation [test]

LBD left border of dullness

LBF *Lactobacillus bulgaricus* factor; limb blood flow; liver blood flow

lbf pound force

lbf-ft pound force foot

LBH length, breadth, height

LBI low serum bound iron

lb/in² pounds per square inch

LBL labeled lymphoblast; lymphoblastic lymphoma

LBM lean body mass; lung basement membrane

LBNP lower body negative pressure

LBO large bowel obstruction

LBP low back pain; low blood pressure

LBPQ Low Back Pain Questionnaire

LBRF louse-borne relapsing fever

LBS low back syndrome

LBSA lipid-bound sialic acid

LBTI lima bean trypsin inhibitor

lb tr pound troy

LBV left brachial vein

LBW low birth weight

LBWI low-birth-weight infant

LBWR lung–body weight ratio

LC Langerhans' cell; late clamped; lecithin cholesterol acyltransferase; lethal concentration; Library of Congress; life care; linguocervical; lipid cytosomes; liquid chromatography; living children; locus ceruleus

LCA left circumflex artery; left coronary artery

LCAO linear combination of atomic orbitals

LCAR late cutaneous anaphylactic reaction

LCAT lecithin cholesterol acyltransferase

LCB Laboratory of Cancer Biology

LCBF local cerebral blood flow

LCC lactose coliform count; left circumflex coronary (artery); liver cell carcinoma

LCCA leukoclastic angiitis

LCCME Liaison Committee on Continuing Medical Education

LCCS lower cervical cesarean section

LCCSCT large cell calcifying Sertoli cell tumor

LCD coal tar solution [liquor carbonis detergens]; liquid crystal diode; localized collagen dystrophy

LCF lymphocyte culture fluid

LCFA long-chain fatty acid

LCGME Liaison Committee on Graduate Medical Education

LCGU local cerebral glucose utilization

LCh Licentiate in Surgery

LCL Levinthal-Coles-Lillie [body]; lower confidence limit; lymphoblastoid cell line; lymphocytic lymphosarcoma; lymphoid cell line

LCM left costal margin; leukocyte-conditioned medium; lymphatic choriomeningitis; lymphocytic choriomeningitis

LCME Liaison Committee on Medical Education

l/cm H_2O liters per centimeter of water

LCMV lymphocytic choriomeningitis virus

LCN left caudate nucleus

LCO low cardiac output

LCOS low cardiac output syndrome

LCP long-chain polysaturated [fatty acid]

LCPS Licentiate of the College of Physicians and Surgeons

LCS life care service; low constant suction; low continuous suction

LCSB Liaison Committee for Specialty Boards

LCT long-chain triglyceride; lymphocytotoxicity; lymphocytotoxin

LCTA lymphocytotoxic antibody

LCV lecithovitellin

LCx left circumflex artery

LD labor and delivery; labyrinthine defect; lactate dehydrogenase; learning disability; learning disorder; left deltoid; Legionnaires' disease; lethal dose; light differentiation; limited disease; linear dichroism; linguodistal; liver disease; living donor; loading dose; Lombard-Dowell [agar]; low density; low dose; lymphocyte-defined; lymphocyte depletion

L-D Leishman-Donovan [body]

L/D light/darkness [ratio]

LD_1 isoenzyme of lactate dehydrogenase found in the heart, erythrocytes, and kidneys

LD_2 isoenzyme of lactate dehydrogenase found in the lungs

LD_3 isoenzyme of lactate dehydrogenase found in the lungs

LD_4 isoenzyme of lactate dehydrogenase found in the liver

LD_5 isoenzyme of lactate dehydrogenase found in the liver and muscles

LD_{50} median infective dose; median lethal dose

$LD_{50/30}$ a dose which is lethal for 50% of the test subjects within 30 days

LD_{100} lethal dose in all exposed subjects

Ld *Leishmania donovani*

LDA left dorso-anterior [fetal position]; linear discriminant analysis; lymphocyte-dependent antibody

LDAR latex direct agglutination reaction

LDB lamb dysentery bacillus; Legionnaires' disease bacillus

LDC lymphoid dendritic cell

LDCC lectin-dependent cellular cytotoxicity

LDCT late distal cortical tubule

LDD late dedifferentiation; light-darkness discrimination

LD-EYA Lombard-Dowell egg yolk agar

LDG lingual developmental groove

LDH lactic dehydrogenase

LDL loudness discomfort level; low density lipoprotein

LDLP low-density lipoprotein

LDM lactate dehydrogenase, muscle

LD-NEYA Lombard-Dowell neomycin egg yolk agar

L-DOPA, L-dopa levodopa, levo–3, 4– dihydroxyphenylalanine

LDP left dorsoposterior [fetal position]

LDS Licentiate in Dental Surgery

LDSc Licentiate in Dental Science

LDUB long double upright brace

LDV lactic dehydrogenase virus; large dense-cored vesicle; laser Doppler velocimetry

LE left ear; left eye; leukoerythrogenic; Long Evans [rat]; lower extremity; lupus erythematosus
LEC leukoencephalitis
LED light-emitting diode; lupus erythematosus disseminatus
LEED low-energy electron diffraction
LEEDS low-energy electron diffraction spectroscopy
LEF lupus erythematosus factor
leg legislation; legal
LeIF leukocyte interferon
LEIS low-energy ion scattering
LEL lowest effect level
LEM lateral eye movement; Leibovitz-Emory medium; leukocyte endogenous mediator
LEMO lowest empty molecular orbital
LEMS Lambert-Eaton myasthenic syndrome
lenit lenitive
LEOPARD lentigines, EKG abnormalities, ocular hypertelorism, pulmonary stenosis, abnormalities of genitalia, retardation of growth, and deafness [syndrome]
LEP lethal effective phase; lipoprotein electrophoresis; low egg passage; lower esophagus
L$_{EPN}$ effective perceived noise level
Leq loudness equivalent
LER lysozomal enzyme release
LERG local electroretinogram
LES Lawrence Experimental Station [agar]; local excitatory state; Locke egg serum; lower esophageal sphincter
les low excitatory state
LESP lower esophageal sphincter pressure
LET linear energy transfer
LEU leucine; leucovorin; leukocyte equivalent unit
Leu leucine
leuc leukocyte
lev light [Lat. *levis*]
LEW Lewis [rat]
l/ext lower extremity
LF labile factor; laryngofissure; Lassa fever; limit of flocculation; low fat [diet]; low forceps
Lf limit of flocculation
lf low frequency

LFA left femoral artery; left fronto-anterior [fetal position]
LFC living female child; low fat and cholesterol [diet]
LFD lactose-free diet; late fetal death; lateral facial dysplasia; least fatal dose; low-fat diet; low forceps delivery
LFER linear free-energy relationship
LFH left femoral hernia
LFL leukocyte feeder layer
LFN lactoferrin
L-[form] a defective bacterial variant that can multiply on hypertonic medium
LFP left frontoposterior [fetal position]
LFPPV low frequency positive pressure ventilation
LFPS Licentiate of the Faculty of Physicians and Surgeons
LFR lymphoid follicular reticulosis
LFT latex flocculation test; left fronto-transverse [fetal position]; liver function test; low-frequency tetanus; low-frequency transduction; low-frequency transfer
LFU lipid fluidity unit
LFV Lassa fever virus
LG laryngectomy; left gluteal; leucyl-glycine; linguogingival; lipoglycopeptide
lg large; leg
LGA large for gestational age
LGB Landry-Guillain-Barré [syndrome]
LGBS Landry-Guillain-Barré syndrome
LGE Langat encephalitis
LGF lateral giant fiber
LGH lactogenic hormone
LGI large glucagon immunoreactivity
LGL large granular leukocyte; large granular lymphocyte; Lown-Ganong-Levin [syndrome]
LGMD limb-girdle muscular dystrophy
LGN lateral geniculate nucleus
LGS limb girdle syndrome
LGT late generalized tuberculosis
LGV lymphogranuloma venereum
LGVHD lethal graft-versus-host disease
LgX lymphogranulomatosis X
LH lateral hypothalamic [syndrome]; left hand; left hemisphere; left hyperphoria; lower half; lues hereditaria; luteinizing hormone
LHBV left heart blood volume
LHC left hypochondrium; Local Health Council

LHF left heart failure
LHG localized hemolysis in gel
LHI lipid hydrocarbon inclusion
LHL left hepatic lobe
LHM lysuride hydrogen maleate
LHMP Life Health Monitoring Program
LHR leukocyte histamine release
l-hr lumen-hour
LHRF luteinizing hormone–releasing factor
LHRH, LH-RH luteinizing hormone–releasing hormone
LHS left hand side; left heart strain; left heelstrike
LHT left hypertropia
LI labeling index; large intestine; leptospirosis icterohaemorrhagica; linguoincisal; low impulsiveness
Li a blood group system; labrale inferius; lithium
LIA Laser Institute of America; leukemia-associated inhibitory activity; lock-in amplifier; lymphocyte-induced angiogenesis; lysine iron agar
LIAFI late infantile amaurotic familial idiocy
lib a pound [Lat. *libra*]
LIBC latent iron-binding capacity
LIC limiting isorrheic concentration
Lic licentiate
LICA left internal carotid artery
LICM left intercostal margin
LicMed Licentiate in Medicine
LID late immunoglobulin deficiency
LIF left iliac fossa; leukocyte inhibitory factor; leukocytosis-inducing factor
LIFO last in, first out
lig ligament
LIH left inguinal hernia
LIHA low impulsiveness, high anxiety
LILA low impulsiveness, low anxiety
lim limit, limited
LIMA left internal mammary artery
Linim liniment
LIP lithium-induced polydipsia; lymphoid interstitial pneumonitis
Lip lipoate
lipoMM lipomyelomeningocele
LIQ low inner quadrant
liq liquid [Lat. *liquor*]
liq dr liquid dram
liq oz liquid ounce
liq pt liquid pint

liq qt liquid quart
LIRBM liver, iron, red bone marrow
LIS laboratory information system; lateral intercellular space; lobular *in situ*; low intermittent suction; low ionic strength
LISP List Processing Language
LISS low-ionic-strength saline
liv live, living
LIV-BP leucine, isoleucine, and valine-binding protein
LIVEN linear inflammatory verrucous epidermal nevus
LJI List of Journals Indexed
LJM limited joint mobility; Lowenstein-Jensen medium
LK left kidney
LKKS liver, kidneys, spleen
LKS liver, kidneys, and spleen
LKV laked kanamycin vancomycin [agar]
LL large lymphocyte; left leg; left lower; left lung; lipoprotein lipase; lower eyelid; lower limb; lower lobe; lumbar length; lymphoid leukemia; lysolecithin
L lat left lateral
LLBCD left lower border of cardiac dullness
LLC liquid-liquid chromatography; lymphocytic leukemia
LLC-MK1 rhesus monkey kidney cells
LLC-MK2 rhesus monkey kidney cells
LLC-MK3 *Cercopithecus* monkey kidney cells
LLC-RK1 rabbit kidney cells
LLD left lateral decubitus [muscle]; long-lasting depolarization
LLE left lower extremity
LLF Laki-Lóránd factor; left lateral femoral
LLL left lower eyelid; left lower lobe
LLM localized leukocyte mobilization
LLO *Legionella*-like organism
LLP late luteal phase; long-lasting potentiation
LLQ left lower quadrant
LLR left lateral rectus [muscle]
LLS lazy leukocyte syndrome
LLT lysolecithin
LLV lymphatic leukemia virus
LLV-F lymphatic leukemia virus, Friend associated
LLVP left lateral ventricular preexcitation

LM lactic acid mineral [medium]; laryngeal muscle; lateral malleolus; legal medicine; lemniscus medialis; Licentiate in Medicine; Licentiate in Midwifery; light microscopy, light microscope, light microscopy; light minimum; lingual margin; linguomesial; lipid mobilization; liquid membrane; longitudinal muscle; lower motor [neuron]

Lm *Listeria monocytogenes*

lm lumen

LMA left mento-anterior [fetal position]; liver cell membrane autoantibody

LMB leiomyoblastoma

LMBB Laurence-Moon-Bardet-Biedl [syndrome]

LMBS Laurence-Moon-Biedl syndrome

LMC lateral motor column; left main coronary [artery]; left middle cerebral [artery]; living male child; lymphocyte-mediated cytotoxicity; lymphomyeloid complex

LMCAD left main coronary artery disease

LMCC Licentiate of the Medical Council of Canada

LMD lipid-moiety modified derivative; local medical doctor; low molecular weight dextran

LMDX low-molecular-weight dextran

LMed&Ch Licentiate in Medicine and Surgery

LMF lymphocyte mitogenic factor

lm/ft^2 lumens per square foot

LMH lipid-mobilizing hormone

lm·h lumen hour

LMI leukocyte migration inhibition

LMIF leukocyte migration inhibition factor

l/min liters per minute

LML large and medium lymphocytes; left mediolateral

LMM *Lactobacillus* maintenance medium; lentigo maligna melanoma; light meromyosin

lm/m^2 lumens per square meter

LMN lower motor neuron

LMO localized molecular orbital

LMP last menstrual period; left mento-posterior [fetal position]

LMR left medial rectus [muscle]

LMRCP Licentiate in Midwifery of the Royal College of Physicians

LMS Licentiate in Medicine and Surgery

lm·s lumen-second

LMSSA Licentiate in Medicine and Surgery of the Society of Apothecaries

LMT left mentotransverse [fetal position]

LMV larva migrans visceralis

LMW low molecular weight

lm/W lumens per watt

LMWD low-molecular-weight dextran

LN lipoid nephrosis; lupus nephritis; lymph node

L/N letter/numerical [system]

ln natural logarithm

LNAA large neutral amino acid

LNC lymph node cell

LNE lymph node enlargement

LNH large number hypothesis

LNL lymph node lymphocyte

LNLS linear-nonlinear least squares

LNMP last normal menstrual period

LNPF lymph node permeability factor

LNS lateral nuclear stratum; Lesch-Nyhan syndrome

LO linguo-occlusal

LOA leave of absence; left occipito-anterior [fetal position]

LOC laxative of choice; liquid organic compound; loss of consciousness

lo cal low calorie

lo calc low calcium

loc dol to the painful spot [Lat. *loco dolenti*]

LOD line of duty

log logarithm

LOH loop of Henle

LOI limit of impurities

LOL left occipitolateral [fetal position]

LOM limitation of motion; loss of motion

LOMSA left otitis media suppurativa acuta

LOMSCh left otitis media suppurativa chronica

long longitudinal

LOP leave on pass; left occipitoposterior [fetal position]

LOPS length of patient's stay

LOQ lower outer quadrant

Lord lordosis, lordotic

LOS length of stay; Licentiate in Obstetrical Science; low cardiac output syndrome; lower [o]esophageal sphincter

LOS(P) lower [o]esophageal sphincter (pressure)

LOT lateral olfactory tract; left occipito-transverse [fetal position]

lot lotion

LP labile peptide; labile protein; laboratory procedure; lactic peroxidase; laryngopharyngeal; latent period, latency period; leukocyte poor; leukocytic pyrogen; lichen planus; light perception; linguopulpal; lipoprotein; low potency; low power; low pressure; low protein; lumbar puncture; lumboperitoneal; lymphoid plasma; lymphomatoid papulosis

L/P lactate/pyruvate [ratio]

Lp sound pressure level

LPA left pulmonary artery

LPAM L-phenylalanine mustard

LPC late positive component; lysophosphatidylcholine

LPCM low placed conus medullaris

LPCT late proximal cortical tubule

LPDF lipoprotein-deficient fraction

LPE lipoprotein electrophoresis

LPF leukocytosis-promoting factor; localized plaque formation; low power field; lymphocytosis-promoting factor

LPH left posterior hemiblock; lipotropic pituitary hormone

LPI left posterior-inferior

LPL lipoprotein lipase

LPM liver plasma membrane

lpm liters per minute

LPN Licensed Practical Nurse

LPO left posterior oblique; light perception only

LPS levator palpebrae superioris [muscle]; lipase; lipopolysaccharide

lps liters per second

LPSR lipopolysaccharide receptor

LPT lipotropin

LPV left pulmonary veins

LPVP left posterior ventricular preexcitation

LPW lateral pharyngeal wall

lpw lumens per watt

LPX, Lp-X lipoprotein-X

LQ longevity quotient; lordosis quotient

LQTS long QT syndrome

LR labeled release; laboratory references; laboratory report; labor room; lactated Ringer's [solution]; latency reaction; latency relaxation; lateral rectus [muscle]; light reaction; light reflex; limit of reachon

L/R left-to-right [ratio]

L&R left and right

Lr lawrencium; Limes reacting dose of diphtheria toxin

LRC lower rib cage

LRCP Licentiate of the Royal College of Physicians

LRCS Licentiate of the Royal College of Surgeons

LRCSE Licentiate of the Royal College of Surgeons, Edinburgh

LRD living related donor

LRDT living related donor transplant

LRE lymphoreticuloendothelial

LRF latex and resorcinol formaldehyde; liver residue factor; luteinizing hormone–releasing factor

LRH luteinizing hormone–releasing hormone

LRI lower respiratory tract illness; lower respiratory tract infection; lymphocyte reactivity index

LROP lower radicular obstetrical paralysis

LRP long-range planning

LRQ lower right quadrant

LRR labyrinthine righting reflex

LRS lactated Ringer's solution; lateral recess syndrome

LRSF lactating rat serum factor; liver regenerating serum factor

LRSS late respiratory systemic syndrome

LRT local radiation therapy; lower respiratory tract

LRTI lower respiratory tract illness; lower respiratory tract infection

LS lateral suspensor; left sacrum; left side; legally separated; leiomyosarcoma; Licentiate in Surgery; life sciences; light sensitivity, light-sensitive; liminal sensation; liver and spleen; low-sodium [diet]; lumbar spine; lumbosacral; lymphosarcoma

L/S lactase/sucrase ratio; lecithin/sphingomyelin ratio

LSA left sacro-anterior [fetal position]; leukocyte-specific activity; lichen sclerosus et atrophicus; lymphosarcoma

LSANA leukocyte-specific antinuclear antibody

LSA/RCS lymphosarcoma–reticulum cell sarcoma
LSB least significant bit; left sternal border; long spike burst
LSC late systolic click; left side colon cancer; lichen simplex chronicus; liquid scintillation counting; liquid-solid chromatography
LScA left scapulo-anterior [fetal position]
LSCL lymphosarcoma cell leukemia
LScP left scapulo-posterior [fetal position]
LSCS lower segment cesarean section
LSD least significant difference; least significant digit; low-sodium diet; lysergic acid diethylamide
LSD-25 lysergic acid diethylamide
LSF lymphocyte-stimulating factor
LSG labial salivary gland
LSH lutein-stimulating hormone; lymphocyte-stimulating hormone
LSHTM London School of Hygiene and Tropical Medicine
LSI large-scale integration; lumbar spine index
LSK liver, spleen, kidneys
LSKM liver-spleen-kidney-megalia
LSL left sacrolateral [fetal position]
LSM late systolic murmur; lymphocyte separation medium; lysergic acid morpholide
LSN left substantia nigra
LSO lateral superior olive
LSP left sacroposterior [fetal position]
LSp life span
L-Spar asparaginase (Elspar)
LSSA lipid-soluble secondary antioxidant
LSR lanthanide shift reagent
LST left sacrotransverse [fetal position]
LSTL laparoscopic tubal ligation
LSU lactose-saccharose-urea [agar]
LSV left subclavian vein
LSVC left superior vena cava
LSWA large amplitude slow wave activity
LT heat-labile toxin; left; left thigh; less than; lethal time; leukotriene; levothyroxine; light; long-term; low temperature; lymphocytotoxin; lymphotoxin
L-T3 L-triiodothyronine
L-T4 L-thyroxine

lt left; light; low tension
LTA leukotriene A; lipoate transacetylase; lipotechoic acid
LTAS lead tetra-acetate Schiff
LTB laryngotracheobronchitis; leukotriene B
LTC large transformed cell; leukotriene C; long-term care
LTCF long-term care facility
LTD Laron-type dwarfism; leukotriene D
LTE leukotriene E
LT-ECG long-term electrocardiography
LTF lipotropic factor; lymphocyte-transforming factor
LTH lactogenic hormone; local tumor hyperthermia; low temperature holding; luteotropic hormone
lt lat left lateral
LTM long-term memory
LTP long-term potentiation
LTPP lipothiamide pyrophosphate
LTR long terminal repeats
LTT limited treadmill test; lymphocyte transformation test
LTW Leydig-cell tumor in Wistar rat
LU left upper [limb]; lytic unit
Lu lutetium
L&U lower and upper
LUE left upper extremity
LUF luteinized unruptured follicle
LUFS luteinized unruptured follicle syndrome
LUL left upper eyelid; left upper lobe
lumb lumbar
LUMO lowest unoccupied molecular orbital
LUO left ureteral orifice
LUOQ left upper outer quadrant
LUQ left upper quadrant
LUSB left upper sternal border
lut yellow [Lat. *luteus*]
LUV large unilamellar vesicle
LV lateral ventricle; lecithovitellin; left ventricle, left ventricular; leucovorin; leukemia virus; live vaccine; live virus; lumbar vertebra
Lv brightness or luminance
lv leave
LVA left ventricular aneurysm
LVAD left ventricular assist device
LVDd left ventricular dimension in end-diastole

LVDI left ventricular dimension
LVDP left ventricular diastolic pressure
LVE left ventricular enlargement
LVED left ventricular end-diastole
LVEDD left ventricular end-diastolic diameter
LVEDP left ventricular end-diastolic pressure
LVEDV left ventricular end-diastolic volume
LVEF left ventricular ejection fraction
LVET left ventricular ejection time
LVETI left ventricular ejection time index
LVF left ventricular failure; left visual field; low-voltage fast; low-voltage foci
LVFP left ventricular filling pressure
LVH large vessel hematocrit; left ventricular hypertrophy
LVL left vastus lateralis
LVLG left ventrolateral gluteal
LVMF left ventricular minute flow
LVN lateral ventricular nerve; lateral vestibular nucleus; Licensed Visiting Nurse; Licensed Vocational Nurse
LVP large volume parenteral [infusion]; left ventricular pressure; lysine-vasopressin
LVPFR left ventricular peak filling rate
LVPW left ventricular posterior wall
LVS left ventricular strain
LVSEMI left ventricular subendocardial ischemia
LVSP left ventricular systolic pressure
LVST lateral vestibulospinal tract
LVSV left ventricular stroke volume
LVSW left ventricular stroke work
LVSWI left ventricular stroke work index
LVT lysine vasotonin
LVV left ventricular volume
LVW left ventricular work
LVWI left ventricular work index
LVWT left ventricular wall thickness
LW lacerating wound; Lee-White [method]
L&W, L/W living and well
Lw lawrencium
LWCT Lee-White clotting time
LX local irradiation
lx lux
LXT left exotopia

LY lactoalbumin and yeastolate [medium]
Ly a T-cell antigen used for grouping T-lymphocytes into different classes
LYDMA lymphocyte-detected membrane antigen
LYG lymphomatoid granulomatosis
lym, lymph lymphocyte, lymphocytic
LyNeF lytic nephritic factor
lyo lyophilized
LYP lactose, yeast, and peptone [agar]
LYS, Lys lysine; lytes electrolytes
LySLk lymphoma syndrome leukemia
LZM lysozyme

–M–

M a blood group in the MNSs blood group system; chin [Lat. *mentum*]; concentration in moles per liter; death [Lat. *mors*]; dullness [of sound] [Lat. *mutitas*]; handful [Lat. *manipulus*]; macerate, macerated [Lat. *macerare*]; macroglobulin; magnetization; male; malignant; married; masculine; mass; massage; maternal contribution; matrix; mature; maximum; mean; median; mediator; medical, medicine; mega-; megohm; memory; mental; mesial; metabolite; meter; methionine; methotrexate; *Micrococcus*; *Microspora*; minim; minute; mix, mixed, mixture; molar [permanent tooth]; molar [solution]; molarity; molecular; moment of force; monkey; monocyte; month; morgan; morphine; mother; motile; mouse; mucoid [colony]; multipara; murmur [cardiac]; muscle; muscular response to an electrical stimulation of its motor nerve [wave]; *Mycobacterium*; *Mycoplasm*; myeloma or macroglobulinemia [component]; myopia; strength of pole; thousand [Lat. *mille*]
M₁ mitral first [sound]; myeloblast; slight dullness
M₂ dose per square meter of body surface; marked dullness; promyelocyte
M₃ absolute dullness; myelocyte at the 3rd stage of maturation

3-M [syndrome] initials for Miller, McKusick, and Malvaux, who first described the syndrome

M/3 middle third

M₄ myelocyte at the 4th stage of maturation

M₅ metamyelocyte

M₆ band form in the 6th stage of myelocyte maturation

M₇ polymorphonuclear neutrophil

M/10 tenth molar solution

M/100 hundredth molar solution

m electron rest mass; electromagnetic moment; magnetic moment; magnetic quantum number; mass; median; melting [temperature]; meter; milli-; minim; minute; molality; molar [deciduous tooth]

m² square meter

m³ cubic meter

m₈ spin quantum number

μ see mu

MA mandelic acid; Master of Arts; mean arterial; medical assistance; medical audit; mega-ampere; membrane antigen; menstrual age; mental age; meter-angle; microagglutination; microscopic agglutination; Miller-Abbott [tube]; milliampere; mitotic apparatus; mixed agglutination; moderately advanced; monoclonal antibody; mutagenic activity

M/A male, altered [animal]; mood and/or affect

MA-104 embryonic rhesus monkey kidney cells

MA-111 embryonic rabbit kidney cells

MA-163 human embryonic thymus cells

MA-184 newborn human foreskin cells

Ma mass of atom

mA, ma milliampere; meter-angle

mÅ milliångström

MAA macroaggregated albumin; Medical Assistance for the Aged; melanoma-associated antigen; monoarticular arthritis

MAACL Multiple Affect Adjective Check List

MAAGB Medical Artists Association of Great Britain

MAb monoclonal antibody

m-AB m-aminobenzamide

MABP mean arterial blood pressure

MAC MacConkey's [broth]; malignancy-associated changes; maximum allowable concentration; maximum allowable cost; medical alert center; membrane attack complex; midarm circumference; minimum alveolar concentration; modulator of adenylate cyclase; *Mycobacterium avium* complex

mac macerate [Lat. *macerare*]

m accur mix very accurately [Lat. *misce accuratissime*]

MACDP Metropolitan Atlanta Congenital Defects Program

macer maceration

mAChR muscarinic acetylcholine receptor

macro macrocyte, macrocytic; macroscopic

MAD maximum allowable dose; methylandrostenediol; mind-altering drug; myoadenylate deaminase

mAD, MADA muscle adenylate deaminase

MADD multiple acyl-Co A dehydrogenation deficiency

MAE medical air evacuation

MAF macrophage activation factor; macrophage agglutinating factor; minimum audible field; mouse amniotic fluid

MAFH macroaggregated ferrous hydroxide

MAG myelin-associated glycoprotein

Mag magnesium

mag, magn large [Lat. *magnus*]; magnification

MAggF macrophage agglutination factor

MAGIC microprobe analysis generalized intensity correction

mAH milliampere-hours

MAHA microangiopathic hemolytic anemia

MAHH malignancy-associated humoral hypercalcemia

MAI microscopic aggregation index; movement assessment of infants; *Mycobacterium avium intracellulare*

MAKA major karyotypic abnormality

MAL midaxillary line

Mal malate; malfunction

Mal-BSA maleated bovine serum albumin

MALiMET Master List of Medical Indexing Terms
MALT male, altered [animal]; mucosa-associated lymphoid tissue
MAM methylazoxymethanol
mam milliampere-minute; myriameter
M+Am compound myopic astigmatism
MAMA monoclonal anti-malignin antibody
MAM Ac methylazoxymethanol acetate
ma-min milliampere-minute
MAN, Man mannose
man handful [Lat. *manipulus*]; manipulate; morning [Lat. *mane*]
mand mandible, mandibular
manifest manifestation
manip handful [Lat. *manipulus*]; manipulation
MANOVA multivariate analysis of variance
man pr early in the morning [Lat. *mane primo*]
MAO Master of the Art of Obstetrics; maximal acid output; monoamine oxidase
MAOI monoamine oxidase inhibitor
MAP mean airway pressure; mean aortic pressure; mean arterial pressure; Medical Audit Program; megaloblastic anemia of pregnancy; mercapturic acid pathway; methyl acceptor protein; methylacetoxyprogesterone; methylaminopurine; microtubule-associated protein; minimum audible pressure; monophasic action potential; mouse antibody production; muscle action potential
MAPA muscle adenosine phosphoric acid
MAPC migrating action potential complex
MAPF microatomized protein food
MAPI microbial alkaline protease inhibitor
MAPS Make a Picture Story [test]
MAR minimal angle resolution
mar margin; marker [chromosome]
MARC multifocal and recurrent choroidopathy
MARS mouse antirat serum
MAS meconium aspiration syndrome; medical advisory service; mesoatrial shunt; milk-alkali syndrome; milliampere-second; mobile arm support; monoclonal antibodies

mA-s, mas milliampere-second
MASA Medical Association of South Africa
masc masculine; mass concentration
MASER microwave amplification by stimulated emission of radiation
MASH mobile Army surgical hospital; multiple automated sample harvester
mas pil pill mass [Lat. *massa pilularum*]
mass massage
massc mass concentration
MAST military antishock trousers
mast mastoid
MASU mobile Army surgical unit
MAT manual arts therapist; methionine adenosyltransferase; multifocal atrial tachycardia; multiple agent therapy
Mat, mat maternal [origin]; mature
matut in the morning [Lat. *matutinus*]
MAV minimum apparent viscosity; myeloblastosis-associated virus
MAVIS mobile artery and vein imaging system
max maxilla, maxillary; maximum
MB Bachelor of Medicine [Lat. *Medicinae Baccalaureus*]; buccal margin; isoenzyme of creatine kinase containing M and B subunits; mammillary body; Marsh-Bender [factor]; mesiobuccal; methyl bromide; methylene blue; microbiological assay
Mb mouse brain; myoglobin
mb millibar; mix well [Lat. *misce bene*]
MBA methyl bovine albumin
MBAC Member of the British Association of Chemists
MBAR myocardial beta adrenergic receptor
mbar millibar
MBAS methylene blue active substance
MBC male breast cancer; maximal bladder capacity; maximal breathing capacity; methylthymol blue complex; microcrystalline bovine collagen; minimum bactericidal concentration
MbCO carbon monoxide myoglobin
MBD methylene blue dye; minimal brain damage; minimal brain dysfunction; Morquio-Brailsford disease
MBDG mesiobuccal developmental groove
MBF muscle blood flow; myocardial blood flow

MBFLB monaural bifrequency loudness balance

MBG morphine-benzedrine scale

MBH medial basal hypothalamus

MBH₂ reduced methylene blue

MBK methyl butyl ketone

MBL Marine Biological Laboratory; menstrual blood loss; minimum bactericidal level

MBLA methylbenzyl linoleic acid; mouse-specific bone marrow-derived lymphocyte antigen

MBM mineral basal medium

MBNOA Member of the British Naturopathic and Osteopathic Association

MBO mesiobucco-occlusal

MBP an antigen from *Brucella bovis, B. melitensis,* and *B. suis*; major basic protein; maltose-binding protein; mean blood pressure; mesiobuccopulpal; myelin basic protein

MBPS multigated blood pool scanning

MBq megabecquerel

MBR methylene blue, reduced

MBRT methylene blue reduction time

MBSA methylated bovine serum albumin

MBT mercaptobenzothiazole

MBTE meningeal tick-borne encephalitis

MBTH 3-methyl-2-benzothiazoline hydrazone

MC mast cell; Master of Surgery [Lat. *Magister Chirurgiae*]; maximum concentration; Medical Corps; megacoulomb; Merkel's cell; mesiocervical; metacarpal; methyl cellulose; mineralocorticoid; minimal change; mitomycin; mixed cellularity; mixed cryoglobulinemia; monkey cell; myocarditis

M/C male, castrated [animal]

M-C mineralocorticoid

M&C morphine and cocaine

Mc megacurie; megacycle

mC millicoulomb

mc millicurie

MCA major coronary artery; Maternity Center Association; methylcholanthrene; middle cerebral artery; monoclonal antibody; multichannel analyzer; multiple congenital abnormalities

MCAB mononuclear antibody

MCA/MR multiple congenital anomalies/mental retardation [syndrome]

MCAR mixed cell agglutination reaction

MCAT Medical College Admission Test

m caute mix with caution [Lat. *misce caute*]

MCB membranous cytoplasmic body

McB McBurney's [point]

mCBF mean cerebral blood flow

MCBM muscle capillary basement membrane

MCBR minimum concentration of bilirubin

MCC mean corpuscular hemoglobin concentration; metacerebral cell; microcrystalline collagen; minimum complete-killing concentration

MCCU mobile coronary care unit

MCD magnetic circular dichroism; mast-cell degranulation; mean cell diameter; mean of consecutive differences; mean corpuscular diameter; medullary collecting duct; medullary cystic disease; metacarpal cortical density; minimal change disease; multiple carboxylase deficiency; muscle carnitine deficiency

MCE multicystic encephalopathy

MCES multiple cholesterol emboli syndrome

MCF macrophage chemotactic factor; median cleft face; microcomplement fixation; myocardial contraction force

MCFA medium-chain fatty acid

MCG magnetocardiogram; membrane coating granule; monoclonal gammopathy

mcg microgram

MCGC metacerebral giant cell

MCGN mesangiocapillary glomerulonephritis; minimal change glomerulonephritis; mixed cryoglobulinemia with glomerulonephritis

MCH Maternal and Child Health; mean corpuscular hemoglobin

MCh Master of Surgery [Lat. *Magister Chirurgiae*]

mc-h, mch millicurie-hour

MCHC mean corpuscular hemoglobin concentration; mean corpuscular hemoglobin count

MChD Master of Dental Surgery

MCHg mean corpuscular hemoglobin

MChir Master in Surgery [Lat. *Magister Chirurgiae*]

MChOrth Master of Orthopaedic Surgery

MChOtol Master of Otology

MCHR Medical Committee for Human Rights

mc-hr millicurie-hour

MCHS Maternal and Child Health Service

MCI mean cardiac index

MCi megacurie

mCi millicurie

MCi-hr millicurie-hour

MCINS minimal change idiopathic nephrotic syndrome

MCL midclavicular line; midcostal line; modified chest lead; most comfortable loudness

MCLS mucocutaneous lymph node syndrome

MClSci Master of Clinical Science

MCMI Millon Clinical Multiaxial Inventory

MCMV murine cytomegalovirus

MCN minimal change nephropathy

MCNS minimal change nephrotic syndrome

MCommH Master of Community Health

mcoul millicoulomb

MCP melphalan, cyclophosphamide, and prednisone; metacarpophalangeal; mitotic-control protein

MCPa Member of the College of Pathologists, Australasia

MCPH metacarpophalangeal

MCPP metacarpophalangeal pattern profile

mCPP m-chlorophenylpiperazine

MCPPP metacarpophalangeal pattern profile plot

MCPS Member of the College of Physicians and Surgeons

Mcps megacycles per second

MCR Medical Corps Reserve; message competition ratio; metabolic clearance rate

MCRA Member of the College of Radiologists, Australasia

MCS mesocaval shunt; methylcholanthrene sarcoma; multiple combined sclerosis

mc/s megacycles per second

MCSA Moloney cell surface antigen

MCSDS Marlowe-Crowne Social Desirability Scale

MCSP Member of the Chartered Society of Physiotherapists

MCT mean cell thickness; mean cell threshold; mean circulation time; mean corpuscular thickness; medium-chain triglyceride; medullary carcinoma of thyroid; medullary collecting tubule; multiple compressed tablet

MCTC metrizamide computed tomography cisternography

MCTD mixed connective tissue disease

MCTF mononuclear cell tissue factor

MCU malaria control unit; micturating cystourethrography; motor cortex unit

MCUG micturating cystogram

MCV mean cell volume; mean clinical value; mean corpuscular volume; median cell volume; motor conduction velocity

MD Doctor of Medicine [Lat. *Medicinae Doctor*]; magnesium deficiency; main duct; malate dehydrogenase; manic-depressive; Mantoux diameter; Marek's disease; maternal deprivation; mean deviation; mediastinal disease; medical department; medium dosage; Ménière's disease; mental deficiency; mental depression; mesiodistal; mitral disease, mixed diet; monocular deprivation; movement disorder; multiple deficiency; muscular dystrophy; myocardial damage; myocardial disease

Md mendelevium

md median

MDA malondialdehyde; 3,4-methylenedioxyamphetamine; monodehydroascorbate; motor discriminative acuity; multivariant discriminant analysis; right mento-anterior [fetal position] [Lat.*mento-dextra anterior*]

MDAD mineral dust airway disease

MDBDF March of Dimes Birth Defect Foundation

MDBK Madin-Darby bovine kidney [cell]

MDC major diagnostic categories; minimum detectable concentration

MDCK Madin-Darby canine kidney

MDD major depressive disorder; mean daily dose

MDentSc Master of Dental Science

MDF mean dominant frequency; myocardial depressant factor

MDG mean diastolic gradient

MDGF macrophage-derived growth factor

MDH malate dehydrogenase; medullary dorsal horn

MDHV Marek's disease herpesvirus
MDI manic-depressive illness; metered dose inhaler; multiple daily injection
m dict as directed [Last. *moro dicto*]
MDM mid-diastolic murmur; minor determinant mix [penicillin]
MDMA 3,4-methylenedioxymethamphetamine
mdn median
MDNB metadinitrobenzene
MDOPA, mdopa alpha-methyl-dopa, alpha-methyl-3,4-dihydroxyphenylalanine
MDP manic-depressive psychosis; methylene diphosphate; muramyldipeptide; muscular dystrophy, progressive; right mentoposterior [fetal position] [Lat. *mento-dextra posterior*]
MDQ minimum detectable quantity
MDR minimum daily requirement
MDRS Mattis Dementia Rating Scale
MDS Master of Dental Surgery; maternal deprivation syndrome; microdilution system; milk drinker's syndrome; Miller-Dieker syndrome; myelodysplastic syndrome
MDT mast cell degeneration test; median detection threshold; right mentotransverse [fetal position] [Lat. *mento-dextra transversa*]
MDTR mean diameter–thickness ratio
MDU Medical Defence Union
MDUO myocardial disease of unknown origin
MDV Marek disease virus; mucosal disease virus
MDY month, date, year
Mdyn megadyne
ME macular edema; malic enzyme; maximum effort; median eminence; medical education; medical examiner; meningoencephalitis; mercaptoethanol; metabolic energy; metabolism; middle ear; mouse embryo; mouse epithelial [cell]
M/E myeloid/erythroid [ratio]
2-ME 2-mercaptoethanol
Me menton; methyl
MEA Medical Exhibition Association; mercaptoethylamine; multiple endocrine adenomatosis
meas measurement
MeB medical board; methylene blue
MeBSA methylated bovine serum albumin

MEC middle ear cell; minimum effective concentration
MeCCNU semustine
MECG mixed essential cryoglobulinemia
MED median erythrocyte diameter; medicine, medical; minimum effective dose; minimum erythema dose; multiple epiphyseal dysplasia
med medial; median; medicine, medical; medium
MEDAC multiple endocrine deficiency, Addison's disease, and candidiasis [syndrome]
MED-ART Medical Automated Records Technology
MEDEX, Medex extension of the physician; a physician assistant program using former military medical corpsmen [Fr. *médicin extension*]
medic military medical corpsman [Lat. *medicus*]
MEDICO Medical International Cooperation
MEDIHC Military Experience Directed Into Health Careers
MEDLARS Medical Literature Analysis and Retrieval System
MEDLINE MEDLARS On-Line
MEDPAR Medical Provider Analysis and Review
MEdREP Medical Education Reinforcement and Enrichment Program
MEDScD Doctor of Medical Science
MedSurg medicine and surgery
MEE methylethyl ether; middle ear effusion
MEF maximal expiratory flow; middle ear fluid; midexpiratory flow; mouse embryo fibroblast
MEFR maximal expiratory flow rate
MEFV maximal expiratory flow volume
MEG magnetoencephalogram, magnetoencephalography; megakaryocyte; mercaptoethylguanidine; multifocal eosinophilic granuloma
mEGF mouse epidermal growth factor
MEGX monoethylglycinexylidide
MEK methyl-ethyl-ketone
MEL metabolic equivalent level; mouse erythroleukemia
MEL B melarsoprol
MELC murine erythroleukemia cell
MEM macrophage electrophoretic

mobility; malic enzyme, mitochondrial; minimal essential medium

memb membrane, membranous

MEMR multiple exostoses–mental retardation [syndrome]

MEN multiple endocrine neoplasia

MEND Medical Education for National Defense

MENI multiple endocrine neoplasia type I

ment mentality, mental

5-MeODMT 5-methoxy-N,N-dimethyltryptamine

MeOH methyl alcohol

MEOS microsomal ethanol oxidizing system

MEP maximum expiratory pressure; mean effective pressure; motor end-plate

mep meperidine

MEPC miniature end-plate current

MEPP miniature end-plate potential

mEQ, mEq, meq milliequivalent

mEq/l milliequivalents per liter

MER mean ejection rate; methanol extraction residue

MERB Medical Examination and Review Board

MERG macular electroretinogram

MES maintenance electrolyte solution; maximal electroshock; maximal electroshock seizures

Mes mesencephalon, mesencephalic

Mesc mescaline

MESCH Multi-Environment Scheme

MeSH Medical Subject Headings

MesPGN mesangial proliferative glomerulonephritis

MET metabolic equivalent of the task; metastasis, metastatic; methionine; midexpiratory time; multistage exercise test

Met methionine

met metallic [chest sounds]

metab metabolism, metabolic

metas metastasis, metastatic

METH methicillin

Meth methedrine

meth methyl

Met-Hb methemoglobin

MeTHF methyltetrahydrofolic acid

MetMb metmyoglobin

m et n morning and night [Lat. *mane et nocte*]

METS metabolic equivalents of oxygen consumption

m et sig mix and write a label [Lat. *misce et signa*]

MEV murine erythroblastosis virus

MeV, mev megaelectron volts

MF medium frequency; merthiolate-formaldehyde [solution]; microscopic factor; midcavity forceps; mitogenic factor; mitomycin-fluorouracil; mitotic figure; mucosal fluid; multiplication factor; mutation frequency; mycosis fungoides; myelin figures; myelofibrosis; myocardial fibrosis; myofibrillar

M/F male/female ratio

Mf maxillofrontale

mF millifarad

mf microfilaria

MFA monofluoroacetate; multifocal functional autonomy; multiple factor analysis

MFB metallic foreign body

MFCM Master, Faculty of Community Medicine

MFD mandibulofacial dysostosis; midforceps delivery; minimum fatal dose

mfd microfarad

MFH malignant fibrous histiocytoma

MFHom Member of the Faculty of Homeopathy

MFID multielectrode flame ionization detector

m flac membrana flaccida [Lat.]

MFOM Master, Faculty of Occupational Medicine

MFP monofluorophosphate; myofascial pain

MFR mean flow rate; mucus flow rate

MFSS Medical Field Service School

MFST Medical Field Service Technician

MFT multifocal atrial tachycardia; muscle function test

m ft let a mixture be made [Lat. *mistura fiat*]

MFW multiple fragment wounds

MG margin; medial gastrocnemius [muscle]; membranous glomerulonephritis; menopausal gonadotropin; mesiogingival; methylglucoside; monoclonal gammopathy; muscle group; myasthenia gravis; myoglobin

Mg magnesium

m⁷G 7-methylguanosine

mg milligram

MGA melengestrol acetate

m γ milligamma
MGBG methylglyoxal-bis-(guanylhydrazone)
MGC minimal glomerular change
MgC magnocellular neuroendocrine cell
MGD maximal glucose disposal; mixed gonadal dysgenesis
mg/dl milligrams per deciliter
MGDS Member in General Dental Surgery
MGES multiple gated equilibrium scintigraphy
MGG May-Grünwald-Giemsa [staining]; molecular and general genetics
MGGH methylglyoxal guanylhydrazone
MGH Massachusetts General Hospital
mgh milligram-hour
mg/kg milligrams per kilogram
MGL minor glomerular lesion
mg/l milligrams per liter
mgm milligram
MGN membranous glomerulonephritis
MGP marginal granulocyte pool; membranous glomerulonephropathy
MGR modified gain ratio
mgr milligram
MGS metric gravitational system
MGUS monoclonal gammopathies of undetermined significance
MGW magnesium sulfate, glycerin, and water
mGy milligray
MH malignant histiocytosis; malignant hyperpyrexia; malignant hypertension; malignant hyperthermia; mammotropic hormone; mannoheptulose; marital history; medical history; melanophore-stimulating hormone; menstrual history; mental health; mental hygiene; mono-symptomatic hypochondriasis; murine hepatitis; mutant hybrid
mH millihenry
MHA May-Hegglin anomaly; Mental Health Association; methemalbumin; microangiopathic hemolytic anemia; microhemagglutination; mixed hemadsorption; Mueller-Hinton agar
MHA-TP microhemagglutination-*Treponema pallidum*
MHB maximum hospital benefit
MHb methemoglobin; myohemoglobin
MHBSS modified Hank's balanced salt solution

MHC major histocompatibility complex; mental health care
MHCS Mental Hygiene Consultation Service
MHCU mental health care unit
MHD maintenance hemodialysis; mean hemolytic dose; mental health department; minimum hemolytic dilution; minimum hemolytic dose
mHg millimeter of mercury
MHLC Multidimensional Health Locus of Control
MHLS metabolic heat load stimulator
MHN massive hepatic necrosis; Mohs hardness number
MHO microsomal heme oxygenase
mho reciprocal ohm, siemens [ohm spelled backwards]
MHP 1-mercuri-2-hydroxypropane; monosymptomatic hypochondriacal psychosis
MHPG 3-methoxy-4-hydroxyphenylglycol
MHR major histocompatibility region; malignant hyperthermia resistance; maximal heart rate; methemoglobin reductase
MHRI Mental Health Research Institute
MHS major histocompatibility system; malignant hypothermia susceptibility; multiple health screening
MHTS Multiphasic Health Testing Services
MHV magnetic heart vector; mouse hepatitis virus
MHyg Master of Hygiene
MHz megahertz
MI maturation index; medical inspection; melanophore index; menstruation induction; mental institution; mercapto-imidazole; mesioincisal; metabolic index; migration index; migration inhibition; mitotic index; mitral incompetence; mitral insufficiency; mononucleosis infectiosa; morphology index; myocardial infarction; myoinositol
mi mile
MIAs multi-institutional arrangements
MIB Medical Impairment Bureau
MIBG metaiodobenzylguanidine
MIBiol Member of the Institute of Biology
MIBK methyl isobutyl ketone

MIBT methyl isatin-beta-thiosemicarbazone

MIC maternal and infant care; Medical Interfraternity Conference; minimal inhibitory concentration; minimal isorrheic concentration; model immune complex

MICG macromolecular insoluble cold globulin

micro microcyte, microcytic; microscopic

microbiol microbiology.

MICU mobile intensive care unit

MID maximum inhibiting dilution; mesioincisodistal; minimum infective dose; minimum inhibitory dose

mid middle

MIDS Management Information Decision System

midsag midsagittal

MIF macrophage inhibitory factor; melanocyte-stimulating hormone–inhibiting factor; merthiolate-iodine-formaldehyde [method]; midinspiratory flow; migration-inhibiting factor; microimmunofluorescence; mixed immunofluorescence

MIFC merthiolate-iodine-formaldehyde concentration

MIFR maximal inspiratory flow rate

MIG measles immune globulin

MIg malaria immunoglobulin; measles immunoglobulin; membrane immunoglobulin

MIH Master of Industrial Health

MIKA minor karyotype abnormalities

MIKE mass-analyzed ion kinetic energy

MILS medication information leaflet for seniors

MIMS medical information management system; medical inventory management system

MIN medial interlaminar nucleus

min mineral; minim; minimum, minimal; minor; minute

MINA monoisonitrosoacetone

MINIA monkey intranuclear inclusion agent

MIO minimum identifiable odor

MIP maximum inspiratory pressure; minimal inspiratory pressure

MIR multiple isomorphous replacement

MIRD medical internal radiation dose

MIRP myocardial infarction rehabilitation program

MIRU myocardial infarction research unit

MIS management information system; medical information service; meiosis-inducing substance

misc miscarriage; miscellaneous

MIST Medical Information Service by Telephone

mist mixture [Lat. *mistura*]

MIT miracidial immobilization test; mitomycin; monoiodotyrosine

mit mitral; send [Lat. *mitte*]

mitt tal send such [Lat. *mitte tales*]

mIU milli-International unit; one-thousandth of an International unit

mix mixture

MJ marijuana; megajoule

MJT Mead Johnson tube

MK monkey kidney; myokinase

Mk monkey

mkat millikatal

mkat/l millikatals per liter

MKC monkey kidney cell

m-kg meter-kilogram

MkK monkey kidney

MKP monobasic potassium phosphate

MKS, mks meter-kilogram-second

MKTC monkey kidney tissue culture

MKV killed measles vaccine

ML Licentiate in Medicine; Licentiate in Midwifery; malignant lymphoma; mesiolingual; middle lobe; midline; mucolipidosis; multiple lentiginosis; myeloid leukemia

M/L monocyte/lymphocyte [ratio]

M-L Martin-Lewis [medium]

mL millilambert

ml milliliter

MLA left mentoanterior [fetal position] [Lat. *mento-laeva anterior*]; Medical Library Association; mesiolabial; monocytic leukemia, acute

mLa millilambert

MLAB Multilingual Aphasia Battery

MLaI mesiolabioincisal

MLAP mean left atrial pressure

MLaP mesiolabiopulpal

MLb macrolymphoblast

MLC minimum lethal concentration; mixed leukocyte culture; mixed ligand chelate; mixed lymphocyte culture; morphine-like compound; multilamellar cytosome; myelomonocytic leukemia, chronic

MLCK myosin light chain kinase

MLCO Member of the London College of Osteopathy

MLCP myosin light-chain phosphatase

MLCT metal-to-ligand charge transfer

MLD median lethal dose; metachromatic leukodystrophy; minimal lesion disease; minimum lethal dose

MLD$_{50}$ median lethal dose

ml/dl milliliters per deciliter

MLE maximum likelihood estimation

MLF medial longitudinal fasciculus; morphine-like factor

MLG mesiolingual groove

MLGN minimal lesion glomerulonephritis

ML-H malignant lymphoma, histiocytic

MLI mesiolinguoincisal; mixed lymphocyte interaction

ml/l milliliters per liter

MLN membranous lupus nephropathy

MLNS mucocutaneous lymph node syndrome

MLO mesiolinguo-occlusal

MLP left mentoposterior [fetal position] [Lat. *mento-laeva posterior*]; mesiolinguopulpal; microsomal lipoprotein

ML-PDL malignant lymphoma, poorly differentiated lymphocytic

MLR mixed lymphocyte reaction

MLS mean lifespan; median life span; median longitudinal section; middle lobe syndrome; myelomonocytic leukemia, subacute

MLT left mentotransverse [fetal position] [Lat. *mento-laeva transversa*]; mean latency time; median lethal time; Medical Laboratory Technician

MLT(ASCP) Medical Laboratory Technician certified by the American Society of Clinical Pathologists

MLTI mixed lymphocyte target interaction

MLU mean length of utterance

MLV Moloney's leukemogenic virus; multilaminar vesicle; murine leukemia virus

MLVDP maximum left ventricular developed pressure

mlx millilux

MM major medical [insurance]; malignant melanoma; Marshall-Marchetti; medial malleolus; metastatic melanoma, melanoma metastasis; minimal medium; morbidity and mortality; mucous membrane; multiple myeloma; muscularis mucosae; myeloid metaplasia; myelomeningocele

mM millimolar; millimole

mm methylmalonyl; millimeter; muscles

mm^2 square millimeter

mm^3 cubic millimeter

MMA mastitis-metritis-agalactia [syndrome]; medical materials account; methylmalonic acid; N6-monomethyl adenosine

MMAD mass median aerodynamic diameter

MMATP methadone maintenance and aftercare treatment program

MMC migrating myoelectric complex; minimum medullary concentration; mitomycin C; mucosal mast cell

MMD mass median diameter; minimum morbidostatic dose; myotonic muscular dystrophy

MME M-mode echocardiography

MMED Master of Medicine

MMEF maximum midexpiratory flow

MMEFR maximum midexpiratory flow rate

MMF maximum midexpiratory flow; mean maximum flow; Member of the Medical Faculty

MMFR maximum midexpiratory flow rate; maximal midflow rate

MMG mean maternal glucose

mmHg millimeters of mercury

mmH$_2$0 millimeters of water

MMI macrophage migration inhibition; methylmercaptoimidazole

MMIHS megacystis-microcolon-intestinal hypoperistalsis syndrome

MMIS Medicaid Management Information System

MML Moloney murine leukemia; monomethyllysine; myelomonocytic leukemia

mM/l millimoles per liter

MMLV Moloney murine leukemia virus

MMM *see 3-M [syndrome]*; microsome-mediated mutagenesis; myelofibrosis with myeloid metaplasia; myelosclerosis with myeloid metaplasia

MMMT malignant mixed Müllerian tumor
MMN morbus maculosus neonatorum
MMNC marrow mononuclear cell
MMO methane monooxygenase
MMOA maxillary mandibular odontectomy alveolectomy
MMoL myelomonoblastic leukemia
mmol millimole
mmol/l millimoles per liter
MMPI Minnesota Multiphasic Personality Inventory
MMPNC Medical Maternal Program for Nuclear Casualties
mmpp millimeters partial pressure
MMPR methylmercaptopurine riboside
MMR mass miniature radiography; maternal mortality rate; measles-mumps-rubella [vaccine]; mild mental retardation; mobile mass x-ray; mono-methylorutin; myocardial metabolic rate
MMS Master of Medical Science; methyl methanesulfonate
MMSA Master of Midwifery, Society of Apothecaries
MMSc Master of Medical Science
mm st muscle strength
MMT manual muscle test
MMTA methylmetatyramine
MMTV mouse mammary tumor virus
MMU medical maintenance unit; mercaptomethyl uracil
mmu millimass unit
mμ millimicron
mμc millimicrocurie
mμg millimicrogram
MMuLV Moloney murine leukemia virus
mμs millimicrosecond
μmμ meson
MMWR Morbidity and Mortality Weekly Report
MN a blood group in the MNSs blood group system; malignant nephrosclerosis; Master of Nursing; meganewton; melena neonatorum; melanocytic nevus; membranous neuropathy; metanephrine; midnight; mononuclear; motor neuron; multinodular; myoneural
Mn manganese
mN micronewton; millinormal
MNA maximum noise area
MNB murine neuroblastoma
5-MNBA 5-mercapto-2-nitrobenzoic acid

MNC mononuclear cell
MNCV motor nerve conduction velocity
MND minimum necrosing dose; minor neurological dysfunction; motor neuron disease
mng morning
MNJ myoneural junction
MNL mononuclear leukocyte
MN/m² meganewtons per square meter
MNMS myonephropathic metabolic syndrome
MNNG N-methyl N'-nitro-N-nitroso-guanidine
MNR marrow neutrophil reserve
MNS medial nuclear stratum; Melnick-Needles syndrome
Mn-SOD manganese-superoxide dismutase
MNSs a blood group system consisting of groups M, N, and MN
MNU N-methyl-N-nitrosourea
MO manually operated; Master of Obstetrics; Master of Osteopathy; medical officer; mesio-occlusal; mineral oil; minute output; molecular orbital
Mo Moloney [strain]; molybdenum; monoclonal
mo mode, month
MoAb monoclonal antibody
mob, mobil mobility, mobilization
MOC maximum oxygen consumption
MOD maturity onset diabetes; Medical Officer of the Day; mesio-occlusodistal
mod moderate, moderation; modification
modem modulator/demodulator
mod praesc in the way directed [Lat. *modo praescripto*]
MODY maturity onset diabetes of the young
MOF marine oxidation/fermentation; methotrexate, Oncovin, and fluorouracil; multiple organ failure
MO&G Master of Obstetrics and Gynaecology
MOH Medical Officer of Health
MOI maximum oxygen intake; multiplicity of infection
mol mole
molc molar concentration
molfr mole fraction
mol/kg moles per kilogram
mol/l moles per liter
moll soft [Lat. *mollis*]
mol/m³ moles per meter cubed

mol/s moles per second
mol wt molecular weight
MOM milk of magnesia
MoM multiples of the median
MOMA methylhydroxymandelic acid
M Ω megohm
m Ω milliohm
MON Mongolian [gerbil]
mono monocyte; mononucleosis
MOOW Medical Officer of the Watch
8-MOP 8-methoxypsoralen
MOPEG 3-methoxy-4-hydroxyphenyl-glycol
MOPP Mustargen, Oncovin, procarba-zine, and prednisone
MOPV monovalent oral poliovirus vaccine
MORC Medical Officers Reserve Corps
MORD magnetic optical rotatory dispersion
mor dict in the manner directed [Lat. *more dicto*]
morphol morphology
mor sol in the usual way [Lat. *more solito*]
mortal mortality
MOS medial orbital sulcus
mOs milliosmolal
MOSFET metal oxide semiconductor field effect transistor
mOsm, MOsm milliosmole
mOsm/kg milliosmoles per kilogram
MOT mouse ovarian tumor
MOUS multiple occurrence of unexplained symptoms
MOVC membranous obstruction of inferior vena cava
MOX moxalactam
MP as directed [Lat. *modo prescripto*]; matrix protein; mean pressure; melphalan and prednisone; melting point; menstrual period; mentum posterior; mercapto-purine; mesial pit; mesiopulpal; metacar-pophalangeal; metatarsophalangeal; methylprednisolone; monophosphate; mucopolysaccharide; multiparous; myco-plasmal pneumonia
6-MP mercaptopurine
mp millipond; melting point
MPA main pulmonary artery; Medical Procurement Agency; medroxyproges-terone acetate; methylprednisolone acetate
MPa megapascal
MPAP mean pulmonary arterial pressure

MPB male pattern baldness
MPC marine protein concentrate; maxi-mum permissible concentration; meperi-dine, promethazine, and chlorpromazine; metallophthalocyanine; minimum myco-plasmacidal concentration
MPCU maximum permissible concen-tration of unidentified radionucleotides
MPD maximum permissible dose; mean population doubling; membrane potential difference; multiple personality disorder; myeloproliferative disease; myofascial pain dysfunction
MPDS mandibular pain dysfunction syndrome
MPE maximum possible error
MPEH methylphenylethylhydantoin
MPF maturation promoting factor; mean power frequency
MPGM monophosphoglycerate mutase
MPGN membranoproliferative glomer-ulonephritis
MPH male pseudohermaphroditism; Master of Public Health; milk protein hydrolysate
MPharm Master of Pharmacy
MPHD multiple pituitary hormone deficiencies
mphot milliphot
MPhysA Member of Physiotherapists' Association
MPI mannose phosphate isomerase; maximum permitted intake; maximum point of impulse; Multiphasic Personality Inventory; myocardial perfusion imaging
MPJ metacarpophalangeal joint
MPL maximum permissible level; melphalan; mesiopulpolingual
MPLa mesiopulpolabial
MPM malignant papillary mesothelioma; multipurpose meal
MPME (5R,8R)-8-(4-p-methoxyphenyl)-1-piperazynylmethyl-6-methylergolene
MPMP 10[(1-methyl-3-piperidinyl)-methyl]-1OH-phenothiazine
MPMV Mason-Pfizer monkey virus
MPN most probable number
MPO minimal perceptible odor; myelo-peroxidase
MPOA medial preoptic area
MPP medical personnel pool; mercapto-pyrazide pyrimidine; metacarpophalangeal profile
MPPH p-tolylphenylhydantoin

MPPN malignant persistent positional nystagmus

MPQ McGill Pain Questionnaire

MPR marrow production rate; myeloproliferative reaction

MPS Member of the Pharmaceutical Society; microbial profile system; mononuclear phagocyte system; Montreal platelet syndrome; movement-produced stimulus; mucopolysaccharide; mucopolysaccharidosis; multiphasic screening; myocardial perfusion scintigraphy

MPSS methylprednisolone sodium succinate

MPSV myeloproliferative sarcoma virus

MPsyMed Master of Psychological Medicine

MPT Michigan Picture Test

MPTP 1-methyl-4-phenyl-1,2,3,6-tetrahydropyridine

MPT-R Michigan Picture Test, Revised

MPU Medical Practitioners Union

MPV mean platelet volume; mitral valve prolapse

mpz millipièze

MR magnetic resonance; may repeat; measles and rubella; medial rectus [muscle]; medical record; megaroentgen; mental retardation; metabolic rate; methyl red; mitral reflux; mitral regurgitation; modulation rate; mortality rate; mortality ratio; muscle receptor; muscle relaxant

M$_r$ relative molecular mass

mR, mr milliroentgen

MRA marrow repopulation activity; medical records administrator

MRAA Mental Retardation Association of America

MRACGP Member of the Royal Australasian College of General Practice

MRACO Member of the Royal Australasian College of Ophthalmologists

MRACP Member of the Royal Australasian College of Physicians

MRACR Member of the Royal Australasian College of Radiologists

MRad Master of Radiology

mrad millirad

MRAP mean right atrial pressure

MRAS main renal artery stenosis

MRBC monkey red blood cell; mouse red blood cell

MRBF mean renal blood flow

MRC maximum recycling capacity; Medical Registration Council; Medical Research Council; Medical Reserve Corps; methylrosaniline chloride

MRCGP Member of the Royal College of General Practitioners

MRCI Medical Registration Council of Ireland; Medical Research Council of Ireland

MRCOG Member of the Royal College of Obstetricians and Gynaecologists

MRCP Member of the Royal College of Physicians

MRCPA Member of the Royal College of Pathologists of Australia

MRCPath Member of the Royal College of Pathologists

MRCPE Member of the Royal College of Physicians of Edinburgh

MRCPsych Member of the Royal College of Psychiatrists

MRCS Member of the Royal College of Surgeons

MRCSE Member of the Royal College of Surgeons of Edinburgh

MRCVS Member of the Royal College of Veterinary Surgeons

MRD minimal reacting dose; minimal residual disease

mrd millirutherford

mrem millirem

mrep milliroentgen equivalent physical

MRF medical record file; melanocyte-stimulating hormone-releasing factor; mesencephalic reticular formation; midbrain reticular formation; mitral regurgitant flow; monoclonal rheumatoid factor; Müllerian regression factor

mRF monoclonal rheumatoid factor

MRFIT Multiple Risk Factor Intervention Trial

MRFT modified rapid fermentation test

MRH melanocyte-stimulating hormone-releasing hormone

MRHA mannose-resistant hemagglutination

mrhm milliroentgens per hour at one meter

MRI machine-readable identifier; magnetic resonance imaging; medical records information; Medical Research Institute; moderate renal insufficiency

MRIF melanocyte-stimulating hormone release–inhibiting factor

MRIH melanocyte-stimulating hormone release–inhibiting hormone

MRIPHH Member of the Royal Institute of Public Health and Hygiene

MRK Mayer-Rokitansky syndrome

MRL medical records librarian; Medical Research Laboratory

mRNA messenger ribonucleic acid

mRNP messenger ribonucleoprotein

MRO minimal recognizable odor; muscle receptor organ

MROD Medical Research and Operations Directorate

MRP medical reimbursement plan

MRR marrow release rate; maximum relation rate

MRS medical receiving station; Melkersson-Rosenthal syndrome

MRSH Member of the Royal Society of Health

MRT median reaction time; median recognition threshold; milk ring test; muscle response test

MRU mass radiography unit; minimal reproductive unit

MRV minute respiratory volume

MRVI mixed virus respiratory infection

MRVP mean right ventricular pressure; methyl red, Voges-Proskauer [medium]

MS maladjustment score; mass spectrometry; Master of Science; Master of Surgery; mechanical stimulation; Meckel syndrome; medical services; medical student; medical supplies; medical survey; menopausal syndrome; mental status; microscope slide; minimal support; mitral stenosis; mobile surgical [unit]; modal sensitivity; molar solution; Mongolian spot; morphine sulfate; motile sperm; mucosubstance; multiple sclerosis; muscle shortening; muscle strength; musculoskeletal

Ms murmurs

ms millisecond; morphine sulfate

m/s meters per second

m/s^2 meters per second squared

MSA male specific antigen; mannitol salt agar; Medical Services Administration; membrane stabilizing action; multiple system atrophy; muscle sympathetic activity

MSAA multiple sclerosis-associated agent

MSB Master of Science in Bacteriology; most significant bit

MSBC maximum specific binding capacity

MSBLA mouse-specific B lymphocyte antigen

MSC Medical Service Corps; Medical Staff Corps

MSc Master of Science

MScD Master of Dental Science

MScMed Master of Science in Medicine

MScN Master of Science in Nursing

MSD mean square deviation; mild sickle cell disease; most significant digit

MSDC Mass Spectrometry Data Centre

MSE medical support equipment; mental status examination; muscle-specific enolase

mse mean square error

MSEA Medical Society Executives Association

msec millisecond

m/sec meters per second

MSER mean systolic ejection rate

MSES medical school environmental stress

MSF macrophage spreading factor

MSG monosodium L-glutamate

MSGV mouse salivary gland virus

MSH medical self-help; melanocyte-stimulating hormone; melanophore-stimulating hormone

MSH-IF melanocyte-stimulating hormone-inhibiting factor

MSHRF melanocyte-stimulating hormone-releasing factor

MSHyg Master of Science in Hygiene

MSI medium-scale integration

MSIS multi-state information system

MSK medullary sponge kidney

MSKCC Memorial Sloan-Kettering Cancer Center

MSKP Medical Sciences Knowledge Profile

MSL midsternal line

MSLR mixed skin cell-leukocyte reaction

MSLT multiple sleep latency test

MSM medial superior olive; mineral salts medium

MSN Master of Science in Nursing; mildly subnormal

MSOF multiple systems organ failure
MSPGN mesangial proliferative glomerulonephritis
MSPH Master of Science in Public Health
MSPhar Master of Science in Pharmacy
MSPS myocardial stress perfusion scintigraphy
MSR Member of the Society of Radiographers; muscle stretch reflex
MSRPP Multidimensional Scale for Rating Psychiatric Patients
MSS massage; Medical Superintendents' Society; Medicare Statistical System; mental status schedule; minor surgery suite; motion sickness susceptibility; muscular subaortic stenosis; mucus-stimulating substance
mss massage
MSSc Master of Sanitary Science
MSSE Master of Science in Sanitary Engineering
MSSG multiple sclerosis susceptibility gene
MSSVD Medical Society for the Study of Venereal Diseases
MST mean survival time; mean swell time
MSTh mesothorium
MSU maple sugar urine; maple syrup urine; medical studies unit; mid-stream urine; monosodium urate
MSUD maple syrup urine disease
MSurg Master of Surgery
MSV maximum sustained level of ventilation; Moloney sarcoma virus; murine sarcoma virus
MSW Master of Social Welfare; Master of Social Work; medical social worker; multiple stab wounds
MSWYE modified sea water yeast extract
MT malignant teratoma; mammary tumor; Martin-Thayer [plate, medium]; maximal therapy; medical technologist; melatonin; membrana tympani; metallothionein; metatarsal; methyltyrosine; microtome; microtubule; minimum threshold; Monroe tidal drainage; more than; multiple tics; multitest [plate]; muscles and tendons; music therapy
M-T macroglobulin-trypsin
Mt megatonne

MTA malignant teratoma, anaplastic; medical technical assistant
MT(ASCP) Medical Technologist certified by the American Society of Clinical Pathologists
MTB methylthymol blue
MTBE meningeal tick-borne encephalitis
MTBF mean time between (or before) failures
MTC maximum tolerated concentration; medical test cabinet; medical training center; medullary thyroid carcinoma; mitomycin C
MTD maximum tolerated dose; mean total dose; metastatic trophoblastic disease; Midwife Teacher's Diploma; send such doses [Lat. *mitte tales doses*]
MT-DN multitest, dermatophytes and *Nocardia* [plate]
mtDNA mitochondrial deoxyribonucleic acid
MTDT modified tone decay test
MTF maximum terminal flow; medical treatment facility; modulation transfer function; mithramycin
5-MTHF 5-methyl-tetrahydrofolate
MTI malignant teratoma, intermediate; minimum time interval
MTLP metabolic toxemia of late pregnancy
MTM Thayer-Martin, modified [agar]
MT-M multitest, mycology [plate]
MTO Medical Transport Officer
MTOC microtubule organizing center; mitotic organizing center
MTP metatarsophalangeal; microtubule protein
MTQ methaqualone
MTR Meinicke turbidity reaction; 5-methylthioribose
MTT malignant teratoma, trophoblastic; meal tolerance test; mean transit time
MTU methylthiouracil
MTV mammary tumor virus; mouse mammary tumor virus
MTX methotrexate
MT-Y multitest yeast [plate]
MU megaunit; mescaline unit; Montevideo unit; motor unit; mouse unit
Mu Mache unit
mU milliunit
μ Greek letter *mu*; chemical potential; electrophoretic mobility; heavy chain of

immunoglobulin M; linear attenuation coefficient; magnetic moment; mean; micro; micrometer; micron; mutation rate; permeability

μ_o permeability of vacuum

μA microampere

MUAP motor unit action potential

μb microbar

μ_B Bohr magneton

μbar microbar

MUC maximum urinary concentration

muc mucilage

μC microcoulomb

μc microcurie

mcg microgram

μch microcurie-hour

$\mu C\text{-hr}$ microcurie-hour

μCi microcurie

$\mu Ci\text{-hr}$ microcurie-hour

$\mu coul$ microcoulomb

$\mu F, \mu f$ microfarad

MUG MUMPS (q.v.) Users' Group

μg microgram

MUGA multiple gated acquisition

$\mu\gamma$ microgamma

MUGEx multigated blood pool image during exercise

$\mu g/kg$ micrograms per kilogram

$\mu g/l$ micrograms per liter

MUGR multigated blood pool image at rest

μGy microgray

μH microhenry

μHg micron of mercury

μin microinch

μIU one-millionth of an International Unit

μkat microkatal

μl microliter

mult multiple

multip multiparous

MuLV, MuLv murine leukemia virus

μM micromolar

μm micrometer; micromilli-

μmg micromilligram [nanogram]

μmHg micrometer of mercury

μmm micromillimeter [nanometer]

μmol micromole

MUMPS Massachusetts General Hospital Utility Multi-Programming System

MuMTv murine mammary tumor virus

$\mu\mu C$ micromicrocurie [picocurie]

$\mu\mu F$ micromicrofarad [picofarad]

$\mu\mu g$ micromicrogram [picogram]

μN nuclear magneton

MUN(WI) Munich Wistar [rat]

MUO myocardiopathy of unknown origin

$\mu\Omega$ microhm

MUP major urinary protein; motor unit potential

$\mu R, \mu r$ microroentgen

μ/ρ mass attenuation coefficient

MURC measurable undesirable respiratory contaminants

MurNAc N-acetylmuramate

μs microsecond

musc muscle, musculature, muscular

μsec microsecond

MUST medical unit, self-contained and transportable

MUU mouse uterine unit

μU microunit

μV microvolt

μW microwatt

MUWU mouse uterine weight unit

MV malignant rabbit fibroma virus; mechanical ventilation; megavolt; minute volume; mitral valve; mixed venous; multivessel; veterinary physician [Lat. *Medicus Veterinarius*]

Mv mendelevium

mV, mv millivolt

MVA mevalonic acid; mitral valve area; motor vehicle accident

MV•A megavolt-ampere

mV•A millivolt-ampere

mval millival

MVB multivesicular body

MVC maximum voluntary contraction

MVD Doctor of Veterinary Medicine; multi-vessel coronary disease

MVE Murray Valley encephalitis

MVI multivitamin infusion

MVLS mandibular vestibulolingual sulcoplasty

MVM microvillose membrane; minute virus of mice

MVMT movement

MVO maximum venous outflow

MVO2, MVO_2 myocardial oxygen consumption

MVOA mitral valve orifice area

MVP mitral valve prolapse

MVPP mustine, vinblastine, procarbazine, and prednisone

MVPS mitral valve prolapse syndrome
MVPT Motor-Free Visual Perception Test
MVR massive vitreous reaction; minimal vascular resistance; mitral valve replacement
mV·s millivolt-second
MVV maximal voluntary ventilation
MW megawatt; microwave; molecular weight
mW miliwatt
mWb milliweber
MWD molecular weight distribution
MWP mean wedge pressure
MWS Marden-Walker syndrome; Moersch-Woltman syndrome
MX matrix
Mx maxwell; MEDEX (*q.v.*)
M$_{xy}$ transverse magnetization
My myopia
my mayer
Myco *Mycobacterium*
Mycol mycology, mycologist
MyD myotonic dystrophy
Myel myelocyte
myel myelin, myelinated
MyG myasthenia gravis
MyMD myotonic muscular dystrophy
MYO myoglobin
MZ mantle zone; monozygotic
M$_z$ longitudinal magnetization
MZA monozygotic twins raised apart
MZT monozygotic twins raised together

–N–

N asparagine; Avogadro's number; a blood group in the MNS blood group system; loudness; nasal; nasion; negative; neper; nerve; neuraminidase; neurology; neuropathy; neutron number; newton; nicotinamide; nitrogen; nodule; normal [solution]; nucleoside; number; number in sample; number of molecules; number of neutrons in an atomic nucleus; population size; radiance; refractive index; spin density
0.02N fiftieth-normal [solution]

0.1N tenth-normal [solution]
0.5N half-normal [solution]
NI-NXII first to twelfth cranial nerves
2N double-normal [solution]
N/2 half-normal [solution]
N/10 tenth-normal [solution]
N/50 fiftieth-normal [solution]
n amount of substance expressed in moles; born [Lat. *natus*]; haploid chromosome number; index of refraction; nano; nerve; neuter; neutron; neutron number density; normal; nostril [Lat. *naris*]; number; number of density of molecule; principle quantum number; refractive index; rotational frequency; sample size
2n haploid chromosome; diploid
3n triploid
4n tetraploid
ν see *nu*
NA Narcotics Anonymous; network administrator; neuraminidase; neutralizing antibody; neutrophil antibody; nicotinic acid; Nomina Anatomica; noradrenalin; not available; nucleic acid; nucleus ambiguus; numerical aperture; nurse's aid; nursing assistant; nursing auxiliary
Na Avogadro's number; sodium [Lat. *natrium*]
nA nanoampere
NAA naphthaleneacetic acid; neutral amino acid; neutron activation analysis; neutrophil aggregation activity; nicotinic acid amide; no apparent abnormalities
NAACLS National Accrediting Agency for Clinical Laboratory Sciences
NAACOG Nurses Association of the American College of Obstetricians and Gynecologists
NAAFA National Association to Aid Fat Americans
NAAP N-acetyl-4-amino-phenazone
NAB novarsenobenzene
NABP National Association of Boards of Pharmacy
NABPLEX National Association of Boards of Pharmacy Licensing Examination
NAC N-acetylcysteine; National Asthma Center; Noise Advisory Council
NACDS North American Clinical Dermatological Society

NACED National Advisory Council on the Employment of the Disabled

NAC-EDTA N-acetylcysteine EDTA

nAChR nicotinic acetylcholine receptor

NACOR National Advisory Committee on Radiation

NAD new antigenic determinant; nicotinamide adenine dinucleotide; nicotinic acid dehydrogenase; no abnormal discovery; no acute distress; no apparent distress; no appreciable disease; normal axis deviation; nothing abnormal detected

NAD⁺ the oxidized form of NAD

NaD sodium dialysate

NADA New Animal Drug Application

NADABA N-adenoxyldiaminobutyric acid

NADG nicotinamide adenine dinucleotide glycohydrolase

NADH reduced nicotinamide adenine dinucleotide

NADL National Association of Dental Laboratories

NaDodSO₄ sodium dedecyl sulfate

NADP nicotinamide adenine dinucleotide phosphate

NADP⁺ oxidized form of nicotinamide adenine dinucleotide phosphate

NADPH reduced nicotinamide adenine dinucleotide phosphate

Naₑ exchangeable body sodium

NAEMT National Association of Emergency Medical Technicians

NAF National Amputation Foundation; National Ataxia Foundation; net acid flux

NAG alpha-N-acetyl-D-glucosaminidase; non-agglutinable

NAGA N-acetyl-beta-glucosaminidase

NAGO neuraminidase and galactose oxidase

NAH 2-hydroxy-3-naphthoic acid hydrazide

NAHA National Association of Health Authorities

NAHCS National Association of Health Center Schools

NAHG National Association of Humanistic Gerontology

NAHI National Athletic Health Institute

NAHPA National Association of Hospital Purchasing Agents

NAHSA National Association for Hearing and Speech Action

NAHSE National Association of Health Services Executives

NAHU National Association of Health Underwriters

NAHUC National Association of Health Unit Clerks-Coordinators

NAI net acid input; non-accident-related injury; nonadherence index

NAIR nonadrenergic inhibitory response

NAL nonadherent leukocyte

NALD neonatal adrenoleukodystrophy

NAM natural actomyosin

NAMCS National Ambulatory Medical Care Survey

NAME National Association of Medical Examiners; nevi, atrial myxoma, myxoid neurofibroma, ephelides [syndrome]

NAMH National Association for Mental Health

NAMRU Navy Medical Reserve Unit

NANA N-acetyl neuraminic acid

NANB non-A, non-B [hepatitis]

NANBH non-A, non-B hepatitis

NAND not-and

NAOO National Association of Optometrists and Opticians

NAOP National Alliance for Optional Parenthood

NAP nasion, point A, pogonion [convexity or concavity of the facial profile]; neutrophil alkaline phosphatase

NAPA N-acetyl-p-aminophenol; N-acetyl procainamide

NAPCA National Air Pollution Control Administration

NaPG sodium pregnanediol glucuronide

NAPH naphthyl; nicotinamide adenine dinucleotide phosphate

NAPHT National Association of Patients on Hemodialysis and Transplantation

NAPM National Association of Pharmaceutical Manufacturers

NAPN National Association of Physicians' Nurses

NAPNAP National Association of Pediatric Nurses Associates and Practitioners

NAPNES National Association for Practical Nursing Education and Services

NAPPH National Association of Private Psychiatric Hospitals

NAPT National Association for the Prevention of Tuberculosis

NAR nasal airway resistance; National Association for Retarded [Children, Citizens]

NARA Narcotics Addict Rehabilitation Act; National Association of Recovered Alcoholics

NARAL National Abortion Rights Action League

NARC narcotic; National Association for Retarded Children

narco narcotic, narcotic addict, drug enforcement agent

NARD National Association of Retail Druggists

NARF National Association of Rehabilitation Facilities

NARMC Naval Aerospace and Regional Medical Center

NARMH National Association for Rural Mental Health

NARS National Acupuncture Research Society

NAS nasal; National Academy of Sciences; National Association of Sanitarians; neuroallergic syndrome; no added salt

NASA National Aeronautics and Space Administration

NASDAD National Association of Seventh-Day Adventist Dentists

NASE National Association for the Study of Epilepsy

NASEAN National Association for State Enrolled Assistant Nurses

NASM Naval Aviation School of Medicine

NAS-NRC National Academy of Science–National Research Council

NASW National Association of Social Workers

NAT N-acetyltransferase; natal; neonatal alloimmune thrombocytopenia; no action taken

Nat native; natural

NB neurometric battery; newborn; nitrous oxide–barbiturate; note well [Lat *nota bene*]

Nb niobium

nb newborn; note well [Lat. *nota bene*]

NBC non-battle casualty

NBCC nevoid basal cell carcinoma

NBCCS nevoid basal cell carcinoma syndrome

NBD neurogenic bladder dysfunction

NBI no bone injury; non-battle injury

NBM no bowel movement; normal bone marrow; normal bowel movement; nothing by mouth

nbM newborn mouse

nbMb newborn mouse brain

NBME National Board of Medical Examiners

NBN newborn nursery

NBO non-bed occupancy

NBP neoplastic brachial plexopathy

NBRT National Board for Respiratory Therapy

NBS National Bureau of Standards; nevoid basal cell carcinoma syndrome; Nijmegen breakage syndrome; normal blood serum; normal bowel sounds; nystagmus blockage syndrome

NBT nitroblue tetrazolium; normal breast tissue

NBTE nonbacterial thrombotic endocarditis

NBTNF newborn, term, normal, female

NBTNM newborn, term, normal, male

NBT PABA N-benzoyl-L-tyrosyl para-aminobenzoic acid

NBTS National Blood Transfusion Service

n-Bu n-butyl

NBW normal birth weight

NC nasal cannula; neural crest; neurologic check; nitrocellulose; no casualty; no change; no charge; no complaints; noise criterion; noncontributory; nose cone; not completed; not cultured; nucleocapsid; nursing coordination

N:C nuclear-cytoplasmic ratio

nC nanocoulomb

nc nanocurie

NCA National Certification Agency; National Council on Aging; National Council on Alcoholism; neurocirculatory asthenia; nodulocystic acne; noncontractile area; nonspecific cross-reacting antigen; nuclear cerebral angiogram

NCAE National Council for Alcohol Education

NCAMI National Committee Against Mental Illness

NCAMLP National Certification Agency for Medical Laboratory Personnel

NC/AT normal cephalic atraumatic

NCC nursing care continuity

NCCDC National Center for Chronic Disease Control

NCCIP National Center for Clinical Infant Program

NCCLS National Committee for Clinical Laboratory Standards

NCCLVP National Coordinating Committee on Large Volume Parenterals

NCCMHC National Council for Community Mental Health Centers

NCCPA National Commission on Certification of Physician Assistants

NCCU newborn convalescent care unit

NCD National Commission on Diabetes; National Council on Drugs; neurocirculatory dystonia; normal childhood disorder; not considered disabling

NCDA National Council on Drug Abuse

NCDV Nebraska calf diarrhea virus

NCE negative contrast echocardiography; new chemical entity; nonconvulsive epilepsy

NCF neutrophil chemotactic factor

NCFA Narcolepsy and Catalepsy Foundation of America

NCF(C) neutrophil chemotactic factor (complement)

NCHC National Council of Health Centers

NCHCA National Commission for Health Certifying Agencies

NCHCT National Center for Health Care Technology

NCHLS National Council of Health Laboratory Services

NCHPD National Council on Health Planning and Development

NCHS National Center for Health Statistics

NCHSR National Center for Health Services Research

NCI National Cancer Institute; nuclear contour index; nursing care integration

nCi nanocurie

NCIB National Collection of Industrial Bacteria

NCIH National Council for International Health

NCJ needle catheter jejunostomy

NCLEX-RN National Council Licensure Examination for Registered Nurses

N/cm^2 newtons per square centimeter

NCMC natural cell-mediated cytotoxicity

NCMH National Committee for Mental Health

NCMHI National Clearinghouse for Mental Health Information

NCMI National Committee Against Mental Illness

NCN National Council of Nurses

NCP noncollagen protein

n-CPAP nasal continuous positive airway pressure

NCPE noncardiac pulmonary edema

NCPPB National Collection of Plant Pathogenic Bacteria

NCR National Research Council; nuclear/cytoplasmic ratio

NCRND National Committee for Research in Neurological Diseases

NCRP National Council on Radiation Protection and Measurements

NCRPM National Committee on Radiation Protection and Measurements

NCRV National Committee for Radiation Victims

NCS no concentrated sweets; noncircumferential stenosis; zinostatis (neocarzinostatin)

NCSN National Council for School Nurses

NCT neural crest tumor

NCTC National Cancer Tissue Culture; National Collection of Type Cultures

NCV nerve conduction velocity; noncholera vibrio

NCYC National Collection of Yeast Cultures

ND Doctor of Naturopathy; natural death; Naval Dispensary; neonatal death; neoplastic disease; neuropsychological deficit; neurotic depression; neutral density; new drug; Newcastle disease; no data; no disease; nondisabling; normal delivery; normal development; not detected; nondetectable; not determined; not diagnosed; not done; nutritionally deprived

N&D nodular and diffuse

N$_D$ refractive index

Nd neodymium

n_D refractive index
NDA National Dental Association; New Drug Application; no data available; no detectable activity; no detectable antibody
NDC National Data Communications; National Drug Code; Naval Dental Clinic; nondifferentiated cell
NDCR National Drug Code Directory
NDD no dialysis days
NDDG National Diabetes Data Group
NDE near-death experience
NDF new dosage form
NDGA nordihydroguaiaretic acid
NDI nephrogenic diabetes insipidus
NDIR nondispersive infrared analyzer
NDMA nitrosodimethylamine
nDNA native deoxyribonucleic acid
NDP net dietary protein
NDS Naval Dental School; normal dog serum
NDSB Narcotic Drugs Supervisory Board
NDT neurodevelopmental treatment; nondestructive test, nondestructive testing
NDTI National Disease and Therapeutic Index
NDV Newcastle disease virus
NE national emergency; nephropathia epidemica; nerve ending; nerve excitation; neurological examination; no effect; nonelastic; norepinephrine; not elevated; not enlarged; not equal; not evaluated; not examined
Ne neon
nebul spray [Lat. *nebula*]
NEC National Electrical Code; necrotizing enterocolitis; not else classified or classifiable
NECHI Northeastern Consortium for Health Information
NED no evidence of disease; no expiration date; normal equivalent deviation
NEEE Near East equine encephalomyelitis
NEF nephritic factor
NEFA nonesterified fatty acid
neg negative
NEHE Nurses for Environmental Health Education
NEI National Eye Institute
NEISS National Electronic Injury Surveillance System

NEJM New England Journal of Medicine
NEM N-ethylmaleimide
nem nutritional milk unit [Ger. *Nahrungs Einheit Milch*]
NEMA National Eclectic Medical Association
nema nematode
NEMD nonspecific esophageal motor dysfunction
Neo neomycin
neo neoarsphenamine
NEP negative expiratory pressure; nephrology
nep nephrectomy
NERHL Northeastern Radiological Health Laboratory
NER no evidence of recurrence
NERD no evidence of recurrent disease
ner nervous
NES not elsewhere specified
NESO Northeastern Society of Orthodontists
NESP Nurse Education Support Program
NET nasoendotracheal tube; nerve excitability test
n et m night and day [Lat. *nocte et mane*]
neu neurilemma
neur, neuro, neurol neurology, neurological, neurologist
neuropath neuropathology
neut neuter, neutral
NEY neomycin egg yolk [agar]
NEYA neomycin egg yolk agar
NF National Formulary; nephritic factor; neurofibromatosis; neutral fraction; noise factor; normal flow; not filtered; not found
nF nanofarad
NFAIS National Federation of Abstracting and Indexing Services
NFB National Foundation for the Blind; nonfermenting bacteria
NFC National Fertility Center
NFD neurofibrillary degeneration
NFDR neurofacial-digitorenal [syndrome]
NFH nonfamilial hematuria
NFIC National Foundation for Ileitis and Colitis
NFID National Foundation for Infectious Diseases

NFLD nerve fiber layer defect

NFLPN National Federation of Licensed Practical Nurses

NFMD National Foundation for Muscular Dystrophy

NFME National Fund for Medical Education

NFND National Foundation for Neuromuscular Diseases

NFNID National Foundation for Non-Invasive Diagnostics

NFPA National Fire Protection Association

NFS National Fertility Study

NFT neurofibrillary tangle

NFTD normal full term delivery

NFW nursed fairly well

NG nasogastric; new growth; nitroglycerin; nodose ganglion

ng nanogram

NGC nucleus reticularis gigantocellularis

NGF nerve growth factor

NGGR nonglucogenic/glucogenic ratio

NGR narrow gauze roll; nasogastric replacement

NGS normal goat serum

NGSA nerve growth stimulating activity

NGSF non-genital skin fibroblast

NGU nongonococcal urethritis

NH natriuretic hormone; Naval Hospital; neonatal hepatitis; nonhuman; nursing home

NHA National Health Association; National Hearing Association; National Hemophilia Association; nonspecific hepatocellular abnormality

NHANES National Health and Nutrition Examination Survey

NHBPCC National High Blood Pressure Coordinating Committee

NHC National Health Council; neighborhood health center; neonatal hypocalcemia; nonhistone chromosomal [protein]

NHCP nonhistone chromosomal protein

NHD normal hair distribution

NHDC National Hansen's Disease Center

NHDF normal human diploid fibroblast

NHDL nonhigh density lipoprotein

NHDS National Hospital Discharge Survey

NHF National Health Federation; National Hemophilia Foundation

NHG normal human globulin

NHGJ normal human gastric juice

NHH neurohypophyseal hormone

NHI National Health Institute; National Health Insurance

NHIS National Health Interview Survey

NHL nodular histiocytic lymphoma; non-Hodgkin's lymphoma

NHLBI National Heart, Lung, and Blood Institute

NHML non-Hodgkin's malignant lymphoma

NHMRC National Health and Medical Research Council

NHP nonhistone protein; normal human pooled plasma; nursing home placement

NHPC National Health Planning Council

NHPF National Health Policy Forum

NHPIC National Health Planning Information Center

NHPPN National Health Professions Placement Network

NHR net histocompatibility ratio

NHRC National Health Research Center

NHS National Health Service; normal horse serum; normal human serum

NHSAS National Health Service Audit Staff

NHSC National Health Service Corps

NHSR National Hospital Service Reserve

NI neuraminidase inhibition; neurological improvement; neutralization index; no information; noise index; not identified; not isolated

Ni nickel

NIA National Institute on Aging; nephelometric inhibition assay; no information available; Nutritional Institute of America

NIAAA National Institute of Alcohol Abuse and Alcoholism

NIADDK National Institute of Arthritis, Diabetes, Digestive and Kidney Diseases

NIAID National Institute of Allergy and Infectious Diseases

NIAMDD National Institute of Arthritis, Metabolism, and Digestive Diseases

NIB National Institute for the Blind

NIBSC National Institute for Biological Standards and Control

NIC neurogenic intermittent claudication

NICHD National Institute of Child Health and Development

NICU neonatal intensive care unit; neurological intensive care unit; neurosurgical intensive care unit

NIDA National Institute of Drug Abuse

NIDD non-insulin-dependent diabetes

NIDDM non-insulin-dependent diabetes mellitus

NIDM National Institute for Disaster Mobilization

NIDR National Institute of Dental Research

NIEHS National Institutes of Environmental Health Sciences

NIF negative inspiratory force

NIGMS National Institute of General Medical Sciences

NIH National Institutes of Health

NIHL noise-induced hearing loss

NIHR National Institute of Handicapped Research

NIHS National Institute of Hypertension Studies

NIIC National Injury Information Clearinghouse

NIIS National Institute of Infant Services

NIMH National Institute of Mental Health

NIMR National Institute for Medical Research

NINCDS National Institute of Neurological and Communicative Disorders and Stroke

NINDB National Institute of Neurological Diseases and Blindness

NIOSH National Institute for Occupational Safety and Health

NIP nipple

NIPH National Institute of Public Health

NIR near infrared

NIRA nitrite reductase

NIRD nonimmune renal disease

NIRMP National Intern and Resident Matching Program

NIRNS National Institute for Research in Nuclear Science

NIRS normal inactivated rabbit serum

NIT National Intelligence Test

NIV nodule-inducing virus

NJ nasojejunal

NJPC National Joint Practice Commission

NK Commission on [Anatomical] Nomenclature [Ger. *Nomenklatur Kommission*]; natural killer [cell]; not known

NKA no known allergies

nkat nanokatal

NKDA no known drug allergies

NKH nonketogenic hyperglycemia; nonketotic hyperosmotic

NL neutral lipid; normal

nl it is not clear [Lat. *non liquet*]; it is not permitted [Lat. *non licet*]; nanoliter; normal [value]

NLA National Leukemia Association; neuroleptanesthesia; normal lactase activity

NLB needle liver biopsy

NLD necrobiosis lipoidica diabeticorum

NLE neonatal lupus erythematosus

Nle norleucine

NLF neonatal lung fibroblast; nonlactose fermentation

NLM National Library of Medicine; noise level monitor

NLN National League for Nursing; no longer needed

NLNE National League for Nursing Education

NLP no light perception; nodular liquefying panniculitis; normal luteal phase

NLS nonlinear least squares; normal lymphocyte supernatant

NLT normal lymphocyte transfer; not less than

NM neuromuscular; nictitating membrane; nitrogen mustard; not measurable, not measured; not mentioned; not motile; nuclear medicine, technologist in nuclear medicine; nuclear membrane

Nm nutmeg [Lat. *nux moschata*]

N/m newtons per meter

N-m newton-meter

N/m² newtons per square meter N/m^2

N x m newtons by meter

nm nanometer

NMA National Malaria Association; National Medical Association; neurogenic muscular atrophy

NMAC National Medical Audio-Visual Center

NM(ASCP) Technologist in Nuclear

Medicine certified by the American Society of Clinical Pathologists

NMC National Medical Care; Naval Medical Center; neuromuscular control; nucleus reticularis magnocellularis

NMCUES National Medical Care Utilization and Expenditure Survey

NME National Medical Enterprises

NMF N-methylformamide; National Medical Fellowship; National Migraine Foundation; nonmigrating fraction

NMFI National Master Facility Inventory

NMJ neuromuscular junction

NMM nodular malignant melanoma

NMN nicotinamide mononucleotide; normetanephrine

NMNRU National Medical Neuropsychiatric Research Unit

nmol nanomole

NMOS N-type metal oxide semiconductor

NMP normal menstrual period

NMPCA non-metric principal component analysis

NMPTP N-methyl-4-phenyl-1,2,3,6-tetrahydropyridine

NMR neonatal mortality rate; nictitating membrane response; nuclear magnetic resonance

NMRDC Naval Medical Research and Development Command

NMRI Naval Medical Research Institute

NMRL Naval Medical Research Laboratory

NMRU Naval Medical Research Unit

NMS Naval Medical School; neuroleptic malignant syndrome; neuromuscular spindle; normal mouse serum

N•m/s newton meters per second

NMSS National Multiple Sclerosis Society

NMT neuromuscular tension; neuromuscular transmission; N-methyltransferase; no more than; nuclear medicine technology

NMTCB Nuclear Medicine Technology Certification Board

NMTD nonmetastatic trophoblastic disease

NMU neuromuscular unit

NN nevocellular nevus

nn nerves; new name [Lat. *nomen novum*]

NNAS neonatal narcotic abstinence syndrome

NNC National Nutrition Consortium

NND neonatal death; New and Nonofficial Drugs; nonspecific nonerosive duodenitis

NNDC National Naval Dental Center

NNE neonatal necrotizing enterocolitis; nonneuronal enolase

NNEB National Nursery Examination Board

NNG nonspecific nonerosive gastritis

NNHS National Nursing Home Survey

NNI noise and number index

NNIS National Nosocomial Infections Study

NNMC National Naval Medical Center

NNN Novy-MacNeal-Nicolle [medium]

NNNMU N-nitroso-N-methylurethane

NNO no new orders

n nov new name [Lat. *nomen novum*]

NNP nerve net pulse

NNR New and Nonofficial Remedies

NNS nonneoplastic syndrome

NNWI Neonatal Narcotic Withdrawal Index

NO nitric oxide; none obtained

No nobelium

No, no number [Lat. *numero*]

NOA National Optometric Association

NOAPP National Organization of Adolescent Pregnancy and Parenting

noc, noct at night [Lat. *nocte*]

noct maneq at night and in the morning [Lat. *nocte maneque*]

NOD nodular melanoma; notify of death

NOEL no observed effect level

NOF National Osteopathic Foundation

NOFT nonorganic failure-to-thrive

NOII non-occlusive intestinal ischemia

nom dub a doubtful name [Lat. *nomen dubium*]

NOMI nonocclusive mesenteric infarction

nom nov new name [Lat. *nomen novum*]

nom nud a name without designation [Lat. *nomen nudum*]

non-REM non-rapid eye movement [sleep]

non rep, non repetat do not repeat [Lat. *non repetatur*]

NOP not otherwise provided for

NOPHN National Organization for Public Health Nursing

NOR nucleolar organizer region

NORC National Opinion Research Center

NOR-EPI norepinephrine

norleu norleucine

norm normal

NOS network operating system; not otherwise specified

NOSIE Nurses' Observation Scale for Inpatient Evaluation

NOSTA Naval Ophthalmic Support and Training Activity

NOTB National Ophthalmic Treatment Board

NOVS National Office of Vital Statistics

nov sp new species [Lat. *novum species*]

NP nasopharynx, nasopharyngeal; near point; neonatal-perinatal; neuropathology; neurophysin; neuropsychiatry; new patient; newly presented; nitrogen-phosphorus; nitrophenol; no pain; normal plasma; normal pressure; nonpracticing; not perceptible; not performed; not pregnant; not present; nucleoplasmic; nucleoprotein; nucleoside phosphorylase; nurse practitioner; nursed poorly; nursing procedure; proper name [Lat. *nomen proprium*]

N-P need-persistence

Np neper; neptunium; neurophysin

NPA National Pharmaceutical Association; National Pituitary Agency; near point accommodation

NPA-NIHHDP National Pituitary Agency–National Institutes of Health Hormone Distribution Program

NPB nodal premature beat; non-protein bound

NPC nasopharyngeal carcinoma; near point of convergence; nodal premature contractions; nonparenchymal liver cell

NPCP National Prostatic Cancer Project

NPD narcissistic personality disorder; negative pressure device; Niemann-Pick disease; nitrogen-phosphorus detector

NPDL nodular poorly differentiated lymphocytic

NPE neurogenic pulmonary edema

NPF National Parkinson Foundation; National Pharmaceutical Foundation; National Psoriasis Foundation

NPFT Neurotic Personality Factor Test

NPH neutral protamine Hagedorn (insulin); normal pressure hydrocephalus

NPhx nasopharynx

NPI Narcissistic Personality Inventory

NPIC neurogenic peripheral intermittent claudication

NPII Neonatal Pulmonary Insufficiency Index

NPJT nonparoxysmal atrioventricular junctional tachycardia

NPL National Physical Laboratory; neoproteolipid

NPM nothing per mouth

NPN nonprotein nitrogen

NPO nothing by mouth [Lat. *nulla per os*]; nucleus preopticus

NPO/HS nothing by mouth at bedtime [Lat. *nulla per os hora somni*]

NPP nitrophenylphosphate; normal pool plasma

NPR net protein ratio

NPRL Navy Prosthetics Research Laboratory

NPSH nonprotein sulhydryl group

NPT neoprecipitin test; nocturnal penile tumescence; normal pressure and temperature

NPU net protein utilization

NPV negative pressure ventilation; nuclear polyhedrosis virus; nucleus paraventricularis

4NQO 4-nitroquinoline 1-oxide

NQR nuclear quadruple resonance

NR do not repeat [Lat. *non repetatur*]; neutral red; nonreactive; nonrebreathing; no radiation; no refill; no response; normal range; normotensive rat; not readable; not recorded; not resolved; nurse; nutrition ratio; Reynold's number

N_R Reynold's number

nr near

NRA nitrate reductase; nucleus retroambigualis

NRB nonrejoining break

NRBC National Rare Blood Club; nucleated red blood cell

NRbc nucleated red blood cell

NRC National Research Council; normal retinal correspondence; Nuclear Regulatory Commission

NRCC National Registry in Clinical Chemistry

NRDL Naval Radiological Defense Laboratory

NREH normal renin essential hypertension

NREM non-rapid eye movement [sleep]

NRF Neurosciences Research Foundation

NRGC nucleus reticularis gigantocellularis

NRH nodular regenerative hyperplasia

NRI non-respiratory infection

NRK normal rat kidney

NRL nucleus reticularis lateralis

NRM National Registry of Microbiologists; nucleus reticularis magnocellularis

NRMP National Residency Matching Plan

nRNA nuclear ribonucleic acid

nRNP nuclear ribonucleoprotein

NRP nucleus reticularis parvocellularis

NRR net reproduction rate

NRRL Northern Regional Research Laboratory

NRS normal rabbit serum; normal reference serum

NRSCC National Reference System in Clinical Chemistry

NRSFPS National Reporting System for Family Planning Services

NRV nucleus reticularis ventralis

NS natural science; nephrosclerosis; nephrotic syndrome; nervous system; neurological surgery, neurosurgery; neurosyphilis; neurotic score; nonspecific; nonstimulation; nonstructural; normal saline; normal serum; normal sodium [diet]; no sample; no specimen; not seen; not significant; not specified; not symptomatic; not sufficient; nuclear sclerosis; nursing services; Nursing Sister

N/S normal saline

Ns nasospinale; nerves

ns nanosecond; no sequelae; no specimen; not significant; nylon suture

NSA Neurological Society of America; normal serum albumin; no significant abnormality; no significant anomaly

nsa no salt added

NSABP National Surgical Adjuvant Breast Project

NSAI non-steroidal anti-inflammatory [drug]

NSAIA nonsteroidal anti-inflammatory agent

NSAID nonsteroidal anti-inflammatory drug

NSAM Naval School of Aviation Medicine

NSC neurosecretory cell; no significant change; non-service connected

NSCC National Society for Crippled Children

NSCD non-service connected disability

NSCLC non-small-cell lung cancer

NSD Nairobi sheep disease; night sleep deprivation; nominal single dose; nominal standard dose; no significant defect; no significant deficiency; no significant deviation; no significant difference; no significant disease; normal spontaneous delivery

NSE neuron-specific enolase

nsec nanosecond

NSF National Science Foundation; nodular subepidermal fibrosis

NSFTD normal spontaneous full-term delivery

NSG neurosecretory granule

nsg nursing

NSH National Society for Histotechnology

NSHD nodular sclerosing Hodgkin's disease

NSI negative self-image

NSIDS near sudden infant death syndrome

NSILA nonsuppressible insulinlike activity

NSM neurosecretory material; neurosecretory motor neuron; nonantigenic specific mediator; nutrient sporulation medium

N·s/m^2 newton seconds per square meter

NSMR National Society for Medical Research

NSN nephrotoxic serum nephritis; nicotine-stimulated neurophysin

NSNA National Student Nurse Association

NSND nonsymptomatic and not disabling

NSO nucleus supraopticus

NSP neuron specific protein

NSPB National Society for the Prevention of Blindness

NSQ Neuroticism Scale Questionnaire; not sufficient quantitiy

NSR nonspecific reaction; normal sinus rhythm; not seen regularly

NSS normal saline solution; not statistically significant

NSSTT nonspecific ST and T [wave]

NST nonshivering thermogenesis; nonstress test; nutritional support team

NSU nonspecific urethritis

NSurg neurosurgery, neurosurgeon

NSV nonspecific vaginosis

NSVD normal spontaneous vaginal delivery

NT nasotracheal; neotetrazolium; neurotensin; neutralization test; nortriptyline; not tested

5'NT 5'-nucleotidase

Nt amino terminal

N&T nose and throat

NTA natural thymocytotoxic autoantibody; nitrilotriacetic acid; Nurse Training Act

NTAB nephrotoxic antibody

NTD neural tube defect; 5'-nucleotidase

NTE not to exceed

NTF normal throat flora

NTG nitroglycerin; nontoxic goiter; normal triglyceridemia

NTIS National Technical Information Service

NTLI neurotensin-like immunoreactivity

NTN nephrotoxic nephritis

NTP National Toxicology Program; normal temperature and pressure; nucleoside triphosphate

NTR nutrition

NTRC National Toxins Research Center

NTS nasotracheal suction; nephrotoxic serum; nucleus tractus solitarius

NTU Navy Toxicology Unit

NU name unknown

nU nanounit

nu nude [mouse]

ν Greek letter *nu*; degrees of freedom; frequency; kinematic velocity; neutrino

NUC sodium urate crystal

nuc nucleated

nucl nucleus

NUG necrotizing ulcerative gingivitis

NUI number user identification

nullip nulliparous

numc number concentration

NURB Neville upper reservoir buffer

NUV near ultraviolet

NV next visit; nonveteran; not vaccinated; not venereal; not volatile

Nv naked vision

N&V nausea and vomiting

NVA near visual acuity

NVB neurovascular bundle

NVD nausea, vomiting, and diarrhea; neck vein distention; no venereal disease, Newcastle virus disease

NVM nonvolatile matter

NVSS normal variant short stature

NW naked weight

NWB non-weight bearing

NWDA National Wholesale Druggists Association

NWR normotensive Wistar rat

NYC New York City [medium]

NYD not yet diagnosed; not yet discovered

nyst nystagmus

NZB New Zealand black [mouse]

NZO New Zealand obese [mouse]

NZR New Zealand red [rabbit]

NZW New Zealand white [mouse]

–O–

O a blood group in the ABO system; eye [Lat. *oculus*]; nonmotile strain of microorganisms [Ger. *ohne Hauch*]; objective findings; observed frequency in a contingency table; obstetrics; obvious; occipital electrode placement in electroencephalography; occiput; occlusal; oculus; often; ohm; old; opening; operator; operon; opium; oral; orale; orange [color]; orderly respirations [anesthesia chart]; ortho-; other; oxygen; pint [Lat. *octarius*]; respirations [anesthesia chart]

O₂ both eyes; diatomic oxygen; molecular oxygen

O₃ ozone

o eye [Lat. *oculus*]; opening; ovary transplant; pint [Lat. *octarius*]; see *omicron*

Ω see *ohm*

Ω   see *omega*
ω   see *omega*
o negative; without
OA occipital artery; occiput anterior; old age; oleic acid; opiate analgesia; optic atrophy; oral alimentation; osteoarthritis; ovalbumin; Overeaters Anonymous
OAA Old Age Assistance; Opticians Association of America; oxaloacetic acid
OAAD ovarian ascorbic acid depletion
OAB ABO blood group; old age benefits
OAD obstructive airway disease; organic anionic dye
OADC oleate-albumin-dextrose-catalase [medium]
OAF open air factor; osteoclast activating factor
OAH ovarian androgenic hyperfunction
OAM outer acrosomal membrane
OAP Office of Adolescent Pregnancy; old age pension, old age pensioner; ophthalmic artery pressure; osteoarthropathy; oxygen at atmospheric pressure
OAS old age security; osmotically active substance
OASDHI Old-Age, Survivors, Disability and Health Insurance
OASDI Old-Age, Survivors, and Disability Insurance
OASI Old Age and Survivors Insurance
OASP organic acid soluble phosphorus
OAT ornithine aminotransferase
OAV oculoauriculovertebral [dysplasia]
OAVD oculoauriculovertebral dysplasia
OB objective benefit; obstetrics, obstetrician; occult bleeding
O&B opium and belladonna
ob he (she) died [Lat. *obiit*]; obese [mouse]
OBD organic brain disease
OBE Office of Biological Education
OBE-CALP placebo capsule or tablet
OBG, ObG obstetrics and gynecology, obstetrician-gynecologist
OBGS obstetrical and gynecological surgery
OB-GYN, ObGyn obstetrics and gyne- cology, obstetrician-gynecologist
obl oblique
ob/ob obese [mouse]
OBS obstetrical service; organic brain syndrome

Obs observation, observed; obstetrics, obstetrician
obs obsolete
Obst obstetrics, obstetrician
obst obstruction, obstructed
OC obstetrical conjugate; occlusocervical; office call; on call; only child; optic chiasma; oral contraceptive; original claim; outer canthal [distance]; oxygen consumed
O&C onset and course
OCA oculocutaneous albinism
O₂cap oxygen capacity
Occ occiput, occipital; occlusion; occlusive
occ, occas occasional
occip occiput, occipital
OccTh occupational therapy, occupational therapist
Occup occupation, occupational
OCD Office of Child Development; Office of Civil Defense; ovarian cholesterol depletion
OCG omnicardiogram; oral cholecystogram
OCH oral contraceptive hormone
OCHS Office of Cooperative Health Statistics
OCIS Oncology Center Information System
OCN oculomotor nucleus
OCP octacalcium phosphate
OCR oculocardiac reflex; optical character recognition
oCRF ovine corticotropin-releasing factor
OCRS oculocerebrorenal syndrome
OCS open canalicular system; oral contraceptive steroid; outpatient clinic substation
OCT optimal cutting temperature; ornithine carbamoyltransferase; oxytocin challenge test
OCU observation care unit
OCV ordinary conversational voice
OD Doctor of Optometry; every day [Lat. *omni die*]; obtained absorbance; occipital dysplasia; occupational disease; oculus dexter; on duty; once a day; optical density; originally derived; out-of-date; outside diameter; overdose, overdosage; right eye [Lat. *oculus dexter*]

O-D obstacle-dominance
ODA right occipito-anterior [fetal position] [Lat. *occipito-dextra anterior*]
ODB opiate-directed behavior
ODC ornithine decarboxylase; oxygen dissociation curve
ODD oculodentodigital [dysplasia]
ODM ophthalmodynamometer, ophthalmodynamometry
ODOD oculo-dento-osseous dysplasia
Odont odontogenic
odorat odoriferous [Lat. *odoratus*]
ODP right occipitoposterior [fetal position] [Lat. *occipito-dextra posterior*]
ODT right occipitotransverse [fetal position] [Lat. *occipito-dextra transversa*]
ODU optical density unit
OE on examination; otitis externa
O&E observation and examination
Oe oersted
OEE osmotic erythrocyte enrichment; outer enamel epithelium
OEF oxygen extraction fraction
OER oxygen enhancement ratio
O2ER oxygen extraction ratio
OERP Office of Education and Regional Programming
OES optical emission spectroscopy
oesoph esophagus [oesophagus]
OF occipitofrontal; orbitofrontal; osmotic fragility; oxidation-fermentation
O/F oxidation-fermentation
OFC occipitofrontal circumference; osteitis fibrosa cystica
OFD object-film distance; oro-facial-digital [syndrome]
ofd object-film distance
Off official
OFM orofacial malformation
OG obstetrics and gynecology; occluso-gingival; optic ganglion; orange green; orogastric
OGF ovarian growth factor
OGH ovine growth hormone
OGS oxygenic steroid
OGTT oral glucose tolerance test
OH every hour [Lat. *omni hora*]; hydroxycorticosteroid; occipital horn; occupational health; occupational history; osteopathic hospital; outpatient hospital
OHA oral hypoglycemic agents
O₂Hb oxyhemoglobin

OHC occupational health center; outer hair cell
OH-Cbl hydroxycobalamin
OHCS hydroxycorticosteroid
OHD hydroxyvitamin D; Office of Human Development; organic heart disease
25-OH-D 25-hydroxyvitamin D
OHDA hydroxydopamine
16-OH-DHAS 16-alpha-hydroxydehydroepiandrosterone sulfate
8-OH-DPAT 8-hydroxy-2-(di-n-propylamino)tetralin
OHDS Office of Human Development Services
OHF Omsk hemorrhagic fever
OHI Occupational Health Institute; oral hygiene index; Oral Hygiene Instruction
OHI-S Oral Hygiene Instruction–Simplified
OHN occupational health nurse
OHP oxygen under high pressure
17-OHP 17-hydroxyprogesterone
OHR Office of Health Research
OHS obesity hypoventilation syndrome; ovarian hyperstimulation syndrome
OHSS ovarian hyperstimulation syndrome
OI opportunistic infection; opsonic index; orgasmic impairment; orientation inventory; osteogenesis imperfecta; oxygen intake
OID Organism Identification Number
OIF observed intrinsic frequency; oil immersion field; Osteogenesis Imperfecta Foundation
OIH Office of International Health; orthoiodohippurate; ovulation-inducing hormone
oint ointment
OIR Office of International Research
OIT organic integrity test
OJ orange juice
OKN optokinetic nystagmus
Ol oil [Lat. *oleum*]
ol left eye [Lat. *oculus laevus*]
OLA left occipito-anterior [fetal position] [Lat. *occipito-laeva anterior*]
OLB open liver biopsy
OLH ovine lactogenic hormone
oLH ovine luteinizing hormone
OLIDS open loop insulin delivery system

ol oliv olive oil [Lat. *oleum olivea*]
OLP left occipitoposterior [fetal position] [Lat. *occipito-laeva posterior*]
ol res oleoresin
OLT left occipitotransverse [fetal position] [Lat. *occipito-laeva transversa*]
OM occipitomental; occupational medicine; oculomotor; Osborne Mendel [rat]; osteomalacia; osteomyelitis; otitis media; outer membrane; ovulation method
om every morning [Lat. *omni mane*]
OMAR Office of Medical Applications of Research
OMAS occupational maladjustment syndrome
OMD ocular muscle dystrophy; oculomandibulodyscephaly
OME office of medical examiner; otitis media with effusions
Ω Greek capital letter *omega*
Ω ohm
Ω -1 ohm^{-1}, siemens
ω Greek lower case letter *omega*; angular velocity
OMH Office of Mental Health
OMI old myocardial infarction
o Greek letter *omicron*
OMN oculomotor nerve
omn bih every two hours [Lat. *omni bihora*]
omn hor every hour [Lat. *omni hora*]
omn 2 hor every second hour [Lat. *omni secunda hora*]
omn man every morning [Lat. *omni mane*]
omn noct every night [Lat. *omni nocte*]
omn quad hor every quarter of an hour [Lat. *omni quadrante hora*]
OMPA octamethyl pyrophosphoramide; otitis media, purulent, acute
om quar hor every quarter of an hour [Lat. *omni quadrante hora*]
OMS organic mental syndrome
OM&S osteopathic medicine and surgery
OMSC otitis media secretory (or suppurative) chronic
ON every night [Lat. *omni nocte*]; office nurse; onlay; optic nerve; orthopedic nurse; overnight
ONC oncology; Orthopaedic Nursing Certificate

OND Ophthalmic Nursing Diploma; other neurological disorders
ONP operating nursing procedure
ONPG o-nitrophenyl-beta-D-galactopyranoside
ONS Oncology Nursing Society
ONTG oral nitroglycerin
ONTR orders not to resuscitate
OO oophorectomy
OOB out of bed
OOLR ophthalmology, otology, laryngology, and rhinology
OP occiput posterior; olfactory peduncle; opening pressure; operation, operative; operative procedure; ophthalmology; osmotic pressure; outpatient; ovine prolactin
O&P ova and parasites
Op opisthocranion
op operation; operator
OPB outpatient basis
OPC outpatient clinic
OPCA olivopontocerebellar atrophy
OPD optical path difference; outpatient department; outpatient dispensary
O'p-DDD mitotane
OpDent operative dentistry
OPDG ocular plethysmodynamography
OPG ocular pneumoplethysmography; oxypolygelatin
opg opening
OPH, Oph ophthalmology; ophthalmoscopy, ophthalmoscope
OphD Doctor of Ophthalmology
Ophth ophthalmology
OPI oculoparalytic illusion
OPK optokinetic
OPL ovine placental lactogen
OPM ophthalmoplegic migraine
OPN ophthalmic nurse
OPP oxygen partial pressure
opp opposite
OPPG oculopneumoplethysmography
OPRR Office of Protection from Research Risks
OPS operations; outpatient service
OpScan optical scanning
OPSI overwhelming post-splenectomy infection
OPT outpatient; outpatient treatment
opt optics, optician
OPV oral polio vaccine

OR a logical binary relation that is true if any argument is true, and false otherwise; [o]estrogen receptor; odds ratio; oil retention [enema]; operating room; optic radiation; orthopedic; orthopedic research

O-R oxidation-reduction

Or orbitale

ORANS Oak Ridge Analytical System

ORBC ox red blood cell

ORD optical rotatory dispersion; oral radiation death

ORDS Office of Research, Demonstration, and Statistics

OREF Orthopedic Research and Education Foundation

Org, org organic

ORIF open reduction with internal fixation

OrJ orange juice

ORL otorhinolaryngology

ORN operating room nurse; orthopedic nurse

Orn ornithine

ORNL Oak Ridge National Laboratory

ORO oil red O

OROS oral osmotic

ORP oxidation-reduction potential

ORPM orthorhythmic pacemaker

ORS olfactory reference syndrome; oral surgery, oral surgeon; Orthopaedic Research Society; orthopedic surgery, orthopedic surgeon

ORT operating room technician; oral rehydration therapy

orth, ortho orthopedics, orthopedic

OS occupational safety; opening snap; oral surgery; orthopedic surgery, orthopedic surgeon; Osgood-Schlatter [disease]; osteogenic sarcoma; osteosarcoma; oxygen saturation

Os osmium

os left eye [Lat. *oculus sinister*]

OSA obstructive sleep apnea; Office of Services to the Aging; Optical Society of America

OSAS obstructive sleep apnea syndrome

OSF outer spiral fiber

OSHA Occupational Safety and Health Adminstration

OSM ovine submaxillary mucin; oxygen saturation meter

osm osmole; osmosis, osmotic

Osm/kg osmoles per kilogram

Osm/l osmoles per liter

osmol osmole

OST object sorting test

osteo osteomyelitis; osteopathy

OSUK Ophthalmological Society of the United Kingdom

OT objective test; oblique talus; occlusion time; occupational therapy, occupational therapist; old term (in anatomy); old tuberculin; olfactory threshold; optic tract; original tuberculin; orotracheal; otology; oxytocin

Ot otolaryngology

OTA ornithine transaminase; orthotoluidine arsenite

OTC ornithine transcarbamylase; oval target cell; over-the-counter; oxytetracycline

OTD oral temperature device; organ tolerance dose

OTE optically transparent electrode

OTF oral transfer factor

OTI ovomucoid trypsin inhibitor

OTM orthotoluidine manganese sulfate

OTO otology; otorhinolaryngology

Otol otology, otologist

OTR Ovarian Tumor Registry; Occupational Therapist, Registered

OTReg Occupational Therapist, Registered

OTS occipital temporal sulcus; orotracheal suction

OTT orotracheal tube

OTU operational taxonomic unit

ou both eyes together [Lat. *oculi unitas*]; each eye [Lat. *oculus uterque*]

OULQ outer upper left quadrant

OURQ outer upper right quadrant

OV office visit; ovalbumin; overventilation; ovulation

ov ovum

OVA ovalbumin

ova ovariectomy

OVD occlusal vertical dimension

OvDF ovarian dysfunction

OVX ovariectomized

O/W oil in water

OWR ovarian wedge resection

OX optic chiasma; oxacillin; oxytocin

os oxymel

OXT oxytocin

OXY oxygen

oz ounce
oz ap apothecaries' ounce (U.S.)
oz apoth apothecaries' ounce (U.K.)
oz t ounce troy (U.S.)
oz tr ounce troy (U.K.)

–P–

P an electrocardiographic wave corresponding to a wave of depolarization crossing the atria; by weight [Lat. *pondere*]; father [Lat. *pater*]; a handful [Lat. *pugilus*]; near [Lat. *proximum*]; near point [Lat. *punctum proximum*]; pain; parietal electrode placement in electroencephalography; part; partial pressure; *Pasteurella*; paternal; patient; percent; percussion; perforation; peta–; pharmacopeia; phenylalanine; phenylphthalein; phosphate group; phosphorus; physiology; pig; pint; placebo; plan; plasma; *Plasmodium*; poise; poison; poisoning; polarity; polarization; pole; polymyxin; population; porcelain; porcine; porphyrin; position; positive; posterior; postpartum; power; precipitin; prednisone; premolar; presbyopia; pressure; primary; primipara; probability; product; progesterone; prolactin; proline; properdin; proprionate; protein; *Proteus*; *Pseudomonas*; psychiatry; pulse; pupil; radiant power; significance probability [value]; sound power

P₁, P-one first parental generation

P₂ pulmonic second sound

³²P radioactive phosphorus

P-50 oxygen half-saturation pressure

p atomic orbital with angular momentum quantum number 1; freeze preservation; the frequency of the more common allele of a pair; momentum; papilla; phosphate; pico–; pint; pond; pressure; probability; proton; pupil; short arm of chromosome; sound pressure

p after

p- para

5p- cri-du-chat syndrome

Π see *pi*

π see *pi*

Ψ see *psi*

Φ see *phi*

PA Paleopathology Association; pantothenic acid; paralysis agitans; paranoia; pathology; periarteritis; periodic acid; pernicious anemia; phakic-aphakic; phosphatidic acid; phosphoarginine; photoallergy; physician assistant; pituitary-adrenal; plasma aldosterone; plasminogen activator; platelet adhesiveness; platelet aggregation; platelet-associated; polyarteritis; polyarthritis; posteroanterior; prealbumin; predictive accuracy; pregnancy-associated; presents again; primary aldosteronism; primary amenorrhea; primary anemia; prior to admission; proactivator; proanthocyanidin; procainamide; prolonged action; protrusio acetabuli; psychoanalysis; pulmonary artery; pulmonary atresia; pulpoaxial; puromycin aminonucleoside; pyrrolizidine alkaloid; yearly [Lat. *per annum*]

P$_A$ alveolar pressure

P-A postero-anterior

P&A percussion and auscultation

Pa arterial pressure; pascal; protactinium; *Pseudomonas aeruginosa*

pA picoampere

PAA phenylacetic acid; plasma angiotensinase activity; polyacrylamide; polyamino acid; pyridineacetic acid

PAB para-aminobenzoate; premature atrial beat; purple agar base

PABA para-aminobenzoic acid

PAC papular acrodermatitis of childhood; parent-adult-child; phenacetin, aspirin, and caffeine; plasma aldosterone concentration; premature atrial contraction

PACE Pacing and Clinical Electrophysiology; personalized aerobics for cardiovascular enhancement

P$_{ACO_2}$ partial pressure of carbon dioxide in alveolar gas

PaCO2 partial pressure of carbon dioxide in arterial blood

PAD phenacetin, aspirin, and desoxyephedrine; photon absorption densitometry; pulmonary artery diastolic

p ae equal parts [Lat. *partes aequales*]

paed pediatrics, pediatric [*paediatrics, paediatric*]

PAEDP pulmonary artery end-diastolic pressure

PAF paroxysmal atrial fibrillation; phosphodiesterase-activating factor; platelet-activating factor; platelet-aggregating factor; pollen adherence factor; premenstrual assessment form; pulmonary arteriovenous fistula

PA&F percussion, auscultation, and fremitus

PAFIB paroxysmal atrial fibrillation

PAFP pre-Achilles fat pad

PAG periaqueductal gray [matter]; polyacrylamide gel; pregnancy-associated globulin

pAg protein A-gold [technique]

PAGE polyacrylamide gel electrophoresis

PAGIF polyacrylamide gel isoelectric focusing

PAGMK primary African green monkey kidney

PAH para-aminohippurate; polycyclic aromatic hydrocarbon; pulmonary artery hypertension; pulmonary artery hypotension

PAHA para-aminohippuric acid

PAHO Pan-American Health Organization

PAIDS pediatric acquired immunodeficiency syndrome

PAIgG platelet-associated immunoglobulin G

PAJ paralysis agitans juvenilis

PAL pathology laboratory; posterior axillary line; pyogenic abscess of the liver

pal palate

palp palpation, palpate

palpi palpitation

PALS prison-acquired lymphoproliferative syndrome

PAM penicillin aluminum monostearate; phenylaline mustard; p-methoxyamphetamine; postauricular myogenic; pralidoxine; primary amebic meningoencephalitis; pulmonary alveolar macrophage; pulmonary alveolar microlithiasis; pyridine aldoxime methiodide

PAMC pterygoarthromyodysplasia congenital

PAME primary amebic meningoencephalitis

PAN periarteritis nodosa; periodic alternating nystagmus; peroxyacylnitrate; polyarteritis nodosa; positional alcohol nystagmus; puromycin aminonucleoside

pan pancreas, pancreatic, pancreatectomy

PAND primary adrenocortical nodular dysplasia

PANS puromycin aminonucleoside

PAO peak acid output; peripheral airway obstruction; plasma amine oxidase; polyamine oxidase

PAo pulmonary artery occlusion pressure

$P_{A O_2}$ partial pressure of oxygen in alveolar gas

$Pa O_2$ partial pressure of oxygen in arterial blood

PAOD peripheral arterial occlusive disease; peripheral arteriosclerotic occlusive disease

PAOP pulmonary artery occlusion pressure

PAP Papanicolaou [test]; peak airway pressure; peroxidase antibody to peroxidase; peroxidase-antiperoxidase [method]; primary atypical pneumonia; positive airway pressure; prostatic acid phosphatase; pulmonary alveolar proteinosis; pulmonary artery pressure

Pap Papanicolaou test

pap papilla

PAPF platelet adhesiveness plasma factor

papova papilloma-polyoma-vacuolating agent [virus]

PAPP p-aminopropiophenone; pregnancy-associated plasma protein

PAPS 3'-phosphoadenosine-5'-phosphosulfate

Paps papillomas

PAPUFA physiologically active polyunsaturated fatty acid

PAPVC partial anomalous pulmonary venous connection

PAPVR partial anomalous pulmonary venous return

PAR passive avoidance reaction; photosynthetically active radiation; physiological aging rate; platelet aggregate ratio; postanesthesia recovery; postanesthesia room; Program for Alcohol Recovery; pulmonary arteriolar resistance

par paraffin; paralysis

PARA, Para, para P–pregnancies, A–abortions, RA–living children
para paraplegic; parathyroid, parathyroidectomy
para 0 nullipara
para I primipara
para II secundipara
para III tripara
para IV quadripara
para 3-2-1 3 pregnancies, 2 abortions, 1 living child
par aff the part affected [Lat. *pars affecta*]
parasit parasitology; parasite, parasitic
parasym parasympathetic
parent parenteral
parox paroxysm, paroxysmal
PARS Personal Adjustment and Role Skills Scale
part aeq equal parts [Lat. *partes aequales*]
part dolent painful parts [Lat. *partes dolentes*]
part vic in divided doses [Lat. *partitis vicibus*]
PARU postanesthetic recovery unit
PAS paraaminosalicylate; patient appointments and scheduling; periodic acid-Schiff [reaction]; peripheral anterior synechia; persistent atrial standstill; photoacoustic spectroscopy; posterior airway space; premature atrial stimulus; Professional Activity Study; progressive accumulated stress; pulmonary arterial stenosis; pulmonary artery systolic
Pa•s pascal-second
Pa x s pascals per second
PASA paraaminosalicylic acid
PAS-C paraaminosalicylic acid crystallized with ascorbic acid
PASD after diastase digestion
PASG pneumatic antishock garment
PASM periodic acid silver methenamine
pass passive
PAST periodic acid-Schiff technique
Past *Pasteurella*
PAT paroxysmal atrial tachycardia; patient; picric acid turbidity; poyamine acetyltransferase; preadmission screening and assessment team; preadmission testing; pregnancy at term
pat paternal origin

PATE psychodynamic and therapeutic education; pulmonary artery thromboembolism
PATH pathology, pathological; pituitary adrenotropic hormone
path pathogenesis, pathogenic; pathology, pathological
PAT-SED pseudoachondroplastic dysplasia
PA-T-SP periodic acid-thiocarbohydrazide-silver proteinate
PAW pulmonary artery wedge
Paw mean airway pressure
PAWP pulmonary arterial wedge pressure
PB British pharmacopeia [*Pharmacopoeia Britannica*]; peripheral blood; phenobarbital; phonetically balanced; premature beat; pressure breathing; protein binding
Pb lead [Lat. *plumbum*]; phenobarbital; presbyopia
P&B phenobarbital and belladona
PBA polyclonal B-cell activity; pressure breathing assist; prolactin-binding assay; prune belly anomaly; pulpobuccoaxial
PBB polybrominated biphenyl
PBC peripheral blood cell; point of basal convergence; pre-bed care; primary biliary cirrhosis
PBD postburn day
PBE tuberculin from *Mycobacterium tuberculosis bovis* [Ger. *Perlsucht Bacillen-emulsion*]
PBF pulmonary blood flow
PBG porphobilinogen
PBG-S porphobilinogen synthase
PBH pulling boat hands
PBHB poly-beta-hydroxybutyrate
PBI parental bonding instrument; protein-bound iodine
PbI lead intoxication
PBL peripheral blood leukocyte; peripheral blood lymphocyte
PBM peripheral blood mononuclear [cell]
PBMC peripheral blood mononuclear cell
PBN paralytic brachial neuritis; polymyxin B sulfate, bacitracin, and neomycin
PBNA partial body neutron activation
PBO penicillin in beeswax; placebo

PBP penicillin-binding protein

PBS phosphate-buffered saline; prune belly syndrome

PBSP prognostically bad signs during pregnancy

PBT profile-based therapy

PBT$_4$ protein-bound thyroxine

PBV predicted blood volume; pulmonary blood volume

PBW posterior bite wing

PBZ phenylbutazone; phenoxybenzamine; pyribenzamine

PC avoirdupois weight [Lat. *pondus civile*]; packed cells; paper chromatography; parent cell; partition coefficient; pentose cycle; peritoneal cell; pharmacology; phosphate cycle; phosphatidyl choline; phosphocreatine; phosphorylcholine; physicians' corporation; pill counter; plasma cortisol; plasmacytoma; platelet concentrate; platelet count; pneumotaxic center; polyposis coli; portacaval; postcoital; posterior cortex; precordial; present complaint; printed circuit; procollagen; professional corporation; prostatic carcinoma; pubococcygeus [muscle]; pulmonary capillary; pulmonic closure; Purkinje cell; pyruvate carboxylase

pc after meals [Lat. *post cibum*]; parsec; percent; picocurie

PCA para-chloramphetamine; passive cutaneous anaphylaxis; patient care assistant/aide; patient-controlled analgesia; portacaval anastomosis; posterior communicating artery; President's Council on Aging; principal components analysis; procoagulant activity; pyrrolidine carboxylic acid

PCB paracervical block; polychlorinated biphenyl; portacaval bypass; procarbazine

PcB near point of convergence to the intercentral base line [*punctum convergens basalis*]

PC-BMP phosphorylcholine-binding myeloma protein

PCC pheochromocytoma; phosphate carrier compound; Poison Control Center; premature chromosome condensation; primary care clinic; prothrombin complex concentration

PCc periscopic concave

PCCU post-coronary care unit

PCD papillary collecting duct; phosphate-citrate-dextrose; posterior corneal deposits; plasma cell dyscrasia; polycystic disease; primary ciliary dyskinesia

PCDC plasma clot diffusion chamber

PCE physical capacity evaluation; pseudocholinesterase

PCF peripheral circulatory failure; pharyngoconjunctival fever; posterior cranial fossa; prothrombin conversion factor

pcf pounds per cubic feet

PCG paracervical ganglion; phonocardiogram; primate chorionic gonadotropin; pubococcygeus [muscle]

PCH paroxysmal cold hemoglobinuria; polycyclic hydrocarbon

pCi picocurie

PCIC Poison Control Information Center

PC-IRV pressure controlled inverted ratio ventilation

PCIS Patient-Care Information System

PCK polycystic kidney

PCKD polycystic kidney disease

PCL pacing cycle length; persistent corpus luteum; posterior cruciate ligament

PCM primary cutaneous melanoma; protein-calorie malnutrition; protein carboxymethylase

PCMO Principal Clinical Medical Officer

PCN penicillin; primary care nursing

PCNA proliferating cell nuclear antigen

PCNV postchemotherapy nausea and vomiting; Provisional Committee on Nomenclature of Viruses

PCO patient complains of; polycystic ovary

P$_{CO2}$, pCO2 partial pressure of carbon dioxide

PCOD polycystic ovarian disease

PCOS polycystic ovary syndrome

PCP parachlorophenate; pentachlorophenol; 1-(1-phenylcyclohexyl)piperidine; persistent cough and phlegm; phencyclidine; *Pneumocytis carinii* pneumonia; primary care physician; procollagen peptide; pulmonary capillary pressure; pulse cytophotometry

PCPA para-chlorophenylalanine

PCPL pulmonary capillary protein leakage

pcpn precipitation

PCR plasma clearance rate

PCS palliative care service; Patient Care System; patterns of care study; pharmacogenic confusional syndrome; portacaval shunt; postconcussion syndrome; primary cancer site; proportional counter spectrometry; pseudotumor cerebri syndrome

pcs preconscious

PCSM percutaneous stone manipulation

PCT plasma clotting time; plasmacrit test; plasmacytoma; polychloroterphenyl; porphyria cutanea tarda; portacaval transposition; prothrombin consumption time; proximal convoluted tubule

pct percent

PCU pain control unit

PCV packed cell volume; polycythemia vera

PCV-M polycythemia vera with myeloid metaplasia

PCW primary capillary wedge; purified cell walls

PCWP pulmonary capillary wedge pressure

PCx periscopic convex

PCZ prochlorperazine

PD Doctor of Pharmacy; Dublin Pharmacopoeia; interpupillary distance; papilla diameter; paralyzing dose; Parkinson disease; parkinsonian dementia; pars distalis; patent ductus; pediatrics; pediatric; peritoneal dialysis; phenyldichlorarsine; phosphate dehydrogenase; photosensitivity dermatitis; plasma defect; poorly differentiated; posterior division; postnasal drainage; potential difference; pressor dose; prism diopter; progression of disease; protein diet; psychotic depression; pulpodistal; pulse duration; pulmonary disease; pupillary distance; pyloric dilator

Pd palladium; pediatrics

PDA patent ductus arteriosus

PdA pediatric allergy

PDAB para-dimethylaminobenzaldehyde

PDB paradichlorobenzene; phosphorus-dissolving bacteria; preventive dental health behavior

PDC penta-decylcatechol; preliminary diagnostic clinic; private diagnostic clinic

PdC pediatric cardiology

PDD cisplatin; pervasive developmental disorder; primary degenerative dementia; pyridoxine-deficient diet

PDE paroxysmal dyspnea on exertion; phosphodiesterase; progressive dialysis encephalopathy; pulsed Doppler echocardiography

PdE pediatric endocrinology

PDF Parkinson's Disease Foundation

PDG parkinsonism-dementia complex of Guam

PDGA pteroyldiglutamic acid

PDGF platelet-derived growth factor

PDH past dental history; phosphate dehydrogenase

PDHC pyruvate dehydrogenase complex

PdHO pediatric hematology-oncology

PDI periodontal disease index; plan-do integration; psychomotor development index

Pdi transdiaphragmatic pressure

PDIE phosphodiesterase

P-diol pregnanediol

PDL periodontal ligament; poorly differentiated lymphocyte; population doubling level

pdl poundal; pudendal

PDLC poorly differentiated lung cancer

PDLD poorly differentiated lymphocytic–diffuse

PDLL poorly differentiated lymphocytic lymphoma

PDLN poorly differentiated lymphocytic–nodular

PDN prednisone

PdNEO pediatric neonatology

PdNEP pediatric nephrology

PDP pattern disruption point; piperidino-pyrimidine; primer-dependent deoxynucleic acid polymerase; Product Development Protocol

PDPI primer-dependent deoxynucleic acid polymerase index

PDQ protocol data query

PDR Physicians' Desk Reference; proliferative diabetic retinopathy

PdR pediatric radiology

pdr powder

PDS pain-dysfunction syndrome; paroxysmal depolarizing shift; patient data system; peritoneal dialysis system

PdS pediatric surgery

PDT population doubling time
PDUR Predischarge Utilization Review
PDW platelet distribution width
PE Edinburgh Pharmacopoeia; paper electrophoresis; penile erection; pericardial effusion; pharyngoesophageal; phenylephrine; phosphatidyl ethanolamine; photographic effect; phycoerythrin; physical education; physical examination; physical exercise; physiological ecology; pigmented epithelium; plasma exchange; pleural effusion; polyethylene; potential energy; powdered extract; preexcitation; probable error; pulmonary edema; pulmonary embolism; pyrogenic exotoxin
Pe pressure on expiration
PEA phenylethyl alcohol; phenylethylamine
PEBG phenethylbiguanide
PEC peritoneal exudate cell; pyrogenic exotoxin C
PED, ped pediatrics
PeDS Pediatric Drug Surveillance
PEEP positive end-expiratory pressure, peak end-expiratory pressure
PEF peak expiratory flow; Psychiatric Evaluation Form; pulmonary edema fluid
PEFR peak expiratory flow rate
PEFV partial expiratory flow volume
PEG Patient Evaluation Grid; pneumoencephalogram, pneumoencephalography; polyethylene glycol
PEI phosphate excretion index; polyethyleneimine; physical efficiency index
PEL peritoneal exudate lymphocyte; permissible exposure limit
pelidisi weight ten line divided sitting height [Lat. *pondus decies linearis divisus sidentis (altitudo)*]
PEM peritoneal exudate macrophage; prescription event monitoring; primary enrichment medium; probable error of measurement; protein energy malnutrition
PEMA phenylethylmalonamide
Pen penicillin
Pent pentothal
PEO progressive external ophthalmoplegia
PEP peptidase; phospho(enol)pyruvate; polyestradiol phosphate; postencephalitic parkinsonism; pre-ejection period; protein electrophoresis
Pep peptidase

PEPA peptidase A
PEPC peptidase C
PEPc corrected pre-ejection period
PEPCK phosphoenolpyruvate carboxykinase
PEPD peptidase D
PEPI pre-ejection period index
PEPP positive expiratory pressure plateau
PEPS peptidase S
PER peak ejection rate; protein efficiency ratio
per perineal; periodicity, periodic
PERF peak expiratory flow rate
perf perforation
PERI Psychiatric Epidemiology Research Interview
periap periapical
Perio periodontics
PERLA pupils equal, react to light and accommodation
per op emet when the action of emetic is over [Lat. *peracta operatione emetici*]
perp perpendicular
PERRLA pupils equal, round, react to light and accommodation
PERT program evaluation and review technique
PES photoelectron spectroscopy; physicians' equity services; postextrasystolic; pre-excitation syndrome
PESP postextrasystolic potentiation
Pess pessary
PET positron emission tomography; pre-eclamptic toxemia
PETH pink-eyed, tan-hooded [rat]
PETN pentaerythritol tetranitrate
petr petroleum
PETT pendular eye-tracking test; positron emission transverse tomography
PF peak flow; pericardial fluid; peritoneal fluid; permeability factor; personality factor; picture-frustration [study]; plantar flexion; plasma factor; platelet factor; pleural fluid; power factor; pulmonary factor; Purkinje fiber; purpura fulminans; push fluids
P-F picture-frustration [test]
PF$_{1-4}$ platelet factors 1 to 4
pF picofarad
PFA p-fluorophenylalanine
PFAS performic acid-Schiff [reaction]

PFC perfluorocarbon; persistent fetal circulation; plaque-forming cell

pFc noncovalently bonded dimer of the C-terminal immunoglobulin of the Fc fragment

PFD polyostotic fibrous dysplasia

PFIB perfluoroisobutylene

PFK phosphofructokinase

PFKL phosphofructokinase, liver type

PFKM phosphofructokinase, muscle type

PFKP phosphofructokinase, platelet type

PFO patent foramen ovale

PFP platelet-free plasma

PFQ personality factor questionnaire

PFR parotid flow rate; peak flow rate

PFS primary fibromyalgia syndrome; protein-free supernatant; pulmonary function score

PFT pancreatic function test; posterior fossa tumor; prednisone, fluororuracil, and taxomifen; pulmonary function test

PFTBE progressive form of tick-borne encephalitis

PFU plaque-forming unit; pock-forming unit

PFV physiologic full value

PG paregoric; pentagastrin; Pharmacopoeia Germanica; phosphate glutamate; phosphatidylglycerol; phosphogluconate; pituitary gonadotropin; plasma glucose; plasma triglyceride; polyfalacturonate; postgraduate; pregnanediol glucuronide; pregnant; propylene glycol; prostaglandin; proteoglycan; pyoderma gangrenosum

Pg nasopharyngeal electrode placement in electroencephalography; pogonion; pregnancy, pregnant

pg picogram

PGA phosphoglyceric acid; polyglandular autoimmune [syndrome]; prosta-glandin A; pteroylglutamic acid

PGA$_{1-3}$ prostaglandins A$_1$ to A$_3$

PGAS persisting galactorrhea-amenorrhea syndrome

PGB prostaglandin B

PGC primordial germ cell

PGD phosphogluconate dehydrogenase; phosphoglyceraldehyde dehydrogenase; prostaglandin D

PGD$_2$ prostaglandin D$_2$

6-PGD 6-phosphogluconate dehydrogenase

PGDH phosphogluconate dehydrogenase

PGDR plasma glucose disappearance rate

PGE, PGE$_1$, PGE$_2$ prostaglandins E, E$_1$, E$_2$

PGF, PGF$_1$, PGF$_2$ prostaglandins F, F$_1$, F$_2$

PG prostaglandin G

PGG$_2$ prostaglandin G$_2$

PGH pituitary growth hormone; prostaglandin H

PGH$_2$ prostaglandin H$_2$

PGI phosphoglucose isomerase; potassium, glucose, and insulin; prostaglandin I

PGI$_2$ prostaglandin I$_2$

PGK phosphoglycerate kinase

PGL persistent generalized lymphadenopathy; phosphoglycolipid

PGlyM phosphoglyceromutase

PGM phosphoglucomutase

PGN proliferative glomerulonephritis

PGO ponto-geniculo-occipital [spike]

PGP postgamma proteinuria; prepaid group practice

PGR progesterone receptor; psychogalvanic response

PgR progesterone receptor

PGS plant growth substance

PGTR plasma glucose tolerance rate

PGTT prednisolone glucose tolerance test

PGU postgonococcal urethritis

PGUT phosphogalactose uridyl transferase

PGV proximal gastric vagotomy

PGX prostacyclin

PGYE peptone, glucose yeast extract

PH partial hepatectomy; past history; personal history; pharmacopeia; previous history; primary hyperparathyroidism; prostatic hypertrophy; public health; pulmonary hypertension

Ph phenyl; phosphate; pharmacopeia

Ph^1 Philadelphia chromosome

pH hydrogen ion concentration

pH$_1$ isoelectric point

ph phial; phot
PHA passive hemagglutination; peripheral hyperalimentation; phytohemagglutinin; phytohemagglutinin antigen; pseudohypoaldosteronism; pulse-height analyzer
pH$_A$ arterial blood hydrogen tension
PHAL phytohemagglutinin-stimulated lymphocyte
phar pharmaceutical; pharmacy
Phar B Bachelor of Pharmacy [Lat. *Pharmaciae Baccalaureus*]
Phar C pharmaceutical chemist
Phar D Doctor of Pharmacy [Lat. *Pharmaciae Doctor*]
PHARM pharmacy
Phar M Master of Pharmacy [Lat. *Pharmaciae Magister*]
pharm pharmacopeia; pharmacy
PHB preventive health behavior
PhB, Phb Pharmacopoeia Britannica
PHBB propylhydroxybenzyl benzimidazole
PHC personal health costs; posthospital care; premolar hypodontia, hyperhidrosis, canities prematura [syndrome]; primary health care; primary hepatic carcinoma; proliferative helper cell
PhC pharmaceutical chemist
Ph^1 c Philadelphia chromosome
PHCC primary hepatocellular carcinoma
PHD photoelectron diffraction
PhD Doctor of Pharmacy [Lat. *Pharmaciae Doctor*]; Doctor of Philosophy [Lat. *Philosophiae Doctor*]
Phe phenylalanine
PhEEM photoemission electron microscopy
Pheo pheochromocytoma
PHF personal hygiene facility
PHFG primary human fetal glia
PhG Graduate in Pharmacy; Pharmacopoeia Germanica
phgly phenylglycine
PHI passive hemagglutination inhibition; phosphohexose isomerase; physiological hyaluronidase inhibitor
PhI Pharmacopoeia Internationalis
φ Greek letter *phi*; magnetic flux; osmotic coefficient
PHIM posthypoxic intention myoclonus
PHK platelet phosphohexokinase; postmortem human kidney

PHLA postheparin lipolytic activity
PHLS Public Health Laboratory Service
PhM Master of Pharmacy [Lat. *Pharmaciae Magister*]
PhmG Graduate in Pharmacy
PHN paaroxysmal noctural hemoglobinuria; passive Heymann nephritis; public health nursing, public health nurse
PH$_2$O partial pressure of water vapor
phos phosphate
PHP postheparin phospholipase; prepaid health plan; primary hyperparathyroidism; pseudohypoparathyroidism
p-HPPO p-hydroxyphenyl pyruvate oxidase
pHPT primary hyperparathyroidism
PHPV persistent hyperplastic primary vitreous
PHR peak heart rate
PHS pooled human serum; posthypnotic suggestion; Public Health Service
pH-stat apparatus for maintaining the pH of a solution
PHT portal hypertension
PhTD Doctor of Physical Therapy
Phx pharynx
PHY pharyngitis; physical; physiology
PHYS physiology
PhyS physiological saline [solution]
phys physical; physician
Phys Ed physical education
physio physiotherapy
Phys Med physical medicine
Phys Ther physical therapy
PI isoelectric point; pacing impulse; patient's interest; performance intensity; perinatal injury; periodontal index; personal injury; personality inventory; Pharmacopoeia Internationalis; phosphatidylinositol; physically impaired; pineal body; plaque index; pneumatosis intestinalis; poison ivy; postictal immobility; postinfection; postinoculation; preinduction [examination]; preparatory interval; present illness; primary infarction; primary infection; prolactin inhibitor; protamine insulin; protease inhibitor; pulmonary incompetence; pulmonary infarction
Pi, P$_i$ inorganic phosphate
Pi parental generation; pressure in inspiration; protease inhibitor
pI isoelectric point

Π Greek capital letter *pi*

π Greek lower case letter *pi*

π the ratio of circumference to diameter, 3.1415926536

PIA plasma insulin activity; preinfarction angina; Phychiatric Institute of America

PIAT Peabody Individual Achievement Test

PIC Personality Inventory for Children

PICA posterior inferior cerebellar artery

PICD primary irritant contact dermatitis

PICU pediatric intensive care unit; pulmonary intensive care unit

PID pain intensity difference [score]; pelvic inflammatory disease; photoionization detector; plasma iron disappearance; prolapsed intervertebral disk

PIDRA portable insulin dosage-regulating apparatus

PIDT plasma iron disappearance time

PIE preimplantation embryo; prosthetic infectious endocarditis; pulmonary infiltration with eosinophilia; pulmonary interstitial emphysema

PIF peak inspiratory flow; proinsulin-free; prolactin-inhibiting factor; proliferation-inhibiting factor

PIFR peak inspiratory flow rate

PIFT platelet immunofluorescence test

pigm pigment, pigmented

PIH pregnancy-induced hypertension; prolactin-inhibiting hormone

PII plasma inorganic iodine; primary irritation index

PIL patient information leaflet

pil pill [Lat. *pilula*]

π pi meson

PINN proposed international nonproprietary name

PINV post-imperative negative variation

PIP paralytic infantile paralysis; peak inflation pressure, peak inspiratory pressure; piperacillin; proximal interphalangeal; Psychotic Inpatient Profile

PIPJ proximal interphalangeal joint

PIQ Performance Intelligence Quotient

PIR postinhibition rebound

PIRS plasma immunoreactive secretion

PIS primary immunodeficiency syndrome; Provisional International Standard

pIs isoelectric point

PISCES percutaneously inserted spinal cord electrical stimulation

PIT picture identification test; pitocin; pitressin; plasma iron turnover

pit pituitary

PITC phenylisothiocyanate

PITR plasma iron turnover rate

PIU polymerase-inducing unit

PIV parainfluenza virus

PIXE particle-induced x-ray emission; proton-induced x-ray emission

PJB premature junctional beat

PJC premature junctional contractions

PJS peritoneojugular shunt; Peutz-Jeghers syndrome

PK pericardial knock; pig kidney; Prausnitz-Küstner [reaction]; psychokinesis; pyruvate kinase

pK negative logarithm of the dissociation constant

pK' apparent value of a pK; negative logarithm of the dissociation constant of an acid

pk peck

pK$_a$ negative logarithm of the acid ionization constant

PKAR protein kinase activation ratio

PKase protein kinase

PKD polycystic kidney disease

PKI potato kallikrein inhibitor

PKK plasma prekallikrein

PKT Prausnitz-Küstner test

PKU phenylketonuria

pkV peak kilovoltage

PL perception of light; phospholipid; photoluminescence; placebo; placental lactogen; plantar; plastic surgery; platelet lactogen; pulpolingual

Pl poiseuille

P$_L$ transpulmonary pressure

pl picoliter

PL/I programming language I (one)

PLA phospholipase A; platelet antigen; polylactic acid; potentially lethal arrhythmia; pulpolinguoaxial

PLa pulpolabial

Pla left atrial pressure

PLB parietal lobe battery; phospholipase B; porous layer bead

PLC proinsulin-like component; pseudolymphocytic choriomeningitis

PLCO postoperative low cardiac output

PLD phospholipase D; platelet defect; posterior latissimus dorsi [muscle]; potentially lethal damage

PLDH plasma lactic dehydrogenase

PLDR potentially lethal damage repair

PLE protein-losing enteropathy

PLED periodic lateralizing epileptiform discharge

PLES parallel-line equal space

PLET polymyxin, lysozyme, EDTA, and thallous acetate [in heart infusion agar]

PLG plasminogen

P-LGV psittacosis-lymphogranuloma venereum

PLH placental lactogenic hormone

PLL peripheral light loss; poly-L-lysine; pressure length loop

PLM percent labeled mitoses; polarized light microscopy

PLN peripheral lymph node

PLO polycystic lipomembranous osteodysplasia

PLP polystyrene latex particles; pyridoxal phosphate

PLS Papillon-Lefèvre syndrome; preleukemic syndrome; primary lateral sclerosis; prostaglandin-like substance

PLT pancreatic lymphocytic infiltration; platelet; primed lymphocyte typing; psittacosis-lymphogranuloma venereum-trachoma [group]

PLUT Plutchnik [geriatric rating scale]

PLV live poliomyelitis vaccine; panleukopenia virus; phenylalanine, lysine, and vasopressin

PLWS Prader-Labhart-Willi [syndrome]

plx plexus

PM after noon [Lat. *post meridiem*]; pacemaker; papillary muscle; papular mucinosis; perinatal mortality; petit mal epilepsy [Fr. *petit mal*]; photomultiplier; physical medicine; plasma membrane; platelet microsome; poliomyelitis; polymorph; polymyositis; porokeratosis of Mibelli; postmortem; premarketing [approval]; premolar; presystolic murmur; pretibial myxedema; preventive medicine; primary motivation; prostatic massage; protein methylesterase; puberal macromastia; pulpomesial

Pm promethium

pm picometer

PMA index of prevalence and severity of gingivitis, where P = papillary gingiva, M = marginal gingiva, and A = attached gingiva; papillary, marginal, attached [gingiva]; para-methoxyamphetamine; Pharmaceutical Manufacturers Association; phenylmercuric acetate; phosphomolybdic acid; primary mental abilities; progressive muscular atrophy; pyridylmercuric acetate

PMB para-hydroxymercuribenzoate; polychrome methylene blue; polymorphonuclear basophil; polymyxin B; postmenopausal bleeding

PMC phenylmercuric chloride; pseudomembranous colitis

PMD primary myocardial disease; programmed multiple development; progressive muscular dystrophy

PMDS primary myelodysplastic syndrome

PME polymorphonuclear eosinophil

PMF progressive massive fibrosis; proton motive force

pmf proton motive force

PMH past medical history; posteromedial hypothalamus

PMHR predicted maximum heart rate

PMI past medical illness; patient medication instruction; perioperative myocardial infarction; point of maximal impulse; point of maximal intensity; posterior myocardial infarction; postmyocardial infarction; present medical illness; previous medical illness

PMIS postmyocardial infarction syndrome; PSRO (*q.v.*) Management Information System

PML polymorphonuclear leukocyte; posterior mitral leaflet; progressive multifocal leukodystrophy; progressive multifocal leukoencephalopathy

PMM protoplast maintenance medium

PMMA polymethylmethacrylate

PMN polymorphonuclear; polymorphonuclear neutrophil

PMNC peripheral blood mononuclear cell

PMNG polymorphonuclear granulocyte

PMNL polymorphonuclear leukocyte

PMNN polymorphonuclear neutrophil

PMNR periadenitis mucosa necrotica recurrens

PMO postmenopausal osteoporosis; Principal Medical Officer
pmol picomole
PMP pain management program; patient medication profile; persistent mento-posterior [fetal position]; previous menstrual period
PMQ phytylmenaquinone
PMR perinatal mortality rate; physical medicine and rehabilitation; polymyalgia rheumatica; prior medical record; proportionate mortality ratio; proton magnetic resonance
PM&R physical medicine and rehabilitation
PMRAFNS Princess Mary's Royal Air Force Nursing Service
PMRS physical medicine and rehabilitation service
PMS patient management system; phenazine methosulfate; postmarketing surveillance; postmitochondrial supernatant; pregnant mare serum; premenstrual syndrome, premenstrual symptoms; postmenstrual stress
PMSC pluripotent myeloid stem cell
PMSG pregnant mare serum gonadotropin
PMT phenol O-methyltransferase; photomultiplier tube; Porteus maze test; premenstrual tension
PMTS premenstrual tension syndrome
PMV prolapse of mitral valve
PN percussion note; peripheral nerve; peripheral neuropathy; plaque neutralization; pneumonia; polyarteritis nodosa; polyneuritis; positional nystagnus; postnatal; practical nurse; psychiatry and neurology; psychoneurotic; pyelonephritis; pyridine nucleotide
P&N psychiatry and neurology
P_{N2} partial pressure of nitrogen
Pn pneumonia
PNA Paris Nomina Anatomica; peanut agglutinin; pentosenucleic acid
P_{Na} plasma sodium
PNAvQ positive-negative ambivalent quotient
PNB premature nodal beat
PNC penicillin; pneumotaxic center
PND paroxysmal nocturnal dyspnea; postnasal drainage; postnasal drip

PNdb perceived noise decibel
PNE plasma norepinephrine
pneu pneumonia
PNF proprioceptive neuromuscular facilitation
PNH paroxysmal nocturnal hemoglobinuria
PNHA Physicians National Housestaff Association
PNI peripheral nerve injury; postnatal infection
PNID Peer Nomination Inventory for Depression
PNK polynucleotide kinase
PNLA percutaneous needle lung aspiration
PNM perinatal mortality; peripheral nerve myelin
PNMT phenyl-ethanolamine-N-methyl-transferase
PNO Principal Nursing Officer
PNP pediatric nurse practitioner; peripheral neuropathy; para-nitrophenol; purine nucleoside phosphorylase
P-NP para-nitrophenol
PNPB positive-negative pressure breathing
PNPP para-nitrophenylphosphate
PNPR positive-negative pressure respiration
PNS parasympathetic nervous system; partial nonprogressive stroke; peripheral nervous system; posterior nasal spine; practical nursing student
PNT partial nodular transformation; patient
Pnt patient
PNU protein nitrogen unit
Pnx pneumothorax
PO by mouth, orally [Lat. *per os*]; period of onset; paarieto-occipital; perioperative; posterior; postoperative
po by mouth [Lat. *per os*]
PO_2, P_{O2}, $pO2$ partial pressure of oxygen
Po polonium; porion
POA pancreatic oncofetal antigen; phalangeal osteoarthritis; preoptic area; primary optic atrophy
POAG primary open-angle glaucoma
POA-HA preoptic anterior hypothalamic area

POB penicillin, oil, beeswax; place of birth

POC particulate organic carbon; postoperative care

pocill small cup [Lat. *pocillum*]

pocul cup [Lat. *poculum*]

POD peroxidase; place of death; polycystic ovary disease; postoperative day

PODx preoperative diagnosis

POE postoperative endophthalmitis; proof of eligibility

POEMS polyneuropathy, organomegaly, endocrinopathy, M protein, skin changes [syndrome]

POF primary ovarian failure; pyruvate oxidation factor

PofE portal of entry

POG polymyositis ossificans generalisata

Pog pogonion

pOH hydroxide ion concentration in a solution

POHI physically or otherwise health-impaired

POHS presumed ocular histoplasmosis syndrome

POI Personal Orientation Inventory

poik poikilocyte, poikilocytosis

POIS Parkland On-Line Information Systems

pois poison, poisoning, poisoned

pol polish, polishing

polio poliomyelitis

Poly polymorphonuclear

poly-A, poly(A) polyadenylic acid

poly-C, poly(C) polycytidylic acid

poly-G, poly(G) polyguanylic acid

poly-I, poly(I) polyinosinic acid

poly-IC, poly-I:C copolymer of polyinosinic and polycytidylic acids; synthetic RNA polymer

polys polymorphonuclear leukocytes

poly-T, poly(T) polythymidylic acid

poly-U, poly(U) polyuridylic acid

POM prescription only medicine

POMC propiomelanocortin

POMP principal outer material protein

POMR problem-oriented medical record

POMS Profile of Mood States

PON paraoxonase; particulate organic nitrogen

pond by weight [Lat. *pondere*]

POP diphosphate group; paroxypropione; persistent occipito-posterior [fetal position]; pituitary opioid peptide; plasma osmotic pressure; plaster of Paris; polymyositis ossificans progressiva

Pop popliteal; population

POPOP 1,4-Bis-(5-phenoxazol-2-yl)benzene

POR postocclusive oscillatory response; problem-oriented record

PORP partial ossicular replacement prosthesis

POS polycystic ovary syndrome; psychoorganic syndrome

pos positive

POSM patient-operated selector mechanism

POSS proximal over-shoulder strap

post posterior

postgangl postganglionic

postop, post-op postoperative

post sing sed liq after very loose stool [Lat. *post singulas sedes liquidas*]

POT periostitis ossificans toxica; postoperative treatment

pot potassium; potential

potass potassium

POU placenta, ovary, and uterus

POW Powassan [encephalitis]

powd powder

PP diphosphate group; emphysema [pink puffers]; near point of accommodation [Lat. *punctum proximum*]; pancreatic polypeptide; paradoxical pulse; partial pressure; perfusion pressure; peritoneal pseudomyxoma; persisting proteinuria; pinprick; placental protein; planned parenthood; plasma protein; polystyrene agglutination plate; population planning; posterior pituitary; postpartum; postprandial; preferred provider; private practice; protoporphyrin; proximal phalanx; pseudomyxoma peritonei; pulse pressure; pyrophosphate

P-5'-P pyridoxal-5'-phosphate

PP$_1$ free pyrophosphate

pp near point of accommodation [Lat. *punctum proximum*]; postprandial; postpartum

PPA first shake well [Lat. *phiala prius agitata*]; pepsin A; phenylpropanolamine; phenylpyruvic acid; Pittsburgh pneumonia agent; polyphosphoric acid;

postpartum amenorrhea; pure pulmonary atresia

Ppa pulmonary artery pressure

pp&a palpation, percussion, and auscultation

PPB positive pressure breathing

ppb parts per billion

PPBS postprandial blood sugar

PPC plasma prothrombin conversion; pneumopericardium; progressive patient care; proximal palmar crease

PPCA plasma prothrombin conversion accelerator; proserum prothrombin conversion accelerator

PPCF plasma prothrombin conversion factor

PPD paraphenylenediamine; phenyldiphenyloxadiazole; postpartum day; progressive perceptive deafness; purified protein derivative; Siebert purified protein derivative of tuberculin

PPD-S purified protein derivative-standard

PPE polyphosphoric ester; porcine pancreatic elastase

PPF pellagra preventive factor; phagocytosis promoting factor; plasma protein fraction

PPFA Planned Parenthood Federation of America

PPG photoplethysmography

ppg picopicogram

PPGF polypeptide growth factor

ppGpp 3'-pyrophosphoryl-guanosine-5'-diphosphate

PPH postpartum hemorrhage; primary pulmonary hypertension; protocollagen proline hydroxylase

pphm parts per hundred million

PPHN persistent pulmonary hypertension of the newborn

PPHP pseudopseudohypoparathyroidism

ppht parts per hundred thousand

PPI patient package insert; present pain intensity

PPi, PP$_i$ inorganic pyrophosphate

PPID peak pain intensity difference [score]

Ppl intrapleural pressure

PPLO pleuropneumonia-like organism

PPM phosphopentomutase; pigmented pupillary membrane

ppm parts per million

PPMA progressive postmyelitis muscular atrophy

PPN partial parenteral nutrition

PPNA peak phrenic nerve activity

PPNG penicillinase-producing *Neisseria gonorrhoeae*

PPO platelet peroxidase; preferred provider organization

PPP palatopharyngoplasty; palmoplantar pustulosis; pentosephosphate pathway; Pickford projective pictures; platelet-poor plasma; polyphoretic phosphate

PPPBL peripheral pulses palpable both legs

PPPI primary private practice insurance

PPR Price precipitation reaction

PPr paraprosthetic

PPRF paramedian pontine reticular formation

PPRWP poor precordial R-wave progression

PPS Personal Preference Scale; polyvalent pneumococcal polysaccharide; postpartum sterilization; postpericardiotomy syndrome; postpump syndrome; primary acquired preleukemic syndrome; prospective payment system

PPSH pseudovaginal perineoscrotal hypospadias

PPT partial prothrombin time; peak-to-peak threshold; plant protease test; pulmonary platelet trapping

ppt precipitation, precipitate; prepared

pptd precipitated

PPTL postpartum tubul ligation

PPV porcine parvovirus; positive pressure ventilation; progressive pneumonia virus

PPVT Peabody Picture Vocabulary Test

PPVT-R Peabody Picture Vocabulary Test, Revised

Ppw pulmonary wedge pressure

PQ permeability quotient; plastoquinone; pyrimethamine-quinine

PR by way of the rectum [Lat. *per rectum*]; far point [of accommodation] [Lat. *punctum remotum*]; parallax and refraction; partial remission; partial response; peer review; peripheral resistance; per rectum; phenol red; photoreactivation; pityriasis rosea; posterior root; potency ratio; preference record;

pregnancy; pregnancy rate; presso-receptor; pressure; prevention; Preyer's reflex; proctology; production rate; profile; progesterone receptor; prolactin; prosthion; protein; public relations; pulse rate; pulse repetition; pyramidal response

P-R the time between the P wave and the beginning of the QRS complex in electrocardiography

P&R pulse and respiration

Pr praseodymium; presbyopia; primary; prism; production rate (of steroid hormones); prolactin; propyl

pr far point of accommodation [Lat. *punctum remotum*]; pair; per rectum

PRA plasma renin activity

prac, pract practice, practice, practitioner

PrA-HPA protein A hemolytic plaque assay

PRAS pre-reduced anaerobically sterilized [medium]

p rat aetat in proportion to age [Lat. *pro ratione aetatis*]

PRB Prosthetics Research Board

PRBC packed red blood cells; placental residual blood volume

PRC packed red cells; peer review committee; phase response curve; plasma renin concentration

PRCA pure red cell aplasia

PRD partial reaction of degeneration; postradiation dysplasia

PRE progressive resistive exercise

pre-AIDS pre-acquired immune deficiency syndrome

pre preliminary

precip precipitate, precipitated, precipitation

PRED prednisone

prefd preferred

preg, pregn pregnancy, pregnant

prelim preliminary

prem prematurity, premature

preop, pre-op preoperative

prep, prepd prepare, prepared

preserv preservation, preserved, preserve

press pressure

prev prevention, preventive; previous

PREVMEDU preventive medicine unit

PRF partial reinforcement; patient report form; pontine reticular formation; prolactin releasing factor

pRF polyclonal rheumatoid factor

PRFM premature rupture of fetal membranes

PRG purge

PRH prolactin releasing hormone

PRI Pain Rating Index; phosphoribose isomerase

PRIAS Packard's radioimmunoassay system

PRIH prolactin release-inhibiting hormone

PRIME Prematriculation Program in Medical Education

primip primipara

prim luc first thing in the morning [Lat. *prima luc*]

prim m first thing in the morning [Lat. *primo mane*]

PRIST paper radioimmunosorbent test

PRK primary rabbit kidney

PRL, Prl prolactin

PRM phosphoribomutase; photoreceptor membrane; Primary Reference Material

PrM preventive medicine

prn as required [Lat. *pro re nata*]

PRNT plaque reduction neutralization test

PRO Professional Review Organization; pronation

Pro proline; prophylactic; prothrombin

pro protein

prob probable

proc proceedings, procedure; process

Proct proctology

prod production, product

prog, progn prognosis

prolong prolongation, prolonged

PROM passive range of motion; premature rupture of fetal membranes; prolonged rupture of fetal membranes; programmable read only memory

PROMIS Problem-Oriented Medical Information System

pron pronator, pronation

PROP propranolol

prop prophylaxis, prophylactic

ProPac Prospective Payment Assessment Commission

pros prostate, prostatic

prosth prosthesis, prosthetic

PROTO protoporphyrin

prov provisional

prox proximal

PRP physiologic rest position; pityriasis rubra pilaris; platelet-rich plasma; polyribosyl ribitol phosphate; postural rest position; pressure rate product; progressive rubella panencephalitis; Psychotic Reaction Profile

PRPP phosphoribosyl pyrophosphate

PRRE pupils round, regular, and equal

PR-RSV Prague Rous sarcoma virus

PRS Personality Rating Scale; plasma renin substrate

PRSIS Prospective Rate Setting Information System

PRT *Penicillium roqueforti* toxin; pharmaceutical research and testing; phosphoribosyl transferase

PRTH-C prothrombin time control

PRU peripheral resistance unit

PRV pseudorabies virus

PRVEP pattern reversal visual evoked potential

PRZF pyrazofurin

PS paradoxical sleep; pathological stage; patient's serum; pediatric surgery; performing scale [I.Q.]; periodic syndrome; pferdestärke; phosphate saline [buffer]; phosphatidyl serine; photosynthesis; physical status; plastic surgery; polystyrene; population sample; Porter-Silber [chromogen]; prescription; psychiatric; pulmonary stenosis; pyloric stenosis

P/S polisher-stimulator; polyunsaturated/ saturated [fatty acid ratio]

P&S paracentesis and suction

Ps prescription; *Pseudomonas*

ps per second; picosecond

PSA polyethylene sulfonic acid; progressive spinal ataxia; prolonged sleep apnea; prostate specific antigen

Psa systemic blood pressure

PSAn psychoanalysis

PSB protected specimen brush

PSbetaG pregnancy-specific beta-1-glycoprotein

PSC patient services coordination; Porter-Silber chromogen; posterior subcapsular cataract; primary sclerosing cholangitis; pulse synchronized contractions

PsChE pseudocholinesterase

Psci pressure at slow component intercept

PSD peptone, starch, and dextrose

PSE penicillin-sensitive enzyme; portal systemic encephalopathy; Present State Examination; purified spleen extract

psec picosecond

PSF pseudosarcomatous fasciitis

PSG peak systolic gradient; phosphate, saline, and glucose; polysomnogram; presystolic gallop

PSGN poststreptococcal glomerulonephritis

PsHD pseudoheart disease

PSI posterior sagittal index; problem solving information; psychosomatic inventory

psi pounds per square inch

Ψ Greek letter *psi*; wave function

PSIFT platelet suspension immunofluorescence test

PSIL preferred frequency speech interference level

PSL potassium, sodium chloride, and sodium lactate [solution]

PSM postmitochondrial supernatant; presystolic murmur

PSMA proximal spinal muscular atrophy

PSMed psychosomatic medicine

PSMF protein-sparing modified fast

PSMT psychiatric services management team

PSP pancreatic spasmolytic peptide; paralytic shellfish poisoning; parathyroid secretory protein; periodic short pulse; phenolsulfonphthalein; positive spike pattern; postsynaptic potential; progressive supranuclear palsy; pseudopregnancy

PSQ Parent Symptom Questionnaire

PSR pain sensitivity range; proliferative sickle retinopathy; pulmonary stretch receptor

PSRC Plastic Surgery Research Council

PSRO Professional Standards Review Organization

PSS physiological saline solution; porcine stress syndrome; progressive systemic scleroderma; progressive systemic sclerosis; Psychiatric Status Schedule

PST penicillin, streptomycin, and tetracycline; peristimulus time; phenolsulfotransferase; poststenotic; poststimulus time; proximal straight tubule

PSTI pancreatic secretory trypsin inhibitor

PSU photosynthetic unit
PSurg plastic surgery
PSVT paroxysmal supraventricular tachycardia
PSW psychiatric social worker
PSWT psychiatric social work training
Psy psychiatry
psych psychology, psychological
psychiat psychiatry, psychiatric
psychoan psychoanalysis, psychoanalytical
psychol psychology, psychological
psychopath psychopathology, psychopathological
PsychosMed psychosomatic medicine
psychother psychotherapy
psy-path psychopathic
PT parathormone; parathyroid; paroxysmal tachycardia; patient; pericardial tamponade; permanent and total; pharmacy and therapeutics; phototoxicity; physical therapy, physical therapist; physical training; physiotherapy; pine tar; pneumothorax; polyvalent tolerance; posterior tibial [artery pulse]; post-transplantation; propylthiouracil; prothrombin time; pulmonary tuberculosis; pyramidal tract; temporal plane
P&T pharmacy and therapeutics
Pt let it be continued [Lat. *perstetur*]; patient; platinum
pt part; patient; pint; point
PTA percutaneous transluminal angioplasty; persistent truncus arteriosus; phosphotungstic acid; plasma thromboplastin antecedent; posttraumatic amnesia; pre-treatment anxiety; prior to admission; prior to arrival
PTAH phosphotungstic acid hematoxylin
PTAP purified diphtheria toxoid precipitated by aluminum phosphate
PTB patellar tendon bearing; prior to birth
PTBE pyretic tick-borne encephalitis
PTC percutaneous transhepatic cholangiography; phase transfer catalyst; phenothiocarbazine; phenylthiocarbamide; phenylthiocarbamoyl; plasma thromboplastin component; premature tricuspid closure; prothrombin complex
PTCA percutaneous transluminal coronary angioplasty

PTD percutaneous transluminal dilatation; permanent total disability
PTE parathyroid extract; proximal tibial epiphysis; pulmonary thromboembolism
PTED pulmonary thromboembolic disease
PteGlu pteroylglutamic acid
PTEN pentaerythritol tetranitrate
pter end of short arm of chromosome
PTF patient treatment file; plasma thromboplastin factor
PTFE polytetrafluoroethylene
PTG parathyroid gland
PTH parathormone; parathyroid; parathyroid hormone; phenylthiohydantoin; plasma thromboplastin component; posttransfusion hepatitis
PTHS parathyroid hormone secretion [rate]
PTI pancreatic trypsin inhibitor; persistent tolerant infection; Pictorial Test of Intelligence
PTLC precipitation thin-layer chromatography
PTM posterior trabecular meshwork; post-transfusion mononucleosis
Ptm pterygomaxillary [fissure]
PTMA phenyltrimethylammonium
PTMDF pupils, tension, media, disc, fundus
pTNM TNM (*q.v.*) staging of tumors as determined by correlation of clinical, pathologic, and residual findings
PTO Klemperer's tuberculin [Ger. *Perlsucht Tuberculin Original*]
PTP post-tetanic potentiation; proximal tubular pressure
Ptp transpulmonary pressure
PTR patient termination record; peripheral total resistance; tuberculin *Mycobacterium tuberculosis bovis* [Ger. *Perlsucht Tuberculin Rest*]
PTr porcine trypsin
PTRIA polystyrene-tube radioimmunoassay
PTS para-toluenesulfonic acid; post-thrombotic syndrome; prior to surgery
Pts, pts patients
PTSD post-traumatic stress disorder
PTSH poststimulus time histogram
PTT partial thromboplastin time; particle transport time; pulmonary transit time; pulse transmission time

PTU propylthiouracil
PTX picrotoxinin
PTx parathyroidectomy
PTZ pentylenetetrazol
PU by way of the urethra [Lat. *per urethra*]; passed urine; peptic ulcer; pregnancy urine; 6-propyluracil
Pu plutonium; purple
pub, publ public
PUD peptic ulcer disease
PuD pulmonary disease
PUFA polyunsaturated fatty acid
PUL, pul, pulm pulmonary
pulv powder [Lat. *pulvis*]
pulv gros coarse powder [Lat. *pulvis grossus*]
pulv subtil smooth powder [Lat. *pulvis subtilis*]
pulv tenu very fine powder [Lat. *pulvis tenuis*]
PUN plasma urea nitrogen
PUO pyrexia of unknown origin
PUPPP pruritic urticarial papules and plaques of pregnancy
Pur purple
purg purgative
PUVA psoralen ultraviolet A-range
PV by way of the vagina [Lat. *per vaginam*]; paraventricular; pemphigus vulgaris; peripheral vascular; peripheral vein; peripheral vessel; pityriasis versicolor; plasma volume; polio vaccine; polycythemia vera; polyoma virus; portal vein; postvoiding; pulmonary vein
P-V pressure-volume [curve]
P&V pyloroplasty and vagotomy
Pv *Proteus vulgaris*; venous pressure
PVA polyvinyl alcohol
PVAc polyvinyl acetate
PVB premature ventricular beat
PVC persistent vaginal cornification; polyvinyl chloride; postvoiding cystogram; premature ventricular contraction; primary visual cortex; pulmonary venous congestion
PVCM paradoxical vocal cord motion
PV$_{CO2}$ partial pressure of carbon dioxide in mixed venous blood
PVD peripheral vascular disease; postural vertical dimension; pulmonary vascular disease
PVF peripheral visual field; portal venous flow

PVI peripheral vascular insufficiency
PVK penicillin V potassium
PVM pneumonia virus of mice; proteins, vitamins, and minerals
PVMed preventive medicine
PVN paraventricular nucleus
PVNPS post-Viet Nam psychiatric syndrome
PVO pulmonary venous obstruction
PV$_{O2}$ partial oxygen pressure in mixed venous blood
PVOD pulmonary vascular obstructive disease; pulmonary veno-occlusive disease
PVP penicillin V potassium; peripheral vein plasma; peripheral venous pressure; polyvinylpyrrolidone; portal venous pressure; pulmonary venous pressure
PVP-I polyvinylpyrrolidone-iodine
PVR peripheral vascular resistance; postvoiding residual; pulmonary vascular resistance; pulse volume recording
PVRI pulmonary vascular resistance index
PVS persistent vegetative state; premature ventricular systole; programmed ventricular stimulation
PVT paroxysmal ventricular tachycardia; portal vein thrombosis; pressure, volume, and temperature; private patient
PW posterior wall [of the heart]; pulmonary wedge [pressure]
Pw progesterone withdrawal
PWB partial weight bearing
PWBC peripheral white blood cell
PWC peak work capacity; physical work capacity
pwd powder
PWE posterior wall excursion
PWI posterior wall infarct
PWM pokeweed mitogen
PWP pulmonary wedge pressure
PWS Prader-Willi syndrome
pwt pennyweight
PX pancreatectomized; physical examination
Px past history; physical examination; pneumothorax; prognosis
PXE pseudoxanthoma elasticum
PXM projection x-ray microscopy
Py phosphopyridoxal; polyoma [virus]; pyridine

PYA psychoanalysis
PyC pyogenic culture
PYE peptone yeast extract
PYG peptone-yeast extract-glucose [broth]
PYGM peptone-yeast-glucose-maltose [broth]
PYLL potential years of life lost
PYM psychosomatic
PYP pyrophosphate
Pyr pyridine; pyruvate
PyrP pyridoxal phosphate
PZ pancreozymin
Pz 4-phenylazobenzylycarbonyl; parietal midline electrode placement in electro-encephalography
pz pièze
PZA pyrazinamide
PZ-CCK pancreozymin-cholecystokinin
PZI protamine zinc insulin
PZP pregnancy zone protein
PZT lead zirconate titanate

–Q–

Q coulomb [electric quantity]; electric charge; 1,4-glucan branching enzyme; glutamine; heat; quantity; quartile; query [fever]; quinacrine; quinone; quotient; radiant energy; reactive power; reaction energy; see QRS [wave]
Q_{10} temperature coefficient

q each, every [Lat. *quaque*]; electric charge; long arm of chromosome; quart; quintal
QAC quaternary ammonium compound
QALE quality-adjusted life expectancy
QALY quality-adjusted life years
qAM every morning
QAP quality assurance program; quinine, atabrine, and pamaquine
QARANC Queen Alexandra's Royal Army Nursing Corps
QARNNS Queen Alexandra's Royal Naval Nursing Service
QAUR quality assurance and utilization review
Q_B total body clearance
QC quality control; quinine colchicine

QCIM Quarterly Cumulative Index Medicus
Q_{CO2} carbon dioxide evoulation by a tissue
qd every day [Lat. *quaque die*]
qds to be taken four times a day [Lat. *quater die sumendum*]
QED quantum electrodynamics
QEF quail embryo fibroblasts
QEONS Queen Elizabeth's Overseas Nursery Service
QEW quick early warning
QF quality factor; quick freeze; relative biological effectiveness
qh every hour [Lat. *quaque hora*]
q2h every two hours [Lat. *quaque secunda hora*]
q3h every three hours [Lat. *quaque tertia hora*]
q4h every four hours [Lat. *quaque quarta hora*]
QHDS Queen's Honorary Dental Surgeon
QHNS Queen's Honorary Nursing Sister
QHP Queen's Honorary Physician
QHS Queen's Honorary Surgeon
qhs every hour of sleep [Lat. *quaque hora somni*]
qid four times daily [Lat. *quater in die*]
QIDN Queen's Institute of District Nursing
ql as much as desired [Lat. *quantum libet*]
QLS Quality of Life Scale
QM quinacrine mustard
qm every morning [Lat. *quaque mane*]
QMWS quasi-morphine withdrawal syndrome
qn every night [Lat. *quaque nocte*]
QNB quinuclidinyl benzilate
QNS quantity not sufficient; Queen's Nursing Sister
qns quantity not sufficient
Q_{O2} oxygen quotient; oxygen utilization
qod every other day [Lat. *quaque die*]
QP quanti-Pirquet [reaction]
qp as much as desired [Lat. *quantum placeat*]
QPEEG quantitative pharmaco-electro-encephalography
qPM every night

qqd every day [Lat. *quoque die*]
qqh every four hours [Lat. *quaque quarta hora*]
qq hor every hour [Lat. *quaque hora*]
QR quality review; quieting response; quinaldine red
qr quantity is correct [Lat. *quantum rectum*]; quarter
QRB Quality Review Bulletin
QRS in electrocardiography, the complex consisting of Q, R, and S waves, corresponding to depolarization of ventricles [complex]; in electrocardiography, the loop traced by QRS vectors, representing ventricular depolarization [interval]
QRS-ST the junction between the QRS complex and the ST segment in the electrocardiogram [junction]
QRS-T the angle between the QRS and T vectors in vectorcardiography [angle]
QRZ wheal reaction time
QS quiet sleep
qs as much as will suffice [Lat. *quantum sufficit*]; sufficient quantity [Lat. *quantum satis*]
QSAR quantitative structure-activity relationship
q sat to a sufficient quantity [Lat. *quantum satis*]
q suff as much as suffices [Lat. *quantum sufficit*]
QT Quick test
Q-T in electrocardiography, the time from the beginning of the QRS complex to the end of the T wave [interval]
qt quart; quiet
QTc Q-T interval corrected for heart rate
qter end of long arm of chromosome
quadrupl four times as much [Lat. *quadruplicato*]
qual quality, qualitative
quant quantity, quantitative
Quat, quat four [Lat. *quattuor*]
QUEST Quality, Utilization, Effectiveness, Statistically Tabulated
QUICHA quantitative inhalation challenge apparatus
quinq five [Lat. *quinque*]
quint fifth, quintan [Lat. *quintus*]
quotid daily, quotidian [Lat. *quotidie*]
qv as much as you desire [Lat. *quantum vis*]; which see [Lat. *quod vide*]

–R–

R arginine; Behnken's unit; Broadbent registration point; a conjugative plasmid responsible for resistance to various elements; any chemical group (particularly an alfyl group); electrical resistance; far point [Lat. *remotum*]; in electrocardiography, the first positive deflection during the QRS complex [wave]; gas constant; organic radical; race; racemic; radioactive; radiology; Rankine [scale]; rate; reaction; Réaumur [scale]; rectal; red; registered trademark; regression coefficient; regular; regular insulin; regulator [gene]; relapse; relaxation; release [factor]; remote; repressor; resistance; respiration; respiratory exchange ratio; response; rest; restricted; reverse [banding]; ribose; *Rickettsia*; right; Rinne [test]; roentgen; rough [colony]; rub; take [Lat. *recipe*]
R' in electrocardiography, the second positive deflection during the QRS complex
+R Rinne's test positive
-R Rinne's test negative
°R degree on the Rankine scale; degree on the Réaumur scale
r correlation coefficient; radius; ribose; ring chromosome; roentgen; sample correlation coefficient
r^2 coefficient of determination
ρ see *rho*
RA radioactive; ragocyte; ragweed antigen; reciprocal asymmetrical; refractory anemia; refractory ascites; renal artery; renin-angiotensin; repeat action; residual air; retinoic acid; rheumatoid arthritis; right angle; right arm; right atrium; right auricle
R_A airway resistance
Ra radium
rA riboadenylate
RAAMC Royal Australian Army Medical Corps
RAAS renin-angiotensin-aldosterone system
Rab rabbit
rac racemate, racemic
RAD radical; right axis deviation; roentgen administered dose
Rad radiotherapy; radium

rad radiation adsorbed dose; radial; radian; radical; radius; root [Lat. *radix*]
RADA rosin amine-D-acetate
RADC Royal Army Dental Corps
RADIO radiotherapy
Radiol radiology
RadLV radiation leukemia virus
RADS reactive airways dysfunction syndrome; retrospective assessment of drug safety
rad/s rad per second; radian per second
RADTS rabbit antidog thymus serum
RAE right atrial enlargement
RAEB refractory anemia with excess blasts
RAEB-T refractory anemia with excess of blasts in transformation
RAEM refractory anemia with excess myeloblasts
RAF rheumatoid arthritis factor
RAFMS Royal Air Force Medical Services
RAG ragweed
Ragg rheumatoid agglutinin
RAH right atrial hypertrophy
RAHTG rabbit antihuman thymocyte globulin
RAI radioactive iodine
RAIS reflection-absorption infrared spectroscopy
RAIU radioactive iodine uptake
RAM random-access memory; rapid alternating movements; research aviation medicine
RAMC Royal Army Medical Corps
RAMT rabbit antimouse thymocyte
RANA rheumatoid arthritis nuclear antigen
RAN resident's admission notes
RAO right anterior oblique
RaONC radiation oncology
RAP regression-associated protein; renal artery pressure; rheumatoid arthritis precipitin; right atrial pressure
RAPO rabbit antibody to pig ovary
RAR rat insulin receptor; right arm reclining; right arm recumbent
RARLS rabbit anti-rat lymphocyte serum
RARTS rabbit anti-rat thymocyte serum
RAS recurrent aphthous stomatitis; renal artery stenosis; renin-angiotensin system; reticular activating system; rheumatoid arthritis serum

ras scrapings or filings [Lat. *rasurae*]
RASS rheumatoid arthritis and Sjögren syndrome
RAST radioallergosorbent test
RAT repeat action tablet
RATG rabbit antithymocyte globulin
RATHAS rat thymus antiserum
RATx radiation therapy
RAV Rous-associated virus
RAVC Royal Army Veterinary Corps
R_{AW} airway resistance
RAZ razoxane
RB rating board; right bundle
Rb rubidium
RBA relative binding affinity; rescue breathing apparatus; right brachial artery; rose bengal antigen
RBAP repetitive bursts of action potential
RBB right bundle branch
RBBB right bundle branch block
RBBsB right bundle branch system block
RBC red blood cell; red blood corpuscle; red blood count
RBCD right border cardiac dullness
RBCM red blood cell mass
RBCV red blood cell volume
RBD right border of dullness
RBE relative biological effectiveness
RBF renal blood flow
Rb Imp rubber base impression
RBL rat basophilic leukemia; Reid's baseline
RBN retrobulbar neuritis
RBNA Royal British Nurses Association
RBOW rupture of the bag of waters
RBP radiation-induced plexopathy; retinol-binding protein; riboflavin-binding protein
RBS random blood sugar; Rutherford backscattering
RbSA rabbit serum albumin
RBV right brachial vein
RBZ rubidazone
RC an electronic circuit containing a resistor and capacitor in series; reaction center; red cell; red cell casts; red corpuscle; Red Cross; referred care; respiration ceases; respiratory care; respiratory center; rest cure; retention catheter; retrograde cystogram; root canal

Rc conditioned response; receptor

RCA red cell agglutination; renal cell carcinoma; right coronary artery

RCAMC Royal Canadian Army Medical Corps

rCBF regional cerebral blood flow

RCBV regional cerebral blood volume

RCC radiological control center; rape crisis center; ratio of cost to charges; receptor-chemoeffector complex; red cell count; renal cell carcinoma

RCCM Regional Committee for Community Medicine

RCD relative cardiac dullness

RCE reasonable compensation equivalent

RCF red cell folate; relative centrifugal field/force; ristocetin cofactor

RCGP Royal College of General Practitioners

RCHMS Regional Committee for Hospital Medical Services

RCI respiratory control index

RCITR red cell iron turnover rate

RCM radiographic contrast medium; red cell mass; reinforced clostridial medium; replacement culture medium; right costal margin; Royal College of Midwives

RCN right caudate nucleus; Royal College of Nursing

RCoF ristocetin cofactor

RCOG Royal College of Obstetricians and Gynaecologists

RCP retrocorneal pigmentation; riboflavin carrier protein; Royal College of Physicians

rcp reciprocal translocation

RCPath Royal College of Pathologists

RCPSGlas Royal College of Physicians and Surgeons, Glasgow

RCR relative consumption rate; respiratory control ratio

RCRA Resource Conservation and Recovery Act

RCS rabbit aorta-contracting substance; reticulum cell sarcoma; Royal College of Science; Royal College of Surgeons

RCSE Royal College of Surgeons, Edinburgh

RCT random controlled trial; retrograde conduction time; root canal therapy; Rorschach content test

rct a marker showing the ability of virulent strains to replicate at 40°C, while vaccine strain shows no replication

RCU respiratory care unit

RCV red cell volume

RCVS Royal College of Veterinary Surgeons

RD rate difference; Raynaud's disease; reaction of degeneration; registered dietician; Reiter's disease; renal disease; resistance determinant; respiratory disease; retinal detachment; Reye's disease; rheumatoid disease; right deltoid; rubber dam; ruptured disk

rd rutherford

R&D research and develpment

RDA recommended daily allowance; recommended dietary allowance; Registered Dental Assistant; right dorsoanterior [fetal position]

RDB random double-blind [trial]

RDC research diagnostic criteria

RDDA recommended daily dietary allowance

RDDP ribonucleic acid-dependent deoxynucleic acid polymerase

RDE receptor-destroying enzyme

RDES remote data entry system

RDFC recurring digital fibroma of childhood

RDH Registered Dental Hygienist

RDHBF regional distribution of hepatic blood flow

RDI rupture-delivery interval

RDLBBB rate-dependent left bundle branch block

rDNA ribosomal deoxyribonucleic acid

RDP right dorsoposterior [fetal position]

RDS reflex sympathetic dystrophy; respiratory distress syndrome

RDT retinal damage threshold; routine dialysis therapy

RDW red blood cell distribution width index

RE radium emanation; rectal examination; regional enteritis; renal and electrolyte; resting energy; reticuloendothelial; retinol equivalent; right ear; right eye

R_E respiratory exchange ratio

R&E research and education

Re rhenium

R_e Reynold's number

REA radiation emergency area; radioenzymatic assay; renal anastomosis; right ear advantage

REAB refractory anemia with excess of blasts

readm readmission

REAS reasonably expected as safe

REAT radiological emergency assistance team

REB roentgen-equivalent biological

rec recombinant chromosome; fresh [Lat. *recens*]; record; recurrent, recurrence

RECG radioelectrocardiography

recip recipient

recon the smallest unit of DNA capable of recombination [recombination + Gr. *on* quantum]

recond reconditioning, reconditioned

recryst recrystallization

rect rectification, rectified; rectum, rectal; rectus [muscle]

recur recurrence, recurrent

RED radiation experience data

redig in pulv let it be reduced to powder [Lat. *redigatur in pulverem*]

red in pulv reduced to powder [Lat. *reductus in pulverem*]

redox oxidation-reduction

REE rapid extinction effect; rare earth element

REEDS retention of tears, ectrodactyly, ectodermal dysplasia, and strange hair, skin and teeth [syndrome]

REEG radioelectroencephalography

ReEND reproductive endocrinology

REF ejection fraction at rest; renal erythropoietic factor

ref reference; reflex

Ref Doc referring doctor

REFI regional ejection fraction image

Refl reflex

REFMS Recreation and Education for Multiple Sclerosis [Victims]

Ref Phys referring physician

REG radiation exposure guide; radioencephalogram, radioencephalography

Reg registered

reg region

regen regeneration, regenerated, regenerating

reg umb umbilical region [Lat. *regio umbilici*]

regurg regurgitation

REH renin essential hypertension

rehab rehabilitation, rehabilitated

REL rate of energy loss

REM rapid eye movement; reticular erythematous mucinosis; return electrode monitor

rem removal; roentgen-equivalent–man

REMA repetitive excess mixed anhydride

REMAB radiation-equivalent–manikin absorption

REMCAL radiation-equivalent–manikin calibration

REMP roentgen-equivalent–man period

REMS rapid eye movement sleep

ren renew [Lat. *renovetur*]

ren sem renew only once [Lat. *renovetum semel*]

REO respiratory enteric orphan [virus]

REP roentgen equivalent–physical

rep let it be repeated [Lat. *repetatur*]; replication; roentgen equivalent–physical

repol repolarization

RER respiratory exchange ratio; rough endoplasmic reticulum

RES reticuloendothelial system

RESNA Rehabilitation Engineering Society of North America

resp respiration, respiratory; response

REST Raynaud's phenomenon, esophageal motor dysfunction, sclerodactyly, and telangiectasis [syndrome]

RET right esotropia

ret rad equivalent therapeutic

retard retardation, retarded

retic reticulocyte

REV reticuloendothelial virus

rev review; revolution

RF radial fiber; radiofrequency; receptive field; Reitland-Franklin [unit]; relative flow; relative fluorescence; release factor; renal failure; resistance factor; respiratory failure; reticular formation; retroperitoneal fibromatosis; rheumatic fever; rheumatoid factor; riboflavin; root canal filling rosette formation

R_F rate of flow

Rf respiratory frequency; rutherfordium

R_f in paper or thin-layer chromatography, the distance that a spot of a substance has moved from the point of application

rf radiofrequency

RFA right femoral artery; right fronto-anterior [fetal position]

RFB retained foreign body
RFC rosette-forming cell
RFE relative fluorescence efficiency
RFI renal failure index
RFL right frontolateral [fetal position]
RFLA rheumatoid-factor-like activity
RFLP restriction fragment length polymorphism
RFLS rheumatoid-factor-like substance
Rfm rifampin
RFP request for proposals; right fronto-posterior [fetal position]
RFPS (Glasgow) Royal Faculty of Physicians and Surgeons of Glasgow
RFR refraction
RFS renal function study
RFT rod-and-frame test; right fronto-transverse [fetal position]
RFW rapid filling wave
RGC radio-gas chromatography; retinal ganglion cell; right giant cell
RG right gluteal
RGE relative gas expansion
RGH rat growth hormone
RGM right gluteus medius
RGN Registered General Nurse
RGR relative growth rate
RH radiant heat; radiological health; reactive hyperemia; regulatory hormone; relative humidity; releasing hormone; retinal hemorrhage; right hand; right hemisphere; right hyperphoria; room humidifier
Rh rhesus [factor]; rhinion; rhodium
Rh+ rhesus positive
Rh- rhesus negative
rh rheumatic
r/h roentgens per hour
RHA Regional Health Authority
RHA(T) Regional Health Authority (Teaching)
RHBF reactive hyperemia blood flow
RHBs Regional Hospital Boards
RHC resin hemoperfusion column; right hypochondrium
RHCSA Regional Hospitals Consultants' and Specialists' Association
RHD radiological health data; relative hepatic dullness; rheumatic heart disease
RHEED reflection high-energy electron diffraction
rheu, rheum rheumatic, rheumatoid
RHF right heart failure

RHI Rural Health Initiative
Rhin rhinology
Rhiz *Rhizobium*
RHJSC Regional Hospital Junior Staff Committee
RHL recurrent herpes labialis; right hepatic lobe
RHLN right hilar lymph node
rhm roentgens per hour at 1 meter
RhMK rhesus monkey kidney
RhMk rhesus monkey
RhMkK rhesus monkey kidney
RHN Rockwell hardness number
RHO right heeloff
ρ Greek letter *rho*; correlation coefficient; electric charge density; electrical resistivity; mass density; reactivity
RHR renal hypertensive rat
r/hr roentgens per hour
RHS right hand side; right heelstrike
RHU registered health underwriter; rheumatology
RI radiation intensity; radioimmunology; recession index; recombinant inbred [strain]; refractive index; regional ileitis; regular insulin; release inhibition; remission induction; renal insufficiency; respiratory illness; respiratory index; retroactive inhibition; retroactive interference; ribosome
RIA radioimmunoassay
RIA-DA radioimmunoassay double antibody [test]
Rib ribose
RIBS Rutherford ion backscattering
RIC Royal Institute of Chemistry
RICM right intercostal margin
RICU respiratory intensive care unit
RID radial immunodiffusion
RIF release-inhibiting factor; rifampin; right iliac fossa
RIFA radioiodinated fatty acid
RIFC rat intrinsic factor concentrate
RIG rabies immune globulin
RIGH rabies immune globulin, human
RIH right inguinal hernia
RIHSA radioactive iodinated human serum albumin
RILT rabbit ileal loop test
RIM radioisotope medicine; recurrent induced malaria; relative-intensity measure
RIMR Rockefeller Institute for Medical Research

RIN rat insulinoma

RIND reversible ischemic neurologic deficit

RINN recommended international non-proprietary name

RIP radioimmunoprecipitation

RIPH Royal Institute of Public Health

RIPHH Royal Institute of Public Health and Hygiene

RIRB radioiodinated rose bengal

RIS rapid immunofluorescence staining

RISA radioactive iodinated serum albumin; radioimmunosorbent assay

RIST radioimmunosorbent test

RIT radioiodinated triolein; rosette inhibition titer

RITC rhodamine isothiocyanate

RIU radioactive iodine uptake

RIVC radionuclide imaging of the inferior vena cava

RK rabbit kidney; right kidney

RKG radiocardiogram

RKV rabbit kidney vacuolating [virus]

RKY roentgen kymography

RL radiation laboratory; reticular lamina; right leg, right lung

RLC residual lung capacity

RLD related living donor; ruptured lumbar disk

RLE right lower extremity

RLF retrolental fibroplasia

RLL right lower lobe

RLN recurrent laryngeal nerve

RLNC regional lymph node cell

RLND regional lymph node dissection

RLP radiation leukemia protection; ribosome-like particle

RLQ right lower quadrant

RLR right lateral rectus [muscle]

RLS restless leg syndrome; Ringer's lactate solution

RLV Rauscher leukemia virus

RM radical mastectomy; range of movement; red marrow; reference material; rehabilitation medicine; respiratory movement

rm room

RMA Registered Medical Assistant; relative medullary area; right mento-anterior [fetal position]

RMBF regional myocardial blood flow

RMC right middle cerebral [artery]

RMD retromanubrial dullness

RME rapid maxillary expansion

RMK rhesus monkey kidney

RML radiation myeloid leukemia; regional medical library; right medio-lateral; right middle lobe

RMLV Rauscher murine leukemia virus

RMM rapid micromedia method

RMN Registered Mental Nurse

RMO Regional Medical Officer; Resident Medical Officer

RMP rapidly miscible pool; regional medical program; resting membrane potential; rifampin; right mentoposterior [fetal position]

RMPA Royal Medico-Psychological Association

RMR resting metabolic rate; right medial rectus [muscle]

RMS rectal morphine sulfate [suppository]; respiratory muscle strength; rheumatic mitral stenosis; root-mean-square

rms root-mean-square

RMSD root-mean-square deviation

RMSF Rocky Mountain spotted fever

RMT registered music therapist; relative medullary thickness; retromolar trigone; right mentotransverse [fetal position]

RMuLV Rauscher murine leukemia virus

RMV respiratory minute volume

RN radionuclide; red nucleus; Registered Nurse

Rn radon

RNA radionuclide angiography; Registered Nurse Anesthetist; ribonucleic acid; rough, non-capsulated, avirulent [bacterial culture]

RNAA radiochemical neutron activation analysis

RNAse, RNase ribonuclease

RND radical neck dissection

RNFP Registered Nurse Fellowship Program

RNIB Royal National Institute for the Blind

RNID Royal National Institute for the Deaf

RNP ribonucleoprotein

RNR ribonucleotide reductase

RNSC radionuclide superior cavography

Rnt roentgenology

RNVG radionuclide ventriculography

RO reverse osmosis; Ritter-Oleson [technique]; rule out
R/O rule out
ROA right occipito-anterior [fetal position]
ROATS rabbit ovarian antitumor serum
rob Robersonian translocation
ROC receiver-operating characteristic; residual organic carbon
roent roentgenology
ROH rat ovarian hyperemia [test]
ROI region of interest; right occipito-lateral [fetal position]
ROM range of motion; read only memory; rupture of membranes
ROP retinopathy of prematurity; right occipitoposterior [fetal position]
Ror Rorschach [test]
ROS review of systems; rod outer segment
RoS rostral sulcus
ROT real oxygen transport; remedial occupational therapy; right occipito-transverse [fetal position]
rot rotating, rotation
ROU recurrent oral ulcer
ROW Rendu-Osler-Weber [syndrome]
RP radial pulse; rapid processing [of film]; Raynaud's phenomenon; reactive protein; readiness potential; refractory period; regulatory protein; respiratory rate; rest pain; resting potential; resting pressure; retinitis pigmentosa; retrograde pyelogram; retroperitoneal; reverse phase; rheumatoid polyarthritis; ribose phosphate
R$_p$ pulmonary resistance
RPA resultant physiologic acceleration; reverse passive anaphylaxis; right pulmonary artery
rPBF regional pulmonary blood flow
RPCF, RPCFT Reiter protein complement fixation [test]
RPCGN rapidly progressive crescenting glomerulonephritis
RPE rate of perceived exertion; retinal pigment epithelium
RPF relaxed pelvic floor; renal plasma flow; retroperitoneal fibrosis
RPG radiation protection guide; retrograde pyelogram
RPGMEC Regional Postgraduate Medical Education Committee

RPGN rapidly progressive glomerulo-nephritis
RPh Registered Pharmacist
RPHA reversed passive hemagglutination
RPHAMFCA reversed passive hemagglutination by miniature centrifugal fast analysis
RP-HPLC reverse phase-high performance liquid chromatography
RPI reticulocyte production index
RPIPP reverse phase ion-pair partition
RPLAD retroperitoneal lymphadenectomy
RPLC reverse phase liquid chromatography
RPM, rpm rapid processing mode; revolutions per minute
RPMD rheumatic pain modulation disorder
RPMI Roswell Park Memorial Institute [medium]
RPO right posterior oblique
RPP heart rate-systolic blood pressure product; retropubic prostatectomy
RPPI role perception picture inventory
RPPR red cell precursor production rate
RPR rapid plasma reagin [test]
RPS renal pressor substance; revolutions per second
rps revolutions per second
RPT refractory period of transmission; Registered Physical Therapist
Rptd ruptured
RPV right portal vein; right pulmonary vein
RPVP right posterior ventricular pre-excitation
RQ recovery quotient; respiratory quotient
RR radiation reaction; radiation response; rate ratio; recovery room; relative response; relative risk; renin release; respiratory rate; response rate; rheumatoid rosette; risk ratio; Riva-Rocci [sphygmomanometer]
R&R rate and rhythm; rest and recuperation
RRA radioreceptor assay; registered record administrator
RRC residency review committee; routine respiratory care; Royal Red Cross
RRE radiation-related eosinophilia

RRE, RR&E round, regular, and equal [pupils]

RR-HPO rapid recompression–high pressure oxygen

RRL Registered Record Librarian

rRNA ribosomal ribonucleic acid

RRP relative refractory period

RRR regular rhythm and rate; renin release ratio

RRS Richards-Rundle syndrome

RRT Registered Respiratory Therapist; relative retention time

RS rating schedule; Raynaud syndrome; recipient's serum; rectal sinus; reinforcing stimulus; Reiter syndrome; renal specialist; respiratory syncytial [virus]; response to stimulus; reticulated siderocyte; review of symptoms; Reye syndrome; right sacrum; right septum; right side; right stellate [ganglion]; Ringer solution; Roberts syndrome

Rs *Rauwolfia serpentina*

R/s roentgens per second

r$_s$ rank correlation coefficient

RSA rabbit serum albumin; relative specific activity; relative standard accuracy; reticulum cell sarcoma; right sacro-anterior [fetal position]; right subclavian artery

RSB reticulocyte standard buffer; right sternal border

RSC rat spleen cell; rested state contraction; reversible sickle-cell

RScA right scapulo-anterior [fetal position]

RSCN Registered Sick Children's Nurse

RScP right scapuloposterior [fetal position]

RSD reflex sympathetic dystrophy; relative standard deviation

RSDS reflex sympathetic dystrophy syndrome

RSES Rosenberg Self-Esteem Scale

RSH Royal Society of Health

RSI repetition strain injury

RSIC Radiation Shielding Information Center

RSIVP rapid-sequence intravenous pyelography

RSL right sacrolateral [fetal position]

RSM Royal Society of Medicine

RSN right substantia nigra

RSNA Radiological Society of North America

RSO Resident Surgical Officer

RSP right sacroposterior [fetal position]

RSPCA Royal Society for the Prevention of Cruelty to Animals

RSPH Royal Society for the Promotion of Health

RSPK recurrent spontaneous psychokinesis

RSR regular sinus rhythm

rSr an electrocardiographic complex

RSS rat stomach strip

RSSE Russian spring-summer encephalitis

RST radiosensitivity test; reagin screen test; right sacrotransverse [fetal position]

R$_{st}$ in paper or thin layer chromatography, the distance that a spot of a substance has moved, relative to a reference standard spot

RSTL relaxed skin tension lines

RSTMH Royal Society of Tropical Medicine and Hygiene

RSV respiratory syncytial virus; right subclavian vein; Rous sarcoma virus

RSVC right superior vena cava

RT radiologic technologist; radiotherapy; radium therapy; reaction time; reading test; reciprocating tachycardia; recreational therapy; reduction time; Registered Technician; relaxation time; resistance transfer; respiratory therapist/therapy; rest tremor; retransformation; right; right thigh; room temperature

RT3, rT$_3$ reverse triiodothyronine

Rt right

rT ribothymidine

rt right

RTA renal tubular acidosis; road traffic accident

RT(ARRT) Radiologic Technologist certified by the American Registry of Radiologic Technologists

RTC random control trial; renal tubular cell; return to clinic

RTD routine test dilution

Rtd retarded

RTECS Registry of Toxic Effects of Chemical Substances

RTF resistance transfer factor; respiratory tract fluid

RTG-2 rainbow trout gonadal tissue cells

RTI respiratory tract infection

rtl rectal

rt lat right lateral

RT(N)(ARRT) Radiologic Technologist (Nuclear Medicine) certified by the American Registry of Radiologic Technologists

RTO right toeoff

RTOG radiation therapy oncology group

RTP reverse transcriptase-producing [agent]

RTR Recreational Therapist, Registered; red blood cell turnover rate

RT (R)(ARRT) Registered Technologist, Radiography certified by the American Registry of Radiologic Technologists)

RTS real time scan; right toestrike

RT(T)(ARRT) Radiologic Technologist (Radiation Therapy) certified by the American Registry of Radiologic Technologists

RTU real-time ultrasound

RTV room temperature vulcanization

RU rat unit; resin uptake; resistance unit; retrograde urogram; right upper; roentgen unit

Ru ruthenium

RU-1 human embryonic lung fibroblasts

rub red [Lat. *ruber*]

RUE right upper extremity

RUL right upper eyelid; right upper lobe

RUOQ right upper outer quadrant

rupt ruptured

RUQ right upper quadrant

RUR resin-uptake ratio

RURTI recurrent upper respiratory tract infection

RUSB right upper sternal border

RUV residual urine volume

RV rat virus; Rauscher virus; rectovaginal; reinforcement value; residual volume; respiratory volume; retroversion; rhinovirus; right ventricle, right ventricular; rubella vaccine; rubella virus; Russell viper

R$_V$ radius of view

RVB red venous blood

RVD relative vertebral density

RVE right ventricular enlargement

RVECP right ventricular endocardial potential

RVEDD right ventricular end-diastolic diameter

RVEDP right ventricular end-diastolic pressure

RVEDV right ventricular end-diastolic volume

RVEF right ventricular ejection fraction; right ventricular end-flow

RVF Rift Valley fever; right ventricular failure; right visual field

RVG right visceral ganglion

RVH renovascular hypertension; right ventricular hypertrophy

RVHD rheumatic valvular heart disease

RVI relative value index; right ventricle infarction

RVL right vastus lateralis

RVLG right ventrolateral gluteal

RVO Regional Veterinary Officer; relaxed vaginal outlet

RVP red veterinary petrolatum; resting venous pressure; right ventricular pressure

RVPFR right ventricular peak filling rate

RVPRA renal vein plasma renin activity

RVR renal vascular resistance; repetitive ventricular response; resistance to venous return

RVRA renal vein reini activity; renal venous renin assay

RVRC renal vein renin concentration

RVS relative value scale/study; reported visual sensation

RVSW right ventricular stroke work

RVT renal vein thrombosis

RVTE recurring venous thromboembolism

RV/TLC residual volume/total lung capacity

RVV Russell viper venom

RW radiological warfare; ragweed

R-W Rideal-Walker [coefficient]

RWAGE ragweed antigen E

RWIS restraint and water immersion stress

RWM regional wall motion

Rx prescribe, prescription, prescription drug; take [Lat. *recipe*]; therapy; treatment;
r(X) right X chromosome
RXLI recessive X-linked ichthyosis
RXN reaction
RXT right exotropia

–S–

S apparent power; half [Lat. *semis*]; in electro- cardiography, a negative deflectsion that follows an R wave [wave]; entropy; left [Lat. *sinister*]; mean dose per unit cumulated activity; the midpoint of the sella turcica [point]; sacral; saline; *Salmonella*; saturated; *Schistosoma*; second; section; sedimentation coefficient; sella [turcica]; semilente [insulin]; senility, senile; sensation; sensitivity; serine; serum; siderocyte; siemens; signature [prescription]; silicate; single; small; smooth [colony]; soft [diet]; solid; soluble; solute; sone [unit]; space; spherical; *Spirillum*; standard normal deviation; *Staphylococcus*; stem [cell]; stimulus; *Streptococcus*; subject; subjective findings; substrate; sulfur; sum of an arithmetic series; supravergence; surface; surgery; Svedberg [unit]; swine; Swiss [mouse]; synthesis; without [Lat. *sine*]; write, let it be written [Lat. *signa*]
S1-S5 first to fifth sacral nerves
$S_1.S_4$ first to fourth heart sounds

s atomic orbital with angular momentum quantum number 0; distance; length of path; sample standard deviation; satellite [chromosome]; scruple; second; section; sensation; series; signed; suckling
s without
s^{-1} cycles per second
s^2 sample variance
Σ see *sigma*
σ see *sigma*
SA according to art [Lat. *secundum artem*]; salicylic acid; salt added; sarcoma; secondary amenorrhea; secondary anemia; self-analysis; semen analysis; serum albumin; serum aldolase; simian adeno-virus; sinoatrial; sleep apnea; slightly active; soluble in alkaline medium; specific activity; spectrum analysis; spiking activity; standard accuracy; stimulus artifact; Stokes-Adams; surface antigen; surface area; sustained action; sympathetic activity; systemic aspergillosis
S-A sino-atrial; sino-auricular
S&A sickness and accident [insurance]; sugar and acetone
Sa the most anterior point of the anterior contour of the sella turcica [point]; saline; *Staphylococcus aureus*
sA statampere
SAA serum amyloid A; severe aplastic anemia
SAARD slow-acting antirheumatic drug
SAB significant asymptomatic bacteriuria; Society of American Bacteriologists
SABP spontaneous acute bacterial peritonitis
SAC saccharin; subarea advisory council
SACD subacute combined degeneration
SACE serum angiotensin converting enzyme
SACH small animal care hospital
SACT sinoatrial conduction time
SAD seasonal affective disorder; source to axis distance; sugar, acetone, and diacetic acid
SADS Schedule for Affective Disorders and Schizophrenia
SADS-C Schedule for Affective Disorders and Schizophrenia–Change
SADT Stetson Auditory Discrimination Test
SAEB sinoatrial entrance block
SAEP *Salmonella abortus equi* pyrogen
SAF self-articulating femoral
SAFA soluble antigen fluorescent antibody
SAG salicyl acyl glucuronide; Swiss agammaglobulinemia
SAH S-adenosyl-L-homocysteine; subarachnoid hemorrhage
SAHS sleep apnea–hypersomnolence [syndrome]
SAI Self-Analysis Inventory; Sexual Arousability Inventory; without other qualification [Lat. *sine altera indicatione*]
SAIDS simian acquired immune deficiency syndrome

Sal salicylate, salicylic; *Salmonella*
sal according to the rules of art [Lat. *secundum artis leges*]; salicylate, salicylic; saliva
Salm *Salmonella*
SAM S-adenosyl-L-methionine; scanning acoustic microscope; sex arousal mechanism; sulfated acid mucopolysaccharide; systolic anterior motion
SAMA Student American Medical Association
SAMD S-adenosyl-L-methionine decarboxylase
SAM-DC S-adenosyl-L-methionine decarboxylase
SAMO Senior Administrative Medical Officer
S-AMY serum amylase
SAN sinoatrial node; sinoauricular node
Sanat sanatorium
SANDR sinoatrial nodal reentry
sang sanguinous
sanit sanitary, sanitation
SAO splanchnic artery occlusion
S$_{AO2}$ oxygen saturation
SAP serum acid phosphatase; serum alkaline phosphatase; serum amyloid P; situs ambiguus with polysplenia; *Staphylococcus aureus* protease; systemic arterial pressure
SAR sexual attitude reassessment; structure-activity relationship
Sar sulfarsphenamine
SAS self-rating anxiety scale; sleep apnea syndrome; small aorta syndrome; sodium amylosulfate; sterile aqueous solution; sterile aqueous suspension; subaortic stenosis; supravalvular aortic stenosis; surface-active substance
SASP salicylazosulfapyridine
SAT satellite; serum antitrypsin; single-agent chemotherapy; subacute thyroiditis; symptomless autoimmune thyroiditis; systematic assertive therapy
Sat, sat saturation, saturated
SATA spatial average, temporal average
SATL surgical Achilles tendon lengthening
SAU statistical analysis unit
SAV sequential atrioventricular [pacing]
SAVD spontaneous assisted vaginal delivery

SB Bachelor of Science; serum bilirubin; shortness of breath; single breath; sinus bradycardia; sodium balance; soybean; spontaneous blastogenesis; Stanford-Binet [Intelligence Scale]; stereotyped behavior; sternal border; stillbirth; surface binding
Sb antimony [Lat. *stibium*]; strabismus
sb stilb
SBA soybean agglutinin
SBB stimulation-bound behavior
S-BD seizure-brain damage
SbDH sorbitol dehydrogenase
SBE breast self-examination; shortness of breath on exertion; subacute bacterial endocarditis
S/ß sickle cell beta-thalassemia
SBF serologic-blocking factor; splanchnic blood flow
SBFT small bowel follow-through
SBG selenite brilliant green
SBH sea-blue histiocyte
SBI soybean trypsin inhibitor
SBL soybean lecithin
SB-LM Stanford-Binet Intelligence Test–From LM
SBN$_2$ single-breath nitrogen [test]
SBNS Society of British Neurological Surgeons
SBO small bowel obstruction
SBOM soybean oil meal
SBP spontaneous bacterial peritonitis; steroid-binding plasma [protein]; sulfobromophthalein; systemic blood pressure; systolic blood pressure
SBR strict bed rest; styrene-butadiene rubber
SBS short bowel syndrome; straight back syndrome
SBSS Seligmann's buffered salt solution
SBT serum bacteriological titer; single-breath test; sulbactam
SBTI soybean trypsin inhibitor
SBTPE State Boards Test Pool Examination
SC conditioned stimulus; sacrococcygeal; Sanitary Corps; Schwann cell; science; secretory component; self care; semilunar valve closure; serum complement; service-connected; sex chromatin; Sézary cell; sick call; sickle cell; silicone-coated;

single chemical; skin conduction; slow component; Snellen's chart; sodium citrate; soluble complex; special care; squamous carcinoma; statistical control; sternoclavicular; stratum corneum; subclavian; subcorneal; subcutaneous; succinylcholine; sugar-coated; systemic candidiasis; systolic click

S-C sickle cell

Sc scandium; scapula; science, scientific

sC statcoulomb

SCA sickle-cell anemia; single-channel analyzer; sperm-coating antigen; steroidal-cell antibody; subclavian artery; suppressor cell activity

SCAA Skin Care Association of America

SCAG Sandoz Clinical Assessment-Geriatric [Rating]

SCAN suspected child abuse and neglect

SCAT sheep cell agglutination test; sickle cell anemia test

SCB strictly confined to bed

SCBA self-contained breathing apparatus

SCBF spinal cord blood flow

SCBG symmetrical calcification of the basal cerebral ganglia

SCBP stratum corneum basic protein

SCC services for crippled children; short course chemotherapy; small cell carcinoma; small cleaved cell; squamous cell carcinoma

SCCH sternocostoclavicular hyperostosis

SCCL small cell carcinoma of the lung

SCCM Sertoli cell culture medium

SCD service-connected disability; sickle-cell disease; spinocerebellar degeneration; subacute combined degeneration; sudden cardiac death; systemic carnitine deficiency

ScD Doctor of Science

ScDA right scapulo-anterior [fetal position] [Lat. *scapulodextra anterior*]

ScDP right scapuloposterior [fetal position] [Lat. *scapulodextra posterior*]

SCE secretory carcinoma of the endometrium; sister chromatid exchange

SCEP sandwich counterelectrophoresis

SCF Skin Cancer Foundation

SCFA short-chain fatty acid

SCG serum chemistry graft; sodium cromoglycate; superior cervical ganglion

SCh succinylchloride

SChE serum cholinesterase

schiz schizophrenia

SCI Science Citation Index; spinal cord injury; structured clinical interview

Sci science, scientific

SCID, SCIDS severe combined immunodeficiency [syndrome]

SCIS spinal cord injury service

SCIV subcutaneous intravenous

SCJ squamocolumnar junction

SCK serum creatine kinase

SCL scleroderma; serum copper level; sinus cycle length; symptom checklist; syndrome checklist

ScLA left scapuloanterior [fetal position] [Lat. *scapulolaeva anterior*]

SCLC small cell lung carcinoma

scler sclerosis, scleroderma

ScLP left scapuloposterior [fetal position] [Lat. *scapulolaeva posterior*]

SCM Society of Computer Medicine; soluble cytotoxic medium; spleen cell–conditioned medium; spondylitic caudal myelopathy; State Certified Midwife; streptococcal cell membrane

SCMC spontaneous cell-mediated cytotoxicity

SCMO Senior Clerical Medical Officer

SCN suprachiasmatic nucleus

SCNS subcutaneous nerve stimulation

SCO somatic crossing-over; subcommissural organ

SCOP scopolamine

SCP single-celled protein; sodium cellulose phosphate; soluble cytoplasmic protein

scp spherical candle power

SCPK serum creatine phosphokinase

SCPNT Southern California Postrotary Nystagmus Test

SCR silicon-controlled rectifier; spondylitic caudal radiculopathy

SCr serum creatinine

scr scruple

SCS Saethre-Chotzen syndrome; silicon-controlled switch; Society of Clinical Surgery

SCT sex chromatin test; sickle-cell trait; staphylococcal clumping test; sugar-coated tablet

SCTAT sex cord tumor with annular tubules
SCU special care unit
SCUBA self-contained underwater breathing apparatus
SCUF slow continuous ultrafiltration
SCV smooth, capsulated, virulent; subclavian vein
SD Sandhoff disease; senile dementia; septal defect; serologically defined; serologically detectable; serologically determined; serum defect; shoulder disarticulation; skin destruction; skin dose; spontaneous delivery; sporadic depression; Sprague-Dawley [rat]; spreading depression; standard deviation; statistical documentation; Still's disease; stone disintegration; streptodornase; sudden death; superoxide dismutase; systolic discharge
S-D sickle-cell hemoglobin D
S/D systolic/diastolic
Sd stimulus drive
S^d discriminative stimulus
SDA right sacro-anterior [fetal position] [Lat.*sacrodextra anterior*]; specific dynamic action; succinic dehydrogenase activity
SDAT senile dementia of Alzheimer type
SDB sleep-disordered breathing
SDBP supine diastolic blood pressure
SDC serum digoxin concentration; sodium deoxycholate; subacute combined degeneration; succinyldicholine
SDCL symptom distress check list
SDDS 2-sulfamoyl-4,4'-diaminodiphenylsulfone
SDE specific dynamic effect
SDF slow death factor
SDG sucrose density gradient
SDH serine dehydrase; sorbitol dehydrogenase; spinal dorsal horn; subdural hematoma; succinate dehydrogenase
SDHD sudden death heart disease
SDI standard deviation interval
SDIHD sudden death ischemic heart disease
SDM sensory detection method; standard deviation of the mean
SDN sexually dimorphic nucleus
SDP right sacroposterior [fetal position] [Lat. *sacrodextra posterior*]

SDR spontaneously diabetic rat
SDS school dental services; self-rating depression scale; sensory deprivation syndrome; sexual differentiation scale; sodium dodecylsulfate; specific diagnosis service; standard deviation score; sudden death syndrome
SD-SK streptodornase-streptokinase
SDS/PAGE, SDS-PGE sodium dodecylsulfate-poly-acrylamide gel electrophoresis
SDT right sacrotransverse [fetal position] [Lat. *sacrodextra transversa*]
SE saline enema; sanitary engineering; side effect; solid extract; sphenoethmoidal; spin-echo; standard error; starch equivalent
S&E safety and efficiency
Se selenium
SEA sheep erythrocyte agglutination; soluble egg antigen; spontaneous electrical activity; staphylococcal enterotoxin A
SEAT sheep erythrocyte agglutination test
SEB staphylococcal enterotoxin B
SEBA staphylococcal enterotoxin B antiserum
SEBM Society of Experimental Biology and Medicine
SEC Singapore epidemic conjunctivitis; soft elastic capsule
sec second; secondary
sec-Bu sec-butyl
SECG stress electrocardiography
SECSY spin-echo correlated spectroscopy
sect section
SED skin erythema dose; spondyloepiphyseal dysplasia; staphylococcal enterotoxin D
sed sedimentation, stool [Lat. *sedes*]
sed rt sedimentation rate
SEE standard error of estimate
SEER Surveillance Epidemiology and End Results [Program]
SEF somatically-evoked field; staphylococcal enterotoxin F
SEG segment; soft elastic gelatin; sonoencephalogram
segm segment, segmented
SEM scanning electron microscopy; secondary enrichment medium; standard error of the mean; systolic ejection murmur

sem one-half [Lat. *semis*]; semen, seminal

SEMDJL spondylo-epimetaphyseal dysplasia with joint laxity

semid half a dram

semih half an hour [Lat. *semihora*]

SEN State Enrolled Nurse

sen sensitivity, sensitive

sens sensation, sensorium, sensory

SEP somatosensory evoked potential; sperm entry point; systolic ejection period

separ separation, separation

sept seven [Lat. *septem*]

seq sequence; sequel, sequela, sequelae; sequestrum

seq luce the following day [Lat. *sequenti luce*]

SER sebum excretion rate; sensory evoked response; service; smooth surface endoplasmic reticulum; somatosensory evoked response; systolic ejection rate

Ser serine

sER smooth endoplasmic reticulum

ser series, serial

SER-IV supination external rotation, type 4 fracture

SERHOLD National Biomedical Serials Holding Database

SERLINE Serials on Line

sero, serol serological, serology

SERT sustained ethanol release tube

serv keep, preserve [Lat. *serva*]; service

SERVHEL Service and Health Records

SES Society of Eye Surgeons; socioeconomic status; subendothelial space

sesquih an hour and a half [Lat. *sesquihora*]

sesunc an ounce and a half [Lat. *sesuncia*]

SET systolic ejection time

sev severe; severed

s expr without expressing [Lat. *sine expressio*]

SF safety factor; scarlet fever; seminal fluid; serosal fluid; serum factor; serum ferritin; serum fibrinogen; sham feeding; shell fragment; sickle cell–hemoglobin F [disease]; simian foam-virus; skin fibroblast; spinal fluid; stable factor; sterile female; stress formula; sugar-free; Svedberg flotation [unit]; symptom-free; synovial fluid

Sf *Streptococcus faecalis*

S$_f$ Svedberg flotation unit

SFA saturated fatty acid; stimulated fibrinolytic activity

SFB Sanfilippo syndrome type B

SFC soluble fibrin complex; soluble fibrin-fibrinogen complex; spinal fluid count

SFD skin-film distance; spectral frequency distribution

SFEMG single fiber electromyography

SFFA serum free fatty acid

SFFF sedimentation field flow fractionation

SFFV spleen focus-forming virus

SFH serum-free hemoglobin; stroma-free hemoglobin

SFL synovial fluid lymphocyte

SFMC soluble fibrin monomer complex

SFP screen filtration pressure; spinal fluid pressure; stopped flow pressure

SPS split function study

SFT skinfold thickness

SFV Semliki Forest virus; shipping fever virus; Shope fibroma virus; squirrel fibroma virus

SFW sexual function of women; shell fragment wound

SG Sachs-Georgi [test]; serum globulin; signs; skin graft; soluble gelatin; specific gravity; substantia gelatinosa; Surgeon General

SGA small for gestational age

SG$_{AW}$ specific airway conductance

SGC spermicide-germicide compound

SGL salivary gland lymphocyte

SGM Society for General Microbiology

SGO Surgeon General's Office

SGOT serum glutamate oxaloacetate transaminase (aspartate aminotransferase)

SGP serine glycerophosphatide; sialoglycoprotein; Society of General Physiologists

SGPT serum glutamate pyruvate transaminase (alanine aminotransferase)

SGR Shwartzman generalized reaction; submandibular gland renin; substantia gelatinosa Rolandi

S-Gt Sachs-Georgi test

SGTT standard glucose tolerance test

SGV salivary gland virus; selective gastric vagotomy

SH Schönlein-Henoch [purpura]; serum hepatitis; sexual harassment; sex hormone; Sherman [rat]; sick in hospital; sinus histiocytosis; social history; somatotropic hormone; spontaneously hypertensive [rat]; sulfhydryl; surgical history

S/H sample and hold

S&H speech and hearing

Sh sheep; *Shigella*

sh shoulder

SHA staphylococcal hemagglutinating antibody

sHa suckling hamster

SHAA serum hepatitis associated antigen; Society of Hearing Aid Audiologists

SHAA-Ab serum hepatitis associated antigen antibody

SHARP school health additional referral program

SHB sequential hemibody [irradiation]

S-Hb sulfhemoglobin

SHBD serum hydroxybutyric dehydrogenase

SHBG sex hormone binding globulin

SHCC State Health Coordinating Council

SHCO sulfated hydrogenated castor oil

SHE Syrian hamster embryo

SHEENT skin, head, eyes, ears, nose, and throat

SHF simian hemorrhagic fever

SHG synthetic human gastrin

SHHD Scottish Home and Health Department

SHHV Society for Health and Human Values

Shig *Shigella*

SHLD shoulder

SHML sinus histiocytosis with massive lymphadenopathy

SHMP Senior Hospital Medical Officer

SHN spontaneous hemorrhagic necrosis; subacute hepatic necrosis

SHO secondary hypertrophic osteoarthropathy; Senior House Officer

SHORT, S-H-O-R-T short stature, hyperextensibility of joints or hernia or both, ocular depression, Rieger anomaly, teething delayed

SHP Schönlein-Henoch purpura; secondary hyperparathyroidism; state health plan

SHPDA State Health Planning and Development Agency

SHR spontaneously hypertensive rat

SHS sheep hemolysate supernatant

SHSP spontaneously hypertensive stroke-prone [rat]

SHT simple hypocalcemic tetany

SHUR System for Hospital Uniform Reporting

SHV simian herpes virus

SI International System of Units [Fr. *le Système International d'Unités*]; sacroiliac; saline infusion; saline injection; saturation index; self-inflicted; serious illness; serum iron; severity index; sex inventory; Singh Index; small intestine; soluble insulin; spirochetosis icterohaemorrhagica; stimulation index; stroke index; suppression index

Si the most anterior point on the lower contour of the sella turcica [point]; silicon

S&I suction and irrigation

SIA stress-induced analgesia; stress-induced anesthesia; subacute infectious arthritis

SIADH syndrome of inappropriate secretion of antidiuretic hormone

SIB self-injurious behavior

sib, sibs sibling, siblings

SIC dry [Lat. *siccus*]; serum insulin concentration

SICD serum isocitrate dehydrogenase

SICU surgical intensive care unit

SID Society for Investigative Dermatology; sucrase-isomaltase deficiency; sudden inexplicable death; sudden infant death

SIDS sudden infant death syndrome

SIECUS Sex Information and Education Council of the United States

SIg surface immunoglobulin

sig let it be labeled [Lat. *signa, signetur*]; sigmoidoscopy; significant

sIg surface immunoglobulin

S-IgA secretory immunoglobulin A

Σ Greek capital letter *sigma*; syphilis; summation of series

σ Greek lower case letter *sigma*; conductivity; cross section; millisecond; molecular type or bond; population standard deviation; stress; surface tension; wave number

sig n pro label with the proper name [Lat. *signa nomine proprio*]

SIH stimulation-induced hypalgesia

SIJ sacroiliac joint
SIM Society of Industrial Microbiology
SIMS secondary ion mass spectroscopy
sin six times a night [Lat. *sex in nocte*]
sing of each [Lat. *singulorum*]
si non val if it is not enough [Lat. *si non valeat*]
si op sit if it is necessary [Lat. *si opus sit*]
SIP slow inhibitory potential
sIPTH serum immunoreactive parathyroid hormone
SIR single isomorphous replacement; specific immune release
SIRA Scientific Instrument Research Association
SIREF specific immune response enhancing factor
SIRS soluble immune response suppressor
SIS social information system; spontaneous interictal spike; sterile injectable solution; sterile injectable suspension
SISI short increment sensitivity index
SISV, SiSV simian sarcoma virus
SIT serum inhibiting titer; Slosson Intelligence Test
SIV Sprague-Dawley-Ivanovas [rat]
si vir perm if the strength will permit [Lat. *si vires permitant*]
SIW self-inflicted wound
SIWIP self-induced water intoxication and psychosis
SIWIS self-induced water intoxication and schizophrenic disorders
SJR Shinowara-Jones-Reinhart [unit]
SJS Stevens-Johnson syndrome
SjS Sjögren syndrome
SK Sloan-Kettering [Institute for Cancer Research]; spontaneous killer [cell]; streptokinase; swine kidney
Sk skin
SKAT Sex Knowledge and Attitude Test
skel skeleton, skeletal
SKI Sloan-Kettering Institute
SKSD, SK-SD streptokinase-streptodornase
SL according to the rules [Lat. *secundum legem*]; sarcolemma; sclerosing leukoencephalopathy; sensation level; Sibley-Lehninger [unit]; small lympho-

cyte; sodium lactate; solidified liquid; streptolysin; sublingual
Sl Steel pmouse]
SLA left sacro-anterior [fetal position] [Lat. *sacrolaeva anterior*]; single cell liquid cytotoxic assay; slide latex agglutination
SLAM scanning laser acoustic microscope
SLB short leg brace
SLD serum lactic dehydrogenase
SLDH serum lactate dehydrogenase
SLE slit lamp examination; St. Louis encephalitis; systemic lupus erythematosus
SLEP short latent evoked potential
SLEV St. Louis encephalitis virus
SLHR sex-linked hypophosphatemic rickets
SLI splenic localization index
SLIR somatostatin-like immunoreactivity
SLKC superior limbic keratoconjunctivitis
SLMC spontaneous lymphocyte-mediated cytotoxicity
SLN superior laryngeal nerve
SLO streptolysin O
SLP left sacroposterior [fetal position] [Lat. *sacrolaeva posterior*]; segmental limb systolic pressure; sex-limited protein; short luteal phase
SLPP serum lipophosphoprotein
SLR Shwartzman local reaction; single lens reflex; straight leg raising
SLRT straight leg raising test
SLS segment long-spacing; Sjögren-Larsson syndrome; Stein-Leventhal syndrome
SLT left sacrotransverse [fetal position] [Lat. *sacrolaeva transversa*]
SM Master of Science; sadomasochism; simple mastectomy; skim milk; smooth muscle; somatomedin; space medicine; sphingomyelin; splenic macrophage; sports medicine; streptomycin; submandibular; submucous; suckling mouse; sucrose medium; suction method; sustained medication; symptoms; synaptic membrane; systolic motion; systolic murmur
Sm samarium; *Serratia marcescens*
sM suckling mouse

SMA sequential multiple analysis; sequential multichannel auto-analyzer; smooth muscle antibody; Society for Medical Anthropology; spinal muscular atrophy; spontaneous motor activity; standard method agar; superior mesenteric artery; supplementary motor area

SMABF superior mesenteric artery blood flow

SMAC sequential multiple analyzer with computer

SMAF smooth muscle activating factor; specific macrophage arming factor

sm an small animal

SMAO superior mesenteric artery occlusion

SMAS superior mesenteric artery syndrome

SMAST Short Michigan Alcoholism Screening Test

SMB standard mineral base

sMb suckling mouse brain

SMC Scientific Manpower Commission; smooth muscle cell; succinylmonocholine

SM-C, Sm-C somatomedin-C

SMCA smooth muscle contracting agent; suckling mouse cataract agent

SM-C/IGF somatomedin-C/insulin-like growth factor

SMD senile macular degeneration; submanubrial dullness

SMDA starch methylenedianiline

SMDC sodium-N-methyl dithiocarbamate

SMEDI stillbirth-mummification, embryonic-death, infertility [syndrome]

SMEM supplemented Eagle's minimum essential medium

SMF streptozocin, mitomycin C, and 5-fluorouracil

SMFP state medical facilities plan

SMH strongyloidiasis with massive hyperinfection

SMI senior medical investigator; small volume infusion; stress myocardial image; Style of Mind Inventory; supplementary medical insurance; sustained maximum inspiration

SmIg surface membrane immunoglobulin

SMMD specimen mass measurement device

SMO Senior Medical Officer

SMOH Senior Medical Officer of Health; Society of Medical Officers of Health

SMON subacute myelo-optico-neuropathy

SMP slowest moving protease

SMR sensorimotor rhythm; severe mental retardation; somnolent metabolic rate; standardized mortality ratio; stroke with minimum residuum; submucosal resection

SMRR submucosal resection and rhinoplasty

SMRV squirrel monkey retrovirus

SMS senior medical student; Shared Medical Systems; stiff-man syndrome; supplemental minimum sodium

SMSA standard metropolitan statistical area

SMSV San Miguel sea lion virus

SMT spontaneous mammary tumor

SMuLV Scripps murine leukemia virus

SMV superior mesenteric vein

SMX, SMZ sulfamethoxazole

SN sclerema neonatorum; sensory neuron; serum neutralization; sinus node; staff nurse; student nurse; subnormal; substantia nigra; supernatant; suprasternal notch

S/N signal/noise [ratio]

Sn subnasale; tin [Lat. *stannum*]

sn according to nature [Lat. *secundum naturam*]

SNA Student Nurses Association

SNa serum sodium concentration

SNagg serum normal agglutinator

SNAP sensory nerve action potential

SNB scalene node biopsy

SNC spontaneous neonatal chylothorax

SNCL sinus node cycle length

SND sinus node dysfunction

SNDA Student National Dental Association

SNDO Standard Nomenclature of Diseases and Operations

SNE sinus node electrogram; subacute necrotizing encephalomyelography

SNF sinus node formation; skilled nursing facility

SNGFR single nephron glomerular filtration rate

SNHL sensorineural hearing loss
SNM Society of Nuclear Medicine; sulfanilamide
SNMA Student National Medical Association
SNMT Society of Nuclear Medical Technologists
SNOBOL String-Oriented Symbolic Language
SNOMED Symmetrical Nomenclature of Medicine
SNOP Systematized Nomenclature of Pathology
SNP school nurse practitioner; sinus node potential
SNR signal-to-noise ratio
snRNA small nuclear ribonucleic acid
snRNP small nuclear ribonucleoprotein
SNRT sinus node recovery time
SNRTd sinus node recovery time, direct measuring
SNRTi sinus node recovery time, indirect measuring
SNS Senior Nursing Sister; Society of Neurological Surgeons; sympathetic nervous system
SNSA seronegative spondyloarthropathy
SNV spleen necrosis virus
SO salpingo-oophorectomy; second opinion; sex offender; spheno-occipital [synchondrosis]; standing orders; supra-optic
S&O salpingo-oophorectomy
SO₂ oxygen saturation

SOA swelling of ankles
SOA-MCA superficial occipital artery to middle cerebral artery
SOAP subjective, objective, assessment, and plan [problem-oriented record]
SOAPIE subjective, objective, assessment, plan, implementation, and evaluation [problem-oriented record]
SOB see order blank; shortness of breath
SOC sequential oral contraceptive; syphilitic osteochondritis
SoC state of consciousness
SocSec Social Security
S-OCT serum ornithine carbamyltransferase
SOD superoxide dismutase
sod sodium
SOH sympathetic orthostatic hypotension

SOHN supraoptic hypothalamic nucleus
SOL solution; space-occupying lesion
sol solution, soluble
solv dissolve [Lat. solve]
SOM secretory otitis media; sensitivity of method; serous otitis media; somatotropin
SOMA Student Osteopathic Medical Association
somat somatic
SOMI sternal occipital mandibular immobilization
SON supraoptic nucleus
SOP standard operating procedure
SOPA syndrome of primary aldosteronism
s op s if it is necessary [Lat. si opus sit]
SOR stimulus-organism response
SOr supraorbitale
Sorb, sorb sorbitol
SOS if it is necessary [Lat. si opus sit]; supplemental oxygen system
SOT systemic oxygen transport
SP sacrum to pubis; salivary progesterone; schizotypal personality; septum pellucidum; serum protein; shunt pressure; shunt procedure; silent period; skin potential; sleep deprivation; solid phase; spleen; standard practice; standard procedure; staphylococcal protease; stool preservative; subliminal perception; suprapubic; symphisis pubis; systolic pressure
Sp the most posterior point on the posterior contour of the sella turcica; species; spine; Spirillum; summation potential
sP senile parkinsonism
sp space; species; specific; spine, spinal; spirit, alcohol [Lat. spiritus];
SPA human albumin [salt-poor albumin]; sheep pulmonary adenomatosis; spinal progressive amyotrophy; spondyloarthropathy; spontaneous platelet aggregation; staphylococcal protein A; suprapubic aspiration
SPAD stenosing peripheral arterial disease
SPAI steroid protein activity index
SPAM scanning photo-acoustic microscopy
SPAT slow paroxysmal atrial tachycardia

SPBI serum protein-bound iodine
SPC salicylamide, phenacetin, and caffeine; single palmar crease; spleen cell; synthetizing protein complex
SPCA serum prothrombin conversion accelerator; Society for Prevention of Cruelty to Animals
sp cd spinal cord
SPD specific paroxysmal discharge; standard peak dilution
SPDC strio-pallido-dentate calcinosis
SPE serum protein electrolytes; serum protein electrophoresis; sucrose polyester
Spec specialist, specialty
spec special; specific; specimen
SPECT single photon emission computed tomography
SPEG serum protein electrophoretogram
SPEP serum protein electrophoresis
SPF skin protection factor; specific-pathogen free; spectrophotofluorometer; split products of fibrin; standard perfusion fluid; sun protection factor
sp fl spinal fluid
SPG serine phosphoglyceride; symmetrical peripheral gangrene
SpG specific gravity
spg sponge
SPGA Bovarnik's solution; sucrose
sp gr specific gravity
SPH secondary pulmonary hemosiderosis; severely and profoundly handicapped; sphingomyelin
Sph sphenoidale; sphingomyelin
sph spherical, spheroid; spherical lens
sp ht specific heat
SPI serum precipitable iodine; Shipley Personal Inventory
SPID summed pain intensity difference
spin spine, spinal
sp indet indeterminate species [Lat. *species indeterminata*]
spir spiral; spirit, alcohol [Lat. *spiritus*]
spiss inspissated, thickened by evaporation [Lat. *spissatus*]
SPK serum pyruvate kinase; superficial punctate keratitis
SPL skin potential level; sound pressure level; spontaneous lesion; staphylococcal phage lysate
SPLV serum parvovirus-like virus
SPM subhuman primate model; suspended particulate matter

SpM spiriformis medialis [nucleus]
SPMA spinal progressive muscular atrophy
SPN sympathetic preganglionic neuron
sp n new species [Lat. *species novum*]
SPOD spouse's perception of disease
spon, spont spontaneous
SPOOL simultaneous peripheral operation on-line
SPP plural of *species*; Sexuality Preference Profile; skin perfusion pressure; suprapubic prostatectomy
spp plural of *species*
SPPP, sppp plural of *subspecies*
SPPS solid phase peptide synthesis; stable plasma protein solution
SPPT superprecipitation response
SPR serial probe recognition; Society for Pediatric Radiology; Society for Pediatric Research
SPRIA solid phase radioimmunoassay
SPROM spontaneous premature rupture of membrane
SPRT sequential probability ratio test
SPS shoulder pain and stiffness; slow-progressive schizophrenia; Society of Pelvic Surgeons; sodium polyanethol sulfonate; sound production sample; stimulated protein synthesis; systemic progressive sclerosis
SPST Symonds Picture-Story Test
Spt spirit, alcohol [Lat. *spiritus*]
Sp tap spinal tap
SPTS subjective posttraumatic syndrome
SPU short procedure unit; Society of Pediatric Urology
SPV Shope papilloma virus; sulfophosphovanillin
SPZ sulfinpyrazone
SQ social quotient; subcutaneous
sq square
sq cell ca squamous cell carcinoma
SQUID superconducting quantum interference device
SR sarcoplasmic reticulum; scanning radiometer; screen; secretion rate; sedimentation rate; seizure resistant; sensitivity response; sensitization response; service record; sex ratio; shorthair [guinea pig]; side rails; sigma reaction; sinus rhythm; skin resistance; slow release; smooth-rough [colony]; specific release; steroid resistance;

stimulus response; stomach rumble; sulfonamide-resistant; superior rectus; sustained release; systemic resistance; systems research; systems review

S-R smooth-rough [bacteria]

Sr strontium

sr steradian

SRA spleen repopulating activity

SRAM static random access memory

SR$_{AW}$, SR$_{aw}$ specific airway resistance

SRBC sheep red blood cells

SRC sedimented red cells; sheep red cells

SRCA specific red cell adherence

SRD Society for the Relief of Distress; Society for the Right to Die; sodium restricted diet

SRDT single radial diffusion test

SRE Schedule of Recent Experiences

SRF skin reactive factor; somatotropin-releasing factor; split renal function; subretinal fluid

SRFS split renal function study

SRH single radial hemolysis; somatotropin-releasing hormone; spontaneously responding hyperthyroidism

SRI severe renal insufficiency; Stanford Research Institute

SRID single radial immunodiffusion

SRIF somatotropin-release inhibiting factor

SRM Standard Reference Material

SMRD stress-related mucosal damage

SRN State Registered Nurse

sRNA soluble ribonucleic acid

SRNG sustained release nitroglycerin

SRNS steroid-responsive nephrotic syndrome

SROM spontaneous rupture of membrane

SRP short rib–polydactyly [syndrome]; Society for Radiological Protection; State Registered Physiotherapist

SRPS short rib–polydactyly syndrome

SRR standardized rate ratio

SR-RSV Schmidt-Ruppin strain Rous sarcoma virus

SRS schizophrenic residual state; Silver-Russell syndrome; slow-reacting substance; Social and Rehabilitation Service

SRSA, SRS-A slow-reacting substance of anaphylaxis

SRT sedimentation rate test; simple reaction time; sinus node recovery time; speech reception threshold; speech reception test

SRU solitary rectal ulcer; structural repeating unit

SRV Schmidt-Ruppin virus

SRVT sustained re-entrant ventricular tachyarrhythmia

SRW short ragweed [test]

SS saline soak; saline solution; saliva sample; saliva substitute; salt substitute; Salmonella-Shigella [agar]; saturated solution; Schizophrenia Subscale; seizure-sensitive; serum sickness; Sézary syndrome; side-to-side; signs and symptoms; single-stranded; Sjögren syndrome; soap suds; Social Security; somatostatin; sparingly soluble; standard score; statistically significant; sterile solution; steroid sensitivity; Stickler syndrome; subaortic stenosis; substernal; suction socket; sum of squares; support and stimulation; Sweet syndrome; systemic sclerosis

Ss *Shigella sonnei*; subjects

ss one half [Lat *semis*]; single-stranded; soap suds; subspinale

SSA salicylsalicylic acid skin-sensitizing antibody; skin sympathetic activity; Smith surface antigen; Social Security Administration; sperm-specific antiserum; sulfosalicylic acid

SSA1 Smallest Space Analysis

SSAV simian sarcoma-associated virus

SSB short spike burst; stereospecific binding

SS-B Sjögren syndrome B

SSBG sex steroid-binding globulin

SSC standard saline citrate; syngeneic spleen cell

SSCCS slow spinal cord compression syndrome

SSCr stainless steel crown

SSD single saturating dose; source-skin distance; source-surface distance; speech-sound discrimination; succinate semialdehyde dehydrogenase; sum of square deviations; syndrome of sudden death

ssDNA single stranded DNA

SSE saline solution enema; skin self-examination; soapsuds enema

SSEA stage-specific embryonic antigen

SSEP somatosensory evoked potential

SSF soluble suppressor factor

SSI small-scale integration; sub-shock insulin; Supplemental Security Income; System Sign Inventory

SSIDS sibling of sudden infant death syndrome [victim]

SSIE Smithsonian Science Information Exchange

SSKI saturated solution of potassium iodide

SSM subsynaptic membrane; superficial spreading melanoma

SSN severely subnormal

SSNS steroid-sensitive nephrotic syndrome

SSO Society of Surgical Oncology

SSP Sanarelli-Shwartzman phenomenon; subacute sclerosing panencephalitis; subspecies; supersensitivity perception

ssp subspecies

SSPE subacute sclerosing panencephalitis

SSPL saturation sound pressure level

SSPP subsynaptic plate perforation

SSPS side-to-side portacaval shunt

SS-PSE Schizophrenic Subscale of the Present State Examination

SSS scalded skin syndrome; sick sinus syndrome; specific soluble substance; Stanford Sleepiness Scale; sterile saline soak; systemic sicca syndrome

sss layer upon layer [Lat. *stratum super stratum*]

SSSS staphylococcal scalded skin syndrome

SSSV superior sagittal sinus velocity

s str in the strict sense [Lat. *sensu stricto*]

SSU self-service unit; sterile supply unit

SSV Schoolman-Schwartz virus; simian sarcoma virus; under a poison label [Lat. *sub signo veneni*]

SSX sulfisoxazole

ST esotropia; scala tympani; sedimentation time; sinus tachycardia; skin test; skin thickness; slight trace; slow twitch; speech therapist; stable toxin; standard test; sternothyroid; stimulus; store; stress test; subtalar; surface tension; survival time; syndrome of the trephined

S-T in electrocardiography, the portion of the segment between the end of the S wave and the beginning of the T wave; sickle-cell thalassemia

St, st let it stand [Lat. *stet*]; let them stand [Lat. *stent*]; stage [of disease]; stere; stokes; stone [unit]; straight; stroke; stomach; stomion; subtype

STA serum thrombotic accelerator

Sta staphylion

stab stabilization; stabnuclear neutrophil

STA-MCA superficial temporal artery to middle cerebral artery

STAI State Trait Anxiety Inventory

StanPsych standard psychiatric [nomenclature]

Staph, staph *Staphylococcus*, staphylococcal

stat immediately [Lat. *statim*]; radiation emanation unit [German]

Stb stillborn

STC soft tissue calcification

STD sexually-transmitted disease; skin-to-tumor distance; skin test dose; standard test dose

std saturated; standardized

STEM scanning transmission electron microscope

sten stenosis, stenosed

stereo stereogram

STESS subject's treatment emergent symptom scale

STET submaximal treadmill exercise test

STF serum thymus factor; special tube feeding

STH somatotropic hormone

STh sickle cell thalassemia

STI Scientific and Technical Information; serum trypsin inhibitor; systolic time interval

STIC serum trypsin inhibition capacity; solid-state transducer intracompartment

stillat drop by drop [Lat. *stillatim*]

stillb stillborn

stim stimulation, stimulated

STK streptokinase

STL status thymicolymphaticus; swelling, tenderness and limited motion

STM scanning tunneling microscope; short-term memory; streptomycin

STN subthalamic nucleus

sTNM TNM (*q.v.*) staging of tumors as determined by surgical procedures

STNR symmetric tonic neck reflex

STNV satellite tobacco necrosis virus
STO store
stom stomach
STORCH syphilis, toxoplasmosis, rubella, cytomegalovirus, and herpesvirus
STP scientifically treated petroleum; standard temperature and pressure; standard temperature and pulse
STPD a volume of gas at standard temperature and pressure that contains no water vapor
STPS specific thalamic projection system
Str, str *Streptococcus*, streptococcal
strab strabismus
Strep *Streptococcus*; streptomycin
struct structure, structural
STS serologic test for syphilis; sodium tetradecyl sulfate; sodium thiosulfate; standard test for syphilis
STSA Southern Thoracic Surgical Association
STSG split-thickness skin graft
STSS staphylococcal toxic shock syndrome
STT serial thrombin time
STU skin test unit
STVA subtotal villose atrophy
STVS short-term visual storage
STX saxitoxin
STZ streptozocin; streptozyme
SU salicyluric acid; sensation unit; spectrophotometric unit; subunit; sulfonamide; sulfonylurea
Su sulfonamide
su let him take [Lat. *sumat*]
SUA serum uric acid; single umbilical artery
subac subacute
subcut subcutaneous
sub fin coct toward the end of boiling [Lat. *sub finem coctionis*]
subling sublingual
SubN subthalamic nucleus
subq subcutaneous
subsp subspecies
substd substandard
suc juice [Lat. *succus*]
Succ succinate, succinic
SUD skin unit dose; sudden unexpected death
SUI stress urinary incontinence
SUID sudden unexplained infant death

sulf sulfate
sulfa sulfonamide
SULF-PRIM sulfamethoxazole and trimethoprim
sum let him take [Lat. *sumat*]; to be taken [Lat. *sumendum*]
SUN standard unit of nomenclature; serum urea nitrogen
SUO syncope of unknown origin
sup above [Lat. *supra*]; superior; supinator; superficial
supin supination, supine
suppl supplement, supplementary
suppos suppository
surg surgery, surgeon, surgical
SURS solitary ulcer of rectum syndrome
SUS solitary ulcer syndrome; stained urinary sediment; suppressor sensitive
susp suspension, suspended
SUUD sudden unexpected unexplained death
SV sarcoma virus; satellite virus; seminal vesicle; severe; simian virus; sinus venosus; snake venom; splenic vein; stroke volume; subclavian vein; subventricular; supravital
S/V surface/volume ratio
SV40 simian vacuolating virus 40
Sv sievert
sv sievert; single vibration; spirit of wine [Lat. *spiritus vini*]
SVA selective visceral angiography; sequential ventriculo-atrial [pacing]
SVAS supraventricular aortic stenosis
SVC slow vital capacity; subclavian vein catheterization; superior vena cava
SVCG spatial vectorcardiogram
SVCO superior vena-caval obstruction
SVCP Special Virus Cancer Program
SVCS superior vena cava syndrome
SVD single vessel disease; singular value decomposition; spontaneous vaginal delivery; spontaneous vertex delivery; swine vesicular disease
SVE slow volume encephalography; soluble viral extract; sterile vaginal examination
SVI stroke volume index
SVL superficial vastus lateralis
SVM syncytiovascular membrane
SVOM sequential volitional oral movement

SVP small volume parenteral [infusion]
SVPB supraventricular premature beat
SVR sequential vascular response; systemic vascular resistance
svr rectified spirit of wine [Lat. *spiritus vini rectificatus*]
SVRI systemic vascular resistance index
SVS slit ventricle syndrome
SVT subclavian vein thrombosis; supraventricular tachycardia
svt proof spirit [Lat. *spiritus vini tenuis*]
SW seriously wounded; slow wave; social worker; spike wave; spiral wound; sterile water; stroke work; Swiss Webster [mouse]
Sw swine
SWD short wave diathermy
SWI sterile water for injection; stroke work index
SWIM sperm washing insemination method
SWM segmental wall motion
SWR serum Wassermann reaction
SWS slow-wave sleep; spike-wave stupor
SWT sine-wave threshold
Sx, S$_x$ signs; symptoms
SY syphilis, syphilitic
SYA subacute yellow atrophy
sym symmetrical; symptom
sympath sympathetic
symph symphysis
sympt symptom
syn synonym
synd syndrome
syph syphilis, syphilitic
SYR Syrian [hamster]
Syr syrup [Lat. *syrupus*]
SYS stretching-yawning syndrome
sys system, systemic
syst system, systemic; systole, systolic
SZ streptozocin
Sz seizure; schizophrenia
SZN streptozocin

–T–

T absolute temperature; an electrocardiographic wave corresponding to the repolarization of the ventricles [wave]; life [time]; period [time]; ribosylthymine; *Taenia*; tamoxifen; telomere or terminal banding; temperature; temporal electrode placement in electroencephalography; temporary; tension [intraocular]; tera; tesla; testosterone; tetra; tetracycline; thoracic; thorax; threonine; threatened [animal]; thymidine; thymine; thymus [cell]; thymus-derived; thyroid; tidal gas; time; topical; torque; total; toxicity; training [group]; transition; transmittance; transverse; *Treponema*; *Trichophyton*; tritium; *Trypanosoma*; tumor; turnkey system; type
τ see *tau*
T$_{1/2}$, t$_{1/2}$ half-life
T1-T12 first to twelfth thoracic vertebrae
T1 spin-lattice or longitudinal relaxation time
T+1, T+2, T+3 first, second, and third stages of increased intraocular tension
T-1, T-2, T-3 first, second, and third stages of decreased intraocular tension
T$_2$ diiodothyronine; spin-spin or transverse relaxation time
2,4,5-T 2,4,5-trichlorophenoxy acetic acid
T$_3$ triiodothyronine
T$_4$ thyroxine
T-7 free thyroxine factor
t duration; student t test; temperature; temporal; terminal; tertiary; three times [Lat. *ter*]; time; tonne; translocation
TA alkaline tuberculin; axillary temperature; tactile afferent; teichoic acid; therapeutic abortion; thermophilic *Actinomyces*; thymocytotoxic autoantibody; titratable acid; total alkaloids; toxic adenoma; toxin-antitoxin; transaldolase; transantral; transplantation antigen; triamcinolone acetonide; tricuspid atresia; true anomaly; truncus arteriosus; tryptamine; tryptose agar; tube agglutination; tumor-associated
T-A toxin-antitoxin
T&A tonsillectomy and adenoidectomy; tonsils and adenoids
Ta tantalum
TAA total ankle arthroplasty; tumor-associated antigen

TAAF thromboplastic activity of the amniotic fluid

TAB typhoid, paratyphoid A, and paratyphoid B [vaccine]

tab tablet

TABC total aerobic bacteria count; typhoid, paratyphoid A, paratyphoid B, and paratyphoid C [vaccine]

TABT typhoid, paratyphoid A, paratyphoid B, and tetanus toxoid [vaccine]

TABTD typhoid, paratyphoid A, paratyphoid B, tetanus toxoid, and diphtheria toxoid [vaccine]

TAC time-activity curve; triamcinolone cream

TACE chlorotrianicene; teichoic acid crude extract

TAD thoracic asphyxiant dystrophy

TADAC therapeutic abortion, dilatation, aspiration, curettage

TAF albumose-free tuberculin [Ger. *Tuberculin Albumose frei*]; tissue angiogenesis factor; toxin-antitoxin floccules; toxoid-antitoxin floccules; trypsin-aldehyde-fuchsin; tumor angiogenesis factor

TAG target attaching globulin; thymine, adenine, and guanine

TAGH triiodothyronine, amino acids, glucagon, and heparin

TAH total abdominal hysterectomy; total artificial heart

TAL tendon of Achilles lengthening; thymic alymphoplasia

tal such a one [Lat. *talis*]

talc talcum

TALH thick ascending limb of Henle's loop

TALL, T-ALL T-cell acute lymphoblastic leukemia

TAM tamoxifen; thermoacidurans agar modified; total active motion; toxin-antitoxoid mixture; transient abnormal myelopoiesis

TAME toluenesulfonylarginine methyl ester

TAMIS Telemetric Automated Microbial Identification System

TAN total ammonia nitrogen

tan tandem translocation; tangent

TANI total axial lymph node irradiation

TAO thromboangiitis obliterans; triacetylole-andomycin

TAPS trial assessment procedure scale

TAPVC total anomalous pulmonary venous connection

TAPVD total anomalous pulmonary venous drainage

TAPVR total anomalous pulmonary venous return

TAR thrombocytopenia with absent radii [syndrome]; tissue-air ratio

TARA total articular replacaement arthroplasty; tumor-associated rejection antigen

TAS therapeutic activities specialist

TASA tumor-associated surface antigen

Tase tryptophan synthetase

TAT tetanus antitoxin; thematic apperception test; thematic aptitude test; thromboplastin activation test; total antitryptic activity; toxin- antitoxin; tumor activity test; turnaround time; tyrosine aminotransferase

TATA Pribnow [box]; tumor-associated transplantation antigen

TATR tyrosine aminotransferase regulator

τ Greek lower case letter *tau*; life [of radioisotope]; relaxation time; shear stress; spectral transmittance; transmission coefficient

TAV trapped air volume

TB thromboxane B; thymol blue; toluidine blue; total base; total bilirubin; total body; tracheal bronchiolar [region]; tracheobronchitis; trapezoid body; tub bath; tubercle bacillus; tuberculin; tuberculosis

Tb terbium; tubercle bacillus; tuberculosis

tb tuberculosis

TBA tertiary butylacetate; testosterone-binding affinity; thiobarbituric acid; to be absorbed; to be added; tubercle bacillus; tumor-bearing animal

TBAB tryptose blood agar base

TBB transbronchial biopsy

TBBM total body bone minerals

TBC thyroxine-binding coagulin

TBD total body density; Toxicology Data Base

TBE tick-borne encephalitis; tuberculin bacillin emulsion

TBF total body fat

TBG testosterone-binding globulin;

thyroxine-binding globulin; tris-buffered Gey's solution

TBGP total blood granulocyte pool

TBH total body hematocrit

TBHT total-body hyperthermia

TBI thyroxine-binding index; toothbrushing instruction; total-body irradiation

TBII thyroid-stimulating hormone-binding inhibitory immunoglobulin

T bili total bilirubin

TBK total body potassium

TBLC term birth, living child

TBM tuberculous meningitis; tubular basement membrane

TBN bacillus emulsion

TBNA transbronchial needle aspiration; treated but not admitted

TBNAA total body neutron activation analysis

TBP bithionol; testosterone-binding protein; thyroxine-binding protein; tributyl phosphate; tuberculous peritonitis

TBPA thyroxine-binding prealbumin

TBPT total body protein turnover

TBR tumor-bearing rabbit

TB-RD tuberculosis and respiratory disease

TBS total body solute; total body surface; total burn size; tribromosalicylanilide; triethanolamine-buffered saline

tbs, tbsp tablespoon

TBSA total body surface area

TBSV tomato bushy stunt virus

TBT tolbutamide test; tracheobronchial toilet

TBV total blood volume

TBW total body water; total body weight

TBX total body irradiation; thromboxane

TC taurocholic acid; temperature compensation; tetracycline; thermal conductivity; thoracic cage; thyrocalcitonin; tissue culture; to contain; total capacity; total cholesterol; total colonoscopy; transcobalamin; transcutaneous; Treacher Collins [syndrome]; true conjugate; tuberculin, contagious; tubocurarine; tumor cell; type and crossmatch

T&C turn and cough; type and crossmatch

T$_4$(C) serum thyroxine measured by column chromatography

Tc technetium; tetracycline; transcobalamin

T$_c$ the generation time of a cell cycle

t(°C) temperature on the Celsius scale

tc transcutaneous; translational control

TCA tetracyclic antidepressant; total cholic acid; total circulating albumin; tricalcium aluminate; tricarboxylic acid; trichloroacetic acid; tricyclic antidepressant

TCAB 3,3',4,4'-tetrachloroazobenzene

TCAD tricyclic antidepressant

TCAOB 3,3',4,4'-tetrachloroazoxybenzene

TCAP trimethyl-cetyl-ammonium pentachlorophenate

TCB tetrachlorobiphenyl; tumor cell burden

TCBS thiosulfate–citrate–bile salts–sucrose [agar]

TCC thromboplastic cell component; transitional-cell carcinoma; trichlorocarbanilide

Tcc triclocarban

TCD thermal conductivity detector; tissue culture dose

TCD$_{50}$ median tissue culture dose

TCDD 2,3,7,8-tetrachlorodibenzo-p-dioxin

TCE tetrachloro-diphenyl ethane; trichloroethylene

TCES transcutaneous cranial electrical stimulation

TCESOM trichloroethylene-extracted soybean oil meal

TCET transcerebral electrotherapy

TCF tissue coding factor; total coronary flow

TCFU tumor colony-forming unit

TCGF T-cell growth factor

TCH thiophen-2-carboxylic acid hydrazide; total circulating hemoglobin; turn, cough, hyperventilate

TChE total cholinesterase

TCI total cerebral ischemia; transient cerebral ischemia

TCi teracurie

TCID tissue culture infective dose; tissue culture inoculated dose

TCID$_{50}$ median tissue culture infective dose

TCIE transient cerebral ischemic episode

TCL thermochemiluminescence; total capacity of the lung

T-CLL T-cell chromic lymphatic leukemia

TCM tissue culture medium; transcutaneous monitor

TCMA transcortical motor aphasia

TCMP thematic content modification program

TCMZ trichloromethiazide

TCN tetracycline

TCP therapeutic continuous penicillin; total circulating protein; tranylcypromine; tricalcium phosphate; trichlorophenol; tricresyl phosphate

tcPCO₂, tcPCO2 transcutaneous carbon dioxide pressure

tcPO₂, tcPO2 transcutaneous oxygen pressure

2,4,5-TCPPA 2-(2,4,5-trichlorophenoxy)-propionic acid

TCR T-cell rosette; thalamocortical relay

tcRNA translational control ribonucleic acid

TCRV total red cell volume

TCSA tetrachlorosalicylanilide

TCT thrombin clotting time; thyrocalcitonin

TCV thoracic cage volume; three concept view

TD tardive dyskinesia; temporary disability; terminal device; tetanus and diphtheria [toxoid]; tetrodotoxin; therapy discontinued; thermal dilution; thoracic duct; three times per day; threshold of detectability; threshold of discomfort; threshold dose; thymus-dependent; time disintegration; to deliver; tone decay; torsion dystonia; total disability, totally disabled; total dose; toxic dose; transdermal; transverse diameter; traveler's diarrhea; treatment discontinued; typhoid dysentery

T_D the time required to double the number of cells in a given population

T₄(D) serum thyroxine measured by displacement analysis

TD₅₀ median toxic dose

td three times daily [Lat. *ter die*]

TDA thyroid-stimulating hormone-displacing antibody

TDB Toxicology Data Bank

TDC taurodeoxycholic acid

TDD telecommunication device for the deaf; tetradecadiene; thoracic duct drainage

TDE tetrachlorodiphenylethane; total digestible energy

TDF thoracic duct fistula; thoracic duct flow

TDH threonine dehydrogenase

TDI toluene 2,4-diisocyanate; total dose infusion

TDL thoracic duct lymph; thymus-dependent lymphocyte

TDM therapeutic drug monitoring

TDN total digestible nutrients

tDNA transfer deoxyribonucleic acid

TDO tricho-dento-osseous [syndrome]

TDP thermal death point; thoracic duct pressure; thymidine diphosphate

TdR thymidine

tds to be taken three times a day [Lat. *ter die sumendum*]

TDT terminal deoxynucleotidyl transferase; thermal death time; tone decay test; tumor doubling time

TdT terminal deoxynucleotidyl transferase

TDZ thymus-dependent zone

TE echo-time; tennis elbow; tetracycline; threshold energy; thromboembolism; thymus epithelium; tissue-equivalent; tooth extracted; total estrogen; *Toxoplasma* encephalitis; tracheoesophageal

T&E trial and error

Te tellurium; tetanic contraction; tetanus

TEA temporal external artery; tetraethylammonium; thermal energy analyzer; thromboendarterectomy; total elbow arthroplasty; triethanolamine

TEAB tetraethylammonium bromide

TEAC tetraethylammonium chloride

TEAE triethylammonioethyl

TEAM Training in Expanded Auxiliary Management

TEBG, TeBG testosterone-estradiol-binding globulin

TEC total eosinophil count; total exchange capacity; transient erythroblastopenia of childhood

T&EC trauma and emergency center

TECV traumatic epiphyseal coxa vara

TED Tasks of Emotional Development;

threshold erythema dose; thromboembolic disease

TEDS anti-embolism stockings

TEE tyrosine ethyl ester

TEF tracheoesophageal fistula; trunk extension-flexion [unit]

TEFRA Tax Equity and Fiscal Responsibility Act

TEFS transmural electrical field stimulation

TEG thromboelastogram

TEIB triethyleneiminobenzoquinone

TEL tetraethyl lead

TEM transmission electron microscope/microscopy; triethylenemelamine

temp temperature; temple, temporal

temp dext to the right temple [Lat. *tempori dextro*]

temp sinist to the left temple [Lat. *tempori sinistro*]

TEN total enteral nutrition; total excretory nitrogen; toxic epidermal necrolysis

TENS transcutaneous electrical nerve stimulation

TEPA triethylenephosphamide

TEPP tetraethyl pyrophosphate; triethylene pyrophosphate

TER total endoplasmic reticulum; transcapillary escape rate

ter terminal or end; ternary; tertiary; three times; threefold

ter in die three times a day

term terminal

tert tertiary

TES thymic epithelial supernatant; toxic epidemic syndrome; transcutaneous electrical stimulation; transmural electrical stimulation; N-tris(hydroxymethyl)methyl-2-aminoethanesulfonic acid

TESPA thiotepa

TET treadmill exercise test

Tet tetralogy of Fallot

tet tetanus

TETD tetraethylthiuram disulfide

TEV tadpole edema virus; talipes equinovarus

TEWL transepidermal water loss

TF tactile fremitus; tail flick [reflex]; temperature factor; testicular feminization; tetralogy of Fallot; thymol flocculation; thymus factor; tissue-damaging factor; to follow; total flow; transfer factor; transferrin; transformation frequency; transfrontal; tube feeding; tuberculin filtrate; tubular fluid; tuning fork

t(°F) temperature on the Fahrenheit scale

Tf transferrin

T$_f$ freezing temperature

TFA total fatty acids; transverse fascicular area; trifluoroacetic acid

TFd dialyzable transfer factor

TFE polytetrafluoroethylene

TFF tube-fed food

TFM testicular feminization male; testicular feminization mutation; transmission electron microscopy

TFN total fecal nitrogen

TFR total fertility rate

TFS testicular feminization syndrome; tube-fed saline

TFT thrombus formation time; thyroid function test; tight filum terminale; trifluorothymidine

TG tetraglycine; thioglucose; thioglycolate; thioguanine; thromboglobulin; thyroglobulin; toxic goiter; treated group; triacylglycerol; trigeminal ganglion; triglyceride; tumor growth

Tg generation time; thyroglobulin

T$_g$ glass transition temperature

6-TG thioguanine

tG$_1$ the time required to complete the G$_1$ phase of the cell cycle

tG$_2$ the time required to complete the G$_2$ phase of the cell cycle

TGA taurocholate gelatin agar; total glycoalkaloids; transient global amnesia; transposition of great arteries; tumor glycoprotein assay

TGAR total graft area rejected

TGBG dimethylglyoxal bis-guanylhydrazone

TGE transmissible gastroenteritis [virus]; tryptone glucose extract

TGF T-cell growth factor; transforming growth factor; tuboglomerular feedback

TGFA triglyceride fatty acid

TGG turkey gamma globulin

TGL triglyceride; triglyceride lipase

6-TGR 6-thioguanine resistance

TGS tincture of green soap

TGT thromboplastin generation test/time

TGV thoracic gas volume; transposition of great vessels

TGY tryptone glucose yeast [agar]
TGYA tryptone glucose yeast agar
TH tetrahydrocortisol; T helper [cell]; thrill; thyrohyoid; thyroid hormone; tyrosine hydroxylase
Th thenar; thoracic, thorax; thorium
th thermie
THA tetrahydroaminoacridine; total hip arthroplasty; total hydroxyapatite; *Treponema* hemagglutination
ThA thoracic aorta
THAM tris(hydroxymethyl)aminomethane
THBP 7,8,9,10-tetrahydrobenzo[a]pyrene
THC tetrahydrocannabinol; tetrahydrocortisol; transhepatic cholangiogram; transplantable hepatocellular carcinoma
THCA alpha-trihydroxy-5-beta-cholestannic acid
Thd ribothymidine
THDOC tetrahydrodeoxycorticosterone
THE tetrahydrocortisone E; tonic hind limb extension; transhepatic embolization; tropical hypereosinophilia
theor theory, theoretical
ther therapy, therapeutic; thermometer
therap therapy, therapeutic
Θ Greek capital letter *theta*; thermodynamic temperature
θ Greek lower case letter *theta*; an angular coordinate variable; customary temperature; temperature interval
THF tetrahydrocortisone F; tetrahydrofolate; tetrahydrofuran; thymic humoral factor
THFA tetrahydrofolic acid; tetrahydrofurfuryl alcohol
THH telangiectasia hereditaria haemorrhagica
THIP tetrahydroisoxazolopyridinol
THM total heme mass
THO titrated water
thor thorax, thoracic
thou thousandth
THP total hip replacement; total hydroxyproline; trihexphenidyl
THPA tetrahydropteric acid
THR targeted heart rate; transhepatic resistance
Thr threonine
thr thyroid, thyroidectomy
THRF thyrotropic hormone-releasing factor

throm, thromb thrombosis, thrombus
THS tetrahydro-compound S
THSC totipotent hematopoietic stem cell
THUG thyroid uptake gradient
Thx thromboxane
Thy thymine
thy thymus, thymectomy
THz terahertz
TI inversion time; thalassemia intermedia; therapeutic index; thoracic index; thymus-independent; time interval; tonic immobility; translational inhibition; transverse inlet; tricuspid incompetence; tricuspid insufficiency; tumor induction
Ti titanium
TIA transient ischemic attack; tumor-induced angiogenesis
TIB tumor immunology bank
TIBC total iron-binding capacity
TIC Toxicology Information Center; trypsin inhibitory capability
TID titrated initial dose
tid three times a day [Lat. *ter in die*]
TIDA tuberoinfundibular dopaminergic system
TIE transient ischemic episode
TIF tumor-inducing factor
TIg tetanus immunoglobulin
TIH time interval histogram
TIM transthoracic intracardiac monitoring
TIMC tumor-induced marrow cytotoxicity
TIN tubulointerstitial nephropathy
tin three times a night [Lat. *ter in nocte*]
tinc, tinct tincture
TIP thermal inactivation point; Toxicology Information Program; translation-inhibiting protein; tumor-inhibiting principle
TIR terminal innervation ratio
TIS trypsin-insoluble segment; tumor in situ
TIT, TITh triiodothyronine
TIU trypsin-inhibiting unit
TIUV total intrauterine volume
TIVC thoracic inferior vena cava
TJ tetrajoule; triceps jerk
TK thymidine kinase; transketolase; triose-kinase
T(°K) absolute temperature on the Kelvin scale
TKA total knee arthroplasty; transketolase activity

TKD thymidine kinase deficiency; tokodynamometer

TKG tokodynagraph

TKLI tachykinin-like immunoreactivity

TKR total knee replacement

TL temporal lobe; terminal limen; thermoluminescence; thymus-leukemia [antigen]; thymus lymphocyte; thymus lymphoma; time lapse; time-limited; total lipids; tubal ligation

T-L thymus-dependent lymphocyte

Tl thallium

TLA translumbar aortogram; transluminal angioplasty

TLAA T-lymphocyte-associated antigen

TLC tender loving care; thin-layer chromatography; total L-chain concentration; total lung capacity; total lung compliance; total lymphocyte count

TLD thermoluminescent dosimeter; thoracic lymphatic duct; tumor lethal dose

T/LD$_{100}$ minimum dose causing 100% deaths or malformations

TLE temporal lobe epilepsy; thin-layer electrophoresis; total lipid extract

TLI thymidine labeling index; total lymphoid irradiation

TLQ total living quotient

TLR tonic labyrinthine reflex

TLT tryptophan load test

TLV threshold limit value; total lung volume

TLW total lung water

TLX trophoblast-lymphocyte cross-reactivity

TM tectorial membrane; temporomandibular; thalassemia major; Thayer-Martin [medium]; time-motion; tobramycin; trademark; transitional mucosa; transmediastinal; transmetatarsal; transport mechanism; transport medium; transverse myelitis; tropical medicine; tympanic membrane

T-M Thayer-Martin [medium]

Tm thulium; tubular maximum excretory capacity of kidneys

T$_m$ temperature midpoint; tubular maximum excretory capacity of kidneys

tM the time required to complete the M phase of the cell cycle

TMA tetramethylammonium; thrombotic microangiopathy; thyroid microsomal antibody; trimellitic anhydride; transmetatarsal amputation; trimethoxyamphetamine; trimethoxyphenyl aminopropane; trimethylamine

TMAH trimethylphenylammonium (anilinium) hydroxide

TMAI trimethylphenylammonium (anilinium) iodide

TMAS Taylor Manifest Anxiety Scale

T$_{max}$ time of maximum concentration

TMBA trimethoxybenzaldehyde

TMC triamcinolone and terramycin capsules

TMD trimethadione

TME total metabolizable energy; transmissible mink encephalopathy

TMET treadmill exercise test

TMF transformed mink fibroblast

TM$_g$ maximum tubular reabsorption rate for glucose

TMH tetramethylammonium hydroxide

TMI transmural infarction

TMIC Toxic Materials Information Center

TMIF tumor-cell migratory inhibition factor

TMIS Technicon Medical Information System

TMJ temporomandibular joint

TML tetramethyl lead

TMP thiamine monophosphate; thymidine monophosphate; thymolphthalein monophosphate; transmembrane potential; trimethoprim

TM$_{PAH}$ maximum tubular excretory capacity for para-aminohippuric acid

TMPD tetramethyl-p-phenylinediamine

TMPDS temporomandibular pain and dysfunction syndrome

TMP-SMX trimethoprim-sulfamethoxazole

TMR topical magnetic resonance

TMS thread mate system; trimethylsilane

TMU tetramethyl urea

TMV tobacco mosaic virus

TMX tamoxifen

TN team nursing; temperature normal; trigeminal nucleus; total negatives; true negative

Tn normal intraocular tension; transposon

TND term normal delivery

TNF tumor necrosing factor

tng tongue

TNI total nodal irradiation

TNM primary tumor, regional nodes, metastasis [tumor staging]

TNMR tritium nuclear magnetic resonance

TNR tonic neck reflex; true negative rate

TNS transcutaneous nerve stimulation; tumor necrosis serum

TNT 2,4,6-trinitrotoluene

TNTC too numerous to count

TNV tobacco necrosis virus

TO old tuberculin; original tuberculin; oral temperature; target organ; telephone order; tincture of opium; tracheo-esophageal; turnover

to tincture of opium

TOA tubo-ovarian abscess

TOAP thioguanine, oncovin, cytosine arabinoside, and prednisone

TOB tobramycin

TobRV tobacco ringspot virus

TOC total organic carbon

TOCP tri-o-cresyl phosphate

TOD Time-Oriented Data Bank

TOE tracheoesophageal

TOES toxic oil epidemic syndrome

TOF tetralogy of Fallot; tracheo-[o]esophageal fistula

TOH transient osteoporosis of hip

TOL trial of labor

tol tolerance, tolerated

tonoc tonight

top topical

TOPV trivalent oral poliovaccine

TORCH toxoplasmosis, rubella, cyto-megalovirus, and herpes simplex [infection]

TORP total ossicular replacement prosthesis

TOS thoracic outlet syndrome

TOT total operating time

tox toxicity, toxic

TOXICON Toxicology Information Conversational On-Line Network

TOXLINE Toxicology Information On-Line

TP temperature and pressure; terminal phalanx; testosterone propionate; threshold potential; thrombocytopenic purpura; thymus polypeptide; thymus protein; total positives; total protein; *Treponema pallidum*; trigger point; triphosphate; true positive; tryptophan; tryptophan pyrrolase; tube precipitin; tuberculin precipitate

T+P temperature and pulse

Tp *Treponema pallidum*; tryptophan

TPA tannic acid, polyphosphomolybdic acid, and amino acid; 12-0-tetradecanoyl-phorbol-13-acetate; tissue plasminogen-activator; total parenteral alimentation; *Treponema pallidum* agglutination; tumor polypeptide antigen

t-PA tissue-type plasminogen activator

TPB tryptone phosphate broth

TPBF total pulmonary blood flow

TPBS three-phase radionuclide bone scanning

TPC thromboplastic plasma component; total patient care; total plasma catechol-amines; *Treponema pallidum* complement

TPCF *Treponema pallidum* complement fixation

TPCV total packed cell volume

TPD thiamine propyl disulfide; tumor-producing dose

TPE therapeutic plasma exchange

TPEY tellurite polymyxin egg yolk [agar]

TPF thymus permeability factor

TPG transmembrane potential gradient; transplacental gradient; tryptophan peptone glucose [broth]

TPGYT trypticase-peptone-glucose-yeast extract-trypsin [medium]

TPH transplacental hemorrhage

TPHA *Treponema pallidum* hemagglu-tination

TPI treponemal immobilization test; *Treponema pallidum* immobilization; triosephosphate isomerase

TPIA *Treponema pallidum* immune adherence

TPL tyrosine phenol-lyase

TPM thrombophlebitis migrans; total passive motion; triphenylmethane

TPN thalamic projection neuron; total parenteral nutrition; triphosphopyridine nucleotide

TPNH reduced triphosphopyridine nucleotide

TPO thyroid peroxidase; tryptophan peroxidase

TPP thiamine pyrophosphate

TPPase thiamine pyrophosphatase

TPPN total peripheral parenteral nutrition
TPR temperature; temperature, pulse, and respiration; testosterone production rate; total peripheral resistance; total pulmonary resistance; true positive rate
TPRI total peripheral resistance index
TPS trypsin; tumor polysaccharide substance
TPSE 2-(p-triphenyl)sulfonylethanol
TPST true positive stress test
TPT tetraphenyl tetrazolium; total protein tuberculin; typhoid-paratyphoid [vaccine]
TPTE 2-(p-triphenyl)thioethanol
TPTX thyro-parathyroidectomized
TPTZ tripyridyltriazine
TPV tetanus-pertussis vaccine
TPVR total peripheral vascular resistance
TQ tocopherolquinone; tourniquet
TR recovery time; rectal temperature; repetition time; residual tuberculin; tetrazolium reduction; therapeutic radiology; time release; total resistance; total response; tricuspid regurgitation; tuberculin R [new tuberculin]; tuberculin residue; turbidity-reducing
T($^\circ$R) absolute temperature on the Rankine scale
Tr tragion; trypsin
T$_r$ retention time
tr tincture; trace; tremor
TRA total renin activity; transaldolase
tra transfer
trach trachea, tracheal, tracheostomy
TRAM Treatment Rating Assessment Matrix; Treatment Response Assessment Method
trans transference; transverse
trans D transverse diameter
transm transmission, transmitted
transpl transplantation, transplanted
traum trauma, traumatic
TRBF total renal blood flow
TRC tanned red cell; total renin concentration; total ridge count
TRCH tanned red cell hemagglutination
TRCHI tanned red cell hemagglutination inhibition
TRCV total red cell volume
TRE true radiation emission

TREA triethanolamine
treat treatment
Trep *Treponema*
TRF T-cell replacing factor; thyrotropin-releasing factor
TRFC total rosette-forming cell
TRH thyrotropin-releasing hormone
TRH-ST thyrotropin-releasing hormone stimulation test
TRI tetrazolium reduction inhibition; Thyroid Research Institute; total response index; tubuloreticular inclusion
tri tricentric
T$_3$RIA, T$_3$(RIA) triiodothyronine radioimmunoassay
T$_4$RIA, T$_4$(RIA) thyroxine radioimmunoassay
TRIC trachoma inclusion conjunctivitis [organism]
TRICB trichlorobiphenyl
Trich *Trichomonas*
Trid three days [Lat. *triduum*]
trig triglycerides
TRIMIS Tri-Service Medical Information System
TRIS tris-hydroxymethyl-amino methane
TRIT triiodothyronine
trit triturate
TRITC tetrarhodamine isothiocyanate
TRK transketolase
TRMC trimethylrhodamino-isothiocyanate
TRML, Trml terminal
TRM-SMX trimethoprim-sulfamethoxazole
tRNA transfer ribonucleic acid
Trop tropical
TRP total refractory period; trichorhinophalangeal [syndrome]; tubular reabsorption of phosphate
Trp tryptophan
TRPA tryptophan-rich prealbumin
TrPl treatment plan
TRPS trichorhinophalangeal syndrome
TRPT theoretical renal phosphorus threshold
TRR total respiratory resistance
TRS total reducing sugars; tubuloreticular structure
TRSV tobacco ringspot virus
TRU turbidity-reducing unit
T$_3$RU triiodothyronine resin uptake

TRV tobacco rattle virus

Try tryptophan

TS temperature sensitivity; temporal stem; test solution; thoracic surgery; total solids [in urine]; Tourette syndrome; toxic substance; toxic syndrome; tracheal sound; transsexual; transverse section; transverse sinus; treadmill score; tricuspid stenosis; triple strength; tropical sprue; trypticase soy [plate]; T suppressor [cell]; tuberous sclerosis; tumor-specific; Turner syndrome; type-specific

tS time required to complete the S phase of the cell cycle

ts, tsp teaspoon

TSA toluene sulfonic acid; total shoulder arthroplasty; toxic shock antigen; trypticase-soy agar; tumor-specific antigen; tumor surface antigen

T₄SA thyroxine-specific activity

TSAb thyroid-stimulating antibody

T's and B's pentazocine and tripelennamine

TSAP toxic-shock-associated protein

TSAS total severity assessment score

TSB trypticase soy broth; tryptone soy broth

TSC technetium sulfur colloid; thiosemicarbazide; transverse spinal sclerosis

TSCA Toxic Substance Control Act

TSD target-skin distance; Tay-Sachs disease; theory of signal detectability

TSE testicular self-examination; total skin examination; trisodium edetate

TSEB total skin electron beam

T sect transverse section

TSF testicular feminization syndrome; thrombopoiesis-stimulating factor; triceps skinfold

TSG tumor-specific glycoprotein

TSH thyroid-stimulating hormone

TSH-RF thyroid-stimulating hormone-releasing factor

TSI thyroid stimulating immunoglobulin; triple sugar iron [agar]

TSIA triple sugar iron agar

TSN type-specific M protein; tryptophan peptone sulfide neomycin

TSP total serum protein; trisodium phosphate

tsp teaspoon

TSPA thiotepa

TSPAP total serum prostatic acid phosphatase

TSR thyroid to serum ratio

TSS toxic shock syndrome; tropical splenomegaly syndrome

TSSA tumor-specific cell surface antigen

TSSE toxic shock syndrome exoprotein

TSST toxic shock syndrome toxin

TST treadmill stress test; tumor skin test

TSTA tumor-specific tissue antigen; tumor-specific transplantation antigen

TSU triple sugar urea [agar]

TSY trypticase soy yeast

TT tablet triturate; tetanus toxin; tetanus toxoid; tetrathionate; tetrazol; thrombin time; thymol turbidity; tibial tubercle; tilt table; total thyroxine; total time; transient tachypnea; transit time; transthoracic; transtracheal; tuberculin test

T&T time and temperature; touch and tone

TT₄ total thyroxine

TTA total toe arthroplasty; transtracheal aspiration

TTC triphenyltetrazolium chloride

TTD tissue tolerance dose

TTFD tetrahydrofurfuryldisulfide

TTG tellurite, taurocholate, and gelatin

TTGA tellurite, taurocholate, and gelatin agar

TTH thyrotropic hormone; tritiated thymidine

TTI tension-time index; time-tension index

TTL transistor-transistor logic

TTP thrombotic thrombocytopenic purpura; thymidine triphosphate

TTPA triethylene thiophosphoramide

TTS tarsal tunnel syndrome; through the skin; temporary threshold shift; transdermal therapeutic system

TTT tolbutamide tolerance test

TTTT test tube turbidity test

TTX tetrodotoxin

TU thiouracil; Todd unit; toxic unit; transmission unit; tuberculin unit; turbidity unit

T₃U triiodothyronine uptake

tuberc tuberculosis

TUD total urethral discharge

TUG total urinary gonadotropin
TUR transurethral resection
TURB, TURBT transurethral resection of bladder [tumor]
turb turbidity, turbid
TURP transurethral prostatectomy
TURV transurethral resection of valves
tus cough [Lat. *tussis*]
TV television; tetrazolium violet; tidal volume; total volume; transvenous; *Trichomonas vaginalis*; tricuspid valve; tuberculin volutin; truncal vagotomy
Tv *Trichomonas vaginalis*
TVC timed vital capacity; total viable cells; total volume capacity; transvaginal cone; triple voiding cystogram
TVD transmissible virus dementia; triple vessel disease
TVF tactile vocal fremitus
TVH total vaginal hysterectomy; turkey virus hepatitis
TVL tenth value layer
TVP transvenous pacemaker; tricuspid valve prolapse
TVR total vascular resistance; tricuspid valve replacement
TVT transmissible venereal tumor; tunica vaginalis testis
TVU total volume of the urine
TW tap water; test weight; total body water
TWA time weighted average
TWD total white and differential [cell count]
TWE tap water enema
TWL transepidermal water loss
TWWD tap water wet dressing
TX a derivative of contagious tuberculin; thromboxane; thyroidectomized; transplantation; treatment
Tx, T$_x$ treatment; therapy, traction
TXA, TxA thromboxane A
TXA2, TXA$_2$ thromboxane A2 (A$_2$)
TXB2, TXB$_2$ thromboxane B2 (B$_{2)}$
Ty type, typhoid; tyrosine
Tymp tympanum, tympanic
TYMV turnip yellow mosaic virus
Tyr tyrosine
TZ zymoplastic tuberculin [the dried residue which is soluble in alcohol] [Ger. *Tuberculin zymoplastische*]

–U–

U in electrocardiography, an undulating deflection that follows the T wave; internal energy; International Unit of enzyme activity; Mann-Whitney rank sum statistic; potential difference (in volts); ultralente [insulin]; unerupted; unit; unknown; upper; uracil; uranium; uridine; uridylic acid; urine; urology; volume velocity
u to be used [Lat. *utendus*]; unified atomic mass unit; velocity
U/3 upper third
UA ultra-audible; unit of analysis; umbilical artery; unauthorized absence; unstable angina; urinalysis; uric acid; uridylic acid; urinary aldosterone; uterine aspiration
U/A urinalysis; uric acid
U-AMY urinary amylase
UAN uric acid nitrogen
UAO upper airway obstruction
UAU uterine activity unit
UB ultimobranchial body
UBA undenaturated bacterial antigen
UBBC unsaturated vitamin B12 binding capacity
UBF uterine blood flow
UBG urobilinogen
UBI ultraviolet blood irradiation
UBL undifferentiated B-cell lymphoma
UC ulcerative colitis; ultracentrifugal; umbilical cord; unchanged; unclassifiable; unit clerk; unsatisfactory condition; urea clearance; urethral catheterization; urinary catheter; urine concentrate; uterine contractions
U&C urethral and cervical; usual and customary
UCD urine collection device; usual childhood diseases
UCG ultrasonic cardiography; urinary chorionic gonadotropin
UCHD usual childhood diseases
UCI urethral catheter in; urinary catheter in
UCL urea clearance
UCLP unilateral cleft of lip and palate
UCO urethral catheter out; urinary catheter out

UCP urinary coproporphyrin; urinary C-peptide
UCPT urinary coproporphyrin test
UCR unconditioned response; usual, customary, and reasonable [fees]
UCS unconditioned stimulus; unconscious
UCTD unclassifiable connective tissue disease
UCV uncontrolled variable
UD ulcerative dermatosis; ulnar deviation; urethral discharge; uridine diphosphate; uroporphyrinogen decarboxylase
ud as directed [Lat. *ud dictum*]
UDC usual diseases of childhood
UDCA ursodeoxycholic acid
UDP uridine diphosphate
UDPG urine diphosphoglucose
UDPGA uridine diphosphate glucuronic acid
UDPGT uridine diphosphate glucuronosyl transferase
UDRP urine diribose phosphate
UDS ultra-Doppler sonography; unscheduled deoxynucleic acid synthesis
UE uncertain etiology; upper esophagus; upper extremity
UEG unifocal eosinophilic granuloma
UEM universal electron microscope
UEMC unidentified endosteal marrow cell
UES upper esophageal sphincter
u/ext upper extremity
UF ultrafiltrate; universal feeder; unknown factor
UFA unesterified fatty acid
UFC urinary free cortisol
UFD ultrasonic flow detector
uFSH urinary follicle-stimulating hormone
UG urogastrone; urogenital
UGDP University Group Diabetes Project
UGF unidentified growth factor
UGH uveitis-glaucoma-hyphema [syndrome]
UGH+ uveitis-glaucoma-hyphema plus vitreous hemorrhage [syndrome]
UGI upper gastrointestinal [tract]
UGS urogenital sinus
UH upper half
UHD unstable hemoglobin disease
UHF ultrahigh frequency

UHR underlying heart rhythm
UHSC university health services clinic
UHT ultrahigh temperature
UI uroporphyrin isomerase
U/I unidentified
UIBC unsaturated iron-binding capacity
UIF undegraded insulin factor
UIP usual interstitial pneumonia
UIQ upper inner quadrant
UIS Utilization Information Service
UJT unijunction transistor
UK unknown; urinary kallikrein; urokinase
UKa urinary kallikrein
UKAEA United Kingdom Atomic Energy Authority
UKCCSG United Kingdom Children's Cancer Study Group
UL Underwriters' Laboratories; upper limb; upper lobe
U&L upper and lower
U/l units per liter
ULBW ultralow birth weight
ULN upper limits of normal
uln ulna, ulnar
ULQ upper left quadrant
ULT ultrahigh temperature
ult praes last prescribed [Lat. *ultimum praescriptus*]
UM upper motor [neuron]; uracil mustard
UMA urinary muramidase activity
umb umbilicus, umbilical
UMN upper motor neuron
UMNL upper motor neuron lesion
UMP uridine monophosphate
UMS urethral manipulation syndrome
UMT units of medical time
UN unilateral neglect; urea nitrogen
UNa urinary sodium
uncomp uncompensated
uncond unconditioned
undet undetermined
UNE urinary norepinephrine
ung ointment [Lat. *unguentum*]
unilat unilateral
univ universal
unk, unkn unknown
unsat unsatisfactory; unsaturated
UNTS unilateral nevoid telangiectasia syndrome
UO urinary output
u/o under observation
UOQ upper outer quadrant

UOsm urinary osmolality
UP upright posture; ureteropelvic; uroporphyrin
U/P urine to plasma [ratio]
UPG uroporphyrinogen
UPI uteroplacental insufficiency; utero-placental ischemia
UPJ ureteropelvic junction
UPL unusual position of limbs
UPPP uvulopalatopharyngoplasty
UPS ultraviolet photoelectron spectros-copy; uninterruptible power supply; uterine progesterone system
Υ   Greek capital letter *upsilon*
υ   Greek lower case letter *upsilon*
UQ ubiquinone; upper quadrant
UR unconditioned reflex; upper respira-tory; urinal; urology; utilization review
Ur urine, urinary
URA, Ura uracil
URC upper rib cage; utilization review committee
URD upper respiratory disease
Urd uridine
ureth urethra
URF uterine relaxing factor
URI upper respiratory infection
URO urology; uroporphyrin; uropor-phyrinogen
URO-GEN urogenital
Urol urology, urologist
URQ upper right quadrant
URS ultrasonic renal scanning
URT upper respiratory tract
URTI upper respiratory tract infection
URVD unilateral renovascular disease
US ultrasound, ultrasonic; ultrasonog-raphy; unconditioned stimulus; unit secretary; Usher syndrome
USAFH United States Air Force Hospital
USAFRHL United States Air Force Radiological Health Laboratory
USAH United States Army Hospital
USAHC United States Army Health Clinic
USAIDR United States Army Institute of Dental Research
USAMEDS United States Army Medical Service
USAN United States Adopted Names
USASI United States of America Stan-dards Institute

USB upper sternal border
USBS United States Bureau of Standards
USD United States Dispensary
USDA United States Department of Agriculture
USDHEW United States Department of Health, Education, and Welfare
USDHHS United States Department of Health and Human Services
USE ultrasonic echography; ultrasonog-raphy
USFMG United States foreign medical graduates
USHL United States Hygienic Laboratory
USHMAC United States Health Manpower Advisory Council
USI urinary stress incontinence
USMG United States medical graduate
USMH United States Marine Hospital
USN ultrasonic nebulizer
USNCHS United States National Center for Health Statistics
USNH United States Naval Hospital
USO unilateral salpingo-oophorectomy
USP United States Pharmacopeia
USP DI United States Pharmacopeia Drug Information
USPHS United States Public Health Service
USPTA United States Phyical Therapy Association
USR unheated serum reagin
ust burnt, calcined [Lat. *ustus*]
USVH United States Veterans Hospital
USVMD urine specimen volume measuring device
UT untested; untreated; urinary tract; urticaria
uT unbound testosterone
UTBG unbound thyroxine-binding globulin
ut dict as directed [Lat. *ut dictum*]
utend to be used [Lat. *utendus*]
UTI urinary tract infection; urinary trypsin inhibitor
UTO upper tibial osteotomy
UTP uridine triphosphate
UTS Ullrich-Turner syndrome
UU urinary urea; urine urobilinogen
UUN urinary urea nitrogen

UV ultraviolet; umbilical vein; urinary volume
UVA ureterovesical angle
UVB ultraviolet B
UVER ultraviolet-enhanced reactivation
UVI ultraviolet irradiation
UVJ ureterovesical junction
UVL ultraviolet light
UVP ultraviolet photometry
UVR ultraviolet radiation
UX uranium X, proactinium

–V–

V in cardiography, unipolar chest lead; coefficient of variation; electrical potential (in volts); in electroencephalography, vertex sharp transient; five; a logical binary relation that is true if any argument is true, and false otherwise; luminous efficiency; potential energy (joules); vaccinated; vagina; valine; valve; vanadium; variation, variable; varnish; vector; vein [Lat. *vena*]; velocity; ventilation; ventral; ventricular [fibrillation]; verbal comprehension [factor]; vertex; *Vibrio*; violet; viral [antigen]; virulence; virus; vision; visual acuity; voice; volt; voltage; volume; vomiting
v rate of reaction catalyzed by an enzyme; see [Lat. *vide*]; specific volume; vein [Lat. *vena*]; velocity; very; virus; volt
VA vacuum aspiration; valproic acid; ventriculoatrial; vertebral artery; Veterans Administration; viral antigen; visual acuity; visual aid; volt-ampere
V$_A$ alveolar ventilation
V/A volt/ampere
V$_a$ alveolar ventilation
VAB vincristine, actinomycin D, and bleomycin
VAC ventriculo-atrial conduction; vincristine, doxorubicin, and cyclophosphamide; virus capsid antigen
vac vacuum
vacc vaccination
VACTERL vertebral abnormalities, anal atresia, cardiac abnormalities, tracheoesophageal fistula and/or esophageal atresia, renal agenesis and dysplasia, and limb defects [association]
VAD ventricular assist device; vitamin A deficiency
vag vagina, vaginal
VAG HYST vaginal hysterectomy
VAH Veterans Administration Hospital; virilizing adrenal hyperplasia
VAHS virus-associated hemophagocytic syndrome
Val valine
val valve
VALE visual acuity, left eye
VAMC Veterans Administration Medical Center
VAMP vincristine, amethopterine, 6-mercaptopurine; and prednisone
vap vapor
V$_A$/Q$_C$ ventilation-perfusion [ratio]
Var, var variant, variety, variation
VARE visual acuity, right eye
VAS vascular; vesicle attachment site; Visual Analogue Scale
VASC Verbal Auditory Screen for Children
vasc vascular
VAS RAD vascular radiology
VAT variable antigen type; ventricular activation time; visual action time; visual apperception test; vocational apperception test
VATER vertebral defects, imperforate anus, tracheoesophageal fistula, and radial and renal dysplasia
VATs surface variable antigen
VB valence bond; venous blood; ventrobasal; Veronal buffer; viable birth; vinblastine
VBC vincristine, bleomycin, and cisplatin
VBD Veronal-buffered diluent
VBI vertebrobasilar insufficiency
VBL vinblastine
VBOS Veronal-buffered oxalated saline
VBP ventricular premature beat
VBR ventricular-brain ratio
VBS Veronal-buffered saline
VBS:FBS Veronal-buffered saline–fetal bovine serum
VC color vision; vasoconstriction; vena cava; ventilatory capacity; ventral column;

Veterinary Corps; videocasette; vincristine; vinyl chloride; visual capacity; visual cortex; vital capacity; vocal cord

V_C pulmonary capillary blood volume

VCA vancomycin, colistin, and anisomycin; viral capsid antibody; viral capsid antigen

VCAP vincristine, cyclophosphamide, Adriamycin, and prednisone

VCC vasoconstrictor center

VCD vibrational circular dichroism

VCE vagina, ectocervix, and endocervix

VCG vectorcardiogram, vectorcardiography

VCM vinyl chloride monomer

VCMP vincristine, cyclophosphamide, melphalan, and prednisone

VCN vancomycin, colistomethane, and nystatin; *Vibrio chloreae* neuraminidase

VCO, V_{CO} endogenous production of carbon monoxide

VCO_2, V_{CO2} carbon dioxide output

VCP vincristine, cyclophosphamide, and prednisone

VCR vincristine; volume clearance rate

VCS vasoconstrictor substance

VCSA viral cell surface antigen

VCT venous clotting time

VCU videocystourethrography; voiding cystourethrogram, voiding cystourethrography

VCUG vesicoureterogram; voiding cystourethrogram

VD vapor density; vascular disease; vasodilation, vasodilator; venereal disease; ventricular dilator; vertical deviation; video-disc; viral diarrhea; voided; volume of distribution

V_D dead space

Vd volume dead space

V_d apparent volume of distribution

VDA visual discriminatory acuity

VDBR volume of distribution of bilirubin

VDC vasodilator center

VDD atrial synchronous ventricular inhibited [pacemaker]

VDEL Venereal Disease Experimental Laboratory

VDEM vasodepressor material

VDF ventricular diastolic fragmentation

VDG, VD-G venereal disease–gonorrhea

vdg voiding

VDH valvular disease of the heart

VDL vasodepressor lipid; visual detection level

VDM vasodepressor material

VDP vincristine, daunorubicin, and prednisone

VDR venous diameter ratio

VDRL Venereal Disease Research Laboratory [test for syphilis]

VDRR vitamin D–resistant rickets

VDRS Verdun Depression Rating Scale

VDRT venereal disease reference test

VDS vasodilator substance; vindesine

VDS, VD-S venereal disease–syphilis

VDT visual display terminal

VE vaginal examination; venous emptying; ventilation; ventricular extrasystole; vertex; vesicular exanthema; viral encephalitis; visual efficiency; volume ejection; voluntary effort

V_E environmental variance; respiratory minute volume

V&E Vinethine and ether

VEA viral envelope antigen

VEB ventricular ectopic beat

VECG vector electrocardiogram

VECP visually evoked cortical potential

VED ventricular ectopic depolarization; vital exhaustion and depression

VEE Venezuelan equine encephalomyelitis

VEF ventricular ejection fraction

vehic vehicle

vel velocity

VEM vasoexcitor material

vent ventilation; ventral; ventricular

ventric ventricle

VEP visual evoked potential

VER visual evoked response

Verc vervet (African green monkey) kidney cells

vert vertebra, vertebral

ves bladder [Lat. *vesica*]; vesicular; vessel

vesic a blister [Lat. *vesicula*]

ves ur urinary bladder [Lat. *vesica urinaria*]

VET vestigial testis

Vet veteran; veterinary, veterinarian

VetMB Bachelor of Veterinary Medicine
Vet Med veterinary medicine
VETS Veterans Adjustment Scale
VF left leg [electrode]; ventricular fibrillation; ventricular fluid; visual field; vocal fremitus
vf visual field
VFA volatile fatty acid
V fib ventricular fibrillation
VFL ventricular flutter
VFP ventricular filling pressure; ventricular fluid pressure
VFT ventricular fibrillation threshold
VG ventricular gallop
V_G genetic variance
VGH very good health
VGP viral glycoprotein
VH vaginal hysterectomy; venous hematocrit; veterans hospital; viral hepatitis
V_H variable domain of heavy chain
VHD valvular heart disease; viral hematodepressive disease
VHF very high frequency; visual half-field
VHN Vickers hardness number
VI six; vaginal irrigation; variable interval; virulence, virulent; viscosity index; visual impairment; visual inspection; volume index
Vi virulence, virulent
VIA virus inactivating agent; virus infection- associated antigen
vib vibration
VIC vasoinhibitory center
VIF virus-induced interferon
VIG, VIg vaccinia immunoglobulin
VIM video-intensification microscopy
VIP vasoactive intestinal polypeptide; vasoinhibitory peptide; venous impedance plethysmography; voluntary interruption of pregnancy
VIQ Verbal Intelligence Quotient
VIR virology
Vir virus, viral
vir virulent
VIS vaginal irrigation smear; visible; visual information storage
vis vision, visual
VISC vitreous infrsion suction cutter
visc viscera, visceral; viscosity
Vit vitamin
vit vital

vit cap vital capacity
vit ov sol dissolved in egg yolk [Lat. *vitello ovis solutus*]
VK vervet (African green monkey) kidney cells
VKH, VKHS Vogt-Koyanagi-Harada [syndrome]
VL left arm [electrode]; vision, left [eye]
V_L variable domain of the light chain
VLBR very low birth rate
VLBW very low birth weight
VLCFA very long chain fatty acid
VLDL, VLDLP very low density lipoprotein
VLF very-low frequency
VLG ventral nucleus of the lateral geniculate body
VLH ventrolateral nucleus of the hypothalamus
VLM visceral larva migrans
VLP vincristine, L-asparaginase, and prednisone; virus-like particle
VLSI very large scale integration
VM vasomotor; ventricular mass; vestibular membrane; viomycin; viral myocarditis; voltmeter
V/m volts per meter
VMA vanillylmandelic acid
VMC vasomotor center
VMCG vector magnetocardiogram
VMD Doctor of Veterinary Medicine
vMDV virulent Marek disease virus
VMF vasomotor flushing
VMH ventromedial hypothalamic [syndrome]
VMI visual motor integration
VMN ventromedial nucleus
VMR vasomotor rhinitis
VMT ventromedial tegmentum
VN virus neutralization; visiting nurse; vocational nurse; vomeronasal
VNA Visiting Nurse Association
VNDPT visual numerical discrimination pre-test
VNO vomeronasal organ
VNS visiting nursing service
VO verbal order; volume overload
VO_2, VO_2 volume of oxygen utilization
VOD veno-occlusive disease; vision, right eye [Lat. *visio, oculus dexter*]
vol volar; volatile; volume; voluntary, volunteer
VOM volt-ohm-milliammeter

VON Victorian Order of Nurses
VOO ventricular asynchronous (competitive, fixed-rate) [pacemaker]
VOP venous occlusion plethysmography
VOR vestibulo-ocular reflex
VOS vision, left eye [Lat. *visio, oculus sinister*]
vos dissolved in egg yolk [Lat. *vitello ovi solutus*]
VOU vision, each eye [Lat. *visio oculus uterque*]
VP vapor pressure; variegate porphyria; vasopressin; venipuncture; venous pressure; ventricular pacing; ventricular premature [beat]; ventriculoperitoneal; vincristine and prednisone; viral protein; Voges-Proskauer [medium or test]; volume-pressure
V/P ventilation and perfusion
V&P vagotomy and pyloroplasty
VPA valproic acid
VPB ventricular premature beat
VPC vapor-phase chromatography; ventricular premature complex; ventricular premature contraction; volume-packed cells; volume percent
VPCMF vincristine, prednisone, cyclophosphamide, methotrexate, and 5-fluorouracil
VPD ventricular premature depolarization
VPF vascular permeability factor
VPG velopharyngeal gap
VPL ventroposterolateral
VPM ventroposteromedial
VPP viral porcine pneumonia
VPRBC volume of packed red blood cells
VPRC volume of packed red cells
vps vibrations per second
V/Q ventilation-perfusion
VR right arm [electrode]; valve replacement; variable ratio; vascular resistance; venous reflux; venous return; ventilation rate; ventilation ratio; ventral root; ventricular rhythm; vesicular rosette; vision, right [eye]; vital records; vocal resonance; vocational rehabilitation
Vr volume of relaxation
VRBC red blood cell volume
VR&E vocational rehabilitation and education
VRI viral respiratory infection
VRL Virus Reference Laboratory
VRNA viral ribonucleic acid

VRR ventral root reflex
VS vaccination scar; vagal stimulation; venesection; ventricular septum; vesicular stomatitis; veterinary surgeon; visual storage; vital sign; volumetric solution; voluntary sterilization
V•s vibration second; volt-second
V x s volts by seconds
vs see above [Lat. *vide supra*]; single vibration; vibration seconds
VSA variant-specific surface antigen
VsB bleeding in the arm [Lat. *venae-sectio brachii*]
VSD ventricular septal defect; virtually safe dose
VSFP venous stop flow pressure
VSG variant surface glycoprotein
VSINC Virus Subcommittee of the International Nomenclature Committee
VSM vascular smooth muscle
VSMS Vineland Social Maturity Scale
vsn vision
VSOK vital signs normal
VSS vital signs stable
VSV vesicular stomatitis virus
VT tetrazolium violet; vacuum tuberculin; vasotonin; venous thrombosis; ventricular tachycardia
V$_T$, Vt tidal volume
V&T volume and tension
VTA ventral tegmental area
VTEC verotoxin-producing *Escherichia coli*
VTG volume thoracic gas
VTI volume thickness index
VTSRS Verdun Target Symptom Rating Scale
VTVM vacuum tube voltmeter
VTX vertex
VU varicose ulcer
VUR vesicoureteral reflex
VV varicose veins; viper venom; vulva and vagina
vv veins
v/v percent volume in volume
VVFR vesicovaginal fistula repair
VVI ventricular inhibited [pacemaker]
vvMDV very virulent Marek disease virus
VVT ventricular triggered [pacemaker]
VW vascular wall; vessel wall; von Willebrand's [disease]
vWD von Willebrand's disease

VWF vibration-induced white finger
vWF, vWf von Willebrand's factor
VIII$_{VWF}$, VIII-vwf von Willebrand factor, factor VIII
vWS von Willebrand syndrome
Vx vertex
VZ varicella-zoster
VZIG,VZIg varicella zoster immunoglobulin
VZV varicella-zoster virus

–W–

W dominant spotting [mouse]; energy; section modulus; a series of small triangular incisions in plastic surgery [plasty]; tryptophan; tungsten [Ger. *wolfram*]; water; watt; Weber [test]; week; wehnelt; weight; white; widowed; width; wife; Wilcoxson rank sum statistic; Wistar [rat]; with; word fluency; work
w velocity (m/s); watt
w̄ with
Wt weakly positive
WA when awake
W/A watt/ampere
WAADA Women's Auxiliary of the American Dental Association
WAGR Wilms' tumor–aniridia, genitourinary abnormalities, and mental retardation
WAIS Wechsler Adult Intelligence Scale
WAIS-R revised Wechsler Adult Intelligence Scale
WAP wandering atrial pacemaker
WARDS Welfare of Animals Used for Research in Drugs and Therapy
WARF warfarin [Wisconsin Alumni Research Foundation]
WAS Wiskott-Aldrich syndrome
Wass Wasserman [reaction]
WB washable base; Wechsler-Bellevue [Scale]; weight-bearing; wet bulb; whole blood; whole body; Willowbrook [virus]
Wb weber
WBA whole body activity
Wb/A webers/ampere
WBAPTT whole blood activated partial thromboplastin time

WBC white blood cell; white blood cell count; whole blood cell count
WBCT whole blood clotting time
WBE whole body extract
WBF whole-blood folate
WBH whole-blood hematocrit
Wb/m^2 weber per square meter
WBPTT whole blood partial thromboplastin time
WBR whole body radiation
WBRT whole blood recalcification time
WBS whole body scan; withdrawal body shakes
WBT wet bulb temperature
WC ward clerk; water closet; wheel chair; white cell; white cell casts; white cell count; whooping cough; wild caught [animal]; work capacity
WC' whole complement
WCC white cell count
WCD Weber-Christian disease
WCE work capacity evaluation
WCL Wenckebach cycle length; whole cell lysate
WD wallerian degeneration; well developed; well differentiated; wet dressing; Whitney Damon [dextrose]; Wilson's disease; with disease; wrist disarticulation
W/D warm and dry
Wd ward
wd well developed; wound, wounded
WDCC well-developed collateral circulation
WDHA watery diarrhea, hypokalemia, achlorhydria [syndrome]
WDL well-differentiated lymphocytic
WDLL well-differentiated lymphatic lymphoma
WDS watery diarrhea syndrome; wet dog shakes [syndrome]
WDWN well developed and well nourished
WE western encephalitis; western encephalomyelitis
WEE western equine encephalitis/encephalomyelitis
WF Weil-Felix reaction; white female; Wistar-Furth [rat]
W/F, wf white female
WFI water for injection
WFOT World Federation of Occupational Therapists

WFR Weil-Felix reaction
WG water gauge; Wegener's granulomatosis
WGA wheat germ agglutinin
WH whole homogenate; wound healing
Wh white
w•h watt-hour
wh white
wh ch wheel chair; white child
WHCOA White House Conference on Aging
WHD Werdnig-Hoffmann disease
WHML Wellcome Historical Medical Library
WHO World Health Organization
whp whirlpool
whr watt-hour
WHRC World Health Research Centre
WHV woodchuck hepatic virus
WHVP wedged hepatic venous pressure
WI human embryonic lung cell line; walk-in [patient]; Wistar [rat]
WIA wounded in action
WIC women, infants, and children
WIS Wechsler Intelligence Scale
WISC Wechsler Intelligence Scale for Children
WISC-R Wechsler Intelligence Scale for Children, Revised
WITT Wittenborn [Psychiatric Rating Scale]
W-J Woodcock-Johnson [Psychoeducational Battery]
WK week; Wernicke-Korsakoff [syndrome]
wk weak: week
WKD Wilson-Kimmelstiel disease
W/kg watts per kilogram
WKY Wistar-Kyoto [rat]
WL waiting list; waterload; wavelength; workload
WM Waldenström's macroglobulinemia; ward manager; white male
W/M white male
wm white male; whole milk; whole mount
w/m² watts per square meter
WMA World Medical Association
WMC weight-matched control
WME Williams' medium E
WMR work metabolic rate; World Medical Relief
WMS Wechsler Memory Scale

WMX whirlpool, massage, exercise
WN, wn well nourished
WNE West Nile encephalitis
WNL within normal limits
WNV West Nile virus
WO wash out; written order
W/O water in oil [emulsion]
w/o without
WOP without pain
WP weakly positive; wet pack; wettable powder; whirlpool; word processor; working point
W/P water/powder ratio
WPB whirlpool bath
WPFM Wright peak flow meter
WPk Ward's pack; wet pack
WPPSI Wechsler Preschool and Primary Scale of Intelligence
WPRS Wittenborn Psychiatric Rating Scale
WPW Wolff-Parkinson-White [syndrome]
WR Wassermann reaction; water retention; weakly reactive; wiping reaction
Wr wrist
WRAMC Walter Reed Army Medical Center
WRAT Wide Range Achievement Test
WRC washed red cells; water retention coefficient
WRE whole ragweed extract
WRK Woodward's reagent K
WRMT Woodcock Reading Mastery Test
WS Waardenburg syndrome; ward secretary; Warthin-Starry [stain]; water soluble; water swallow; Werner syndrome; West syndrome; Williams syndrome
W•s watt-second
WSI Waardenburg syndrome type I
WSA water-soluble antibiotic
WSL Wesselsbron [virus]
W/sr watts per steradian
WT wild type [strain]; Wilms' tumor
wt weight; white
WTF weight transferral frequency
W/U workup
W/V, w/v percent weight in volume, weight/volume
W^v variable dominant spotting [mouse]
WW wet weight
WxP wax pattern

W/W, w/w percent weight in weight, weight/weight
WxB wax bite
WZa wide zone alpha

–X–

X androgenic [zone]; cross; crossbite; exophoria distance; extra; female sex chromosome; ionization exposure; Kienböck's unit of x-ray exposure; multiplication times; reactance; removal of; respirations [anesthesia chart]; start of anesthesia; "times"; translocation between two X chromosomes; transverse; unknown quantity; X unit
X̄ sample mean
X ionization exposure rate
x the horizontal axis of a rectangular coordinate system; mole fraction; multiplication times; roentgen [rays]
x except; sample mean
X3 orientation as to time, place, and person
XA xanthurenic acid
X-A xylene and alcohol
Xa chiasma
Xaa unknown amino acid
Xan xanthine
Xanth xanthomatosis
Xao xanthosine
Xc excretory cystogram
XDH xanthine dehydrogenase
XDP xanthine diphosphate; xeroderma pigmentosum
XDR transducer
Xe xenon
XEF excess ejection fraction
XES x-ray energy spectrometry
XGP xanthogranulomatous pyelonephritis
Ξ Greek capital letter *xi*
ξ Greek lower case letter *xi*
XL xylose-lysine [agar base]
X-LA X-linked agammaglobulinemia
XLD xylose-lysine-deoxycholate [agar]
XLH X-linked hypophosphatemia
XLMR X-linked mental retardation
XLP X-linked lymphoproliferative [syndrome]

XM crossmatch
XMP xanthine monophosphate
XO presence of only one sex chromosome; xanthine oxidase
XOR exclusive operating room
XP xeroderma pigmentosum
Xp short arm of chromosome X
Xp- deletion of short arm of chromosome X
XPA xeroderma pigmentosum group A
XPC xeroderma pigmentosum group C
Xq long arm of chromosome X
Xq- deletion of long arm of chromosome X
XR x-ray
XRD x-ray diffraction
XRT x-ray therapy
XS cross-section; excessive; xiphisternum
XT exotropia
Xta chiasmata
Xtab cross-tabulating
XTE xeroderma, talipes, and enamel defect [syndrome]
XTP xanthosine triphosphate
XU excretory urogram; X unit
Xu x-unit
XX female chromosome type
46, XX 46 chromosomes, 2 X chromosomes (normal female)
47, XXY 47 chromosomes, 2 X and 1 Y chromosomes (Klinefelter syndrome)
47, XYY 47 chromosomes, 1 X and 2 Y chromosomes (XYY syndrome)
49, XXXXY 49 chromosomes, 4 X and 1 Y chromosomes (XXXXY syndrome)
XY male chromosome type
46, XY 46 chromosomes, 1 X and 1 Y chromosome (normal male)
47, XY, +21 47 chromosomes, male, additional No. 21 chromosome (Down syndrome)
Xyl xylose

–Y–

Y a coordinate axis in a plane; male sex chromosome; tyrosine; year; yellow; yttrium; *Yersinia*

y the vertical axis of a rectangular coordinate system

Υ   see *upsilon*

υ   see *upsilon*

YA *Yersinia* arthritis

YACP young adult chronic patient

YADH yeast alcohol dehydrogenase

YAG yttrium aluminum garnet [laser]

Yb ytterbium

YCB yeast carbon base

yd yard

YE yellow enzyme

YEH$_2$ reduced yellow enzyme

Yel yellow

YF yellow fever

YLC youngest living child

YM yeast and mannitol

YNB yeast nitrogen base

y/o years old

YOB year of birth

YP yield pressure

YPA yeast, peptone, and adenine sulfate

yr year

ys yellow spot; yolk sac

–Z–

Z acoustic impedance; atomic number; complex impedance; contraction [Ger. *Zuckung*]; the disk that separates sarcomeres [Ger. *Zwischenscheibe*, intermediate disk]; glutamine; impedance; ionic charge number; a point formed by a line perpendicular to the nasion-menton line through the anterior nasal spine; proton number; section modulus; standard score; standardized deviate; zero; zone; a Z-shaped incision in plastic surgery

Z',Z" increasing degrees of contraction

z algebraic unknown or space coordinate; axis of a three-dimensional rectangular coordinate system; catalytic amount; standard normal deviate

ZAP zymosan-activated plasma [rabbit]

ZB zebra body

ZD zero defects; zero discharge

ZDDP zinc dialkyldithiophosphate

ZDO zero differential overlap

ZDS zinc depletion syndrome

ZE Zollinger-Ellison [syndrome]

ZEEP zero end-expiratory pressure

Z-ERS zeta erythrocyte sedimentation rate

ZES Zollinger-Ellison syndrome

Ζ   Greek capital letter *zeta*

ζ   Greek lower case letter *zeta*

ZF zona fasciculata

ZG zona glomerulosa

ZIG, ZIg zoster immunoglobulin

ZIP zoster immune plasma

Zm zygomaxillare

Zn zinc

ZnOE zinc oxide and eugenol

ZOE zinc oxide-eugenol

Zool zoology

ZPA zone of polarizing activity

ZPG zero population growth

ZPO zinc peroxide

ZR zona reticularis

Zr zirconium

ZSR zeta sedimentation ratio

Z-TSP zephiran-trisodium phosphate

Zy zygion

Zz ginger [Lat. *zingibar*]

READER ENTRIES

A_____

_____

_____

_____

B_____

_____

_____

_____

C_____

_____

_____

_____

D_____

_____

_____

_____

E_____

_____

_____

READER ENTRIES

F_____

_____

_____

_____

G_____

_____

_____

_____

H_____

_____

_____

_____

I_____

_____

_____

_____

J_____

_____

_____

READER ENTRIES

K_____

_____

_____

_____

L_____

_____

_____

_____

M_____

_____

_____

_____

N_____

_____

_____

_____

_____

_____

READER ENTRIES

O_____

_____

_____

_____

_____

P_____

_____

_____

_____

_____

_____

_____

Q_____

_____

R_____

_____

_____

_____

READER ENTRIES

S_____

_____

_____

_____

_____

_____

T_____

_____

_____

_____

U_____

_____

_____

_____

_____

V_____

_____

_____

_____

READER ENTRIES

W_____

_____

_____

_____

_____

_____

X_____

_____

_____

_____

Y_____

_____

_____

_____

_____

Z_____

_____

_____

SUGGESTIONS

_____

_____

_____

_____

_____

_____

_____

_____

_____

_____

_____

_____

_____

_____

_____

_____

_____

_____

_____

_____

_____

_____

Clip and mail to the Publisher:
HANLEY & BELFUS, INC., 210 S. 13th Street, Philadelphia, PA 19107